Ethnopharmacology of Medicinal Plants

Ethnopharmacology of Medicinal Plants

Asia and the Pacific

Christophe Wiart, PharmD

HUMANA PRESS ✱ TOTOWA, NEW JERSEY

999 Riverview Drive, Suite 208
Totowa, New Jersey 07512

www.humanapress.com

This publication is printed on acid-free paper. ∞
ANSI Z39.48-1984 (American Standards Institute)
Permanence of Paper for Printed Library Materials.

Production Editor: Jennifer Hackworth

Cover illustration: Photo 15

Cover design by Patricia F. Cleary

For additional copies, pricing for bulk purchases, and/or information about other Humana titles, contact Humana at the above address or at any of the following numbers: Tel.: 973-256-1699; Fax: 973-256-8341; E-mail: orders@humanapr.com; or visit our Website: www.humanapress.com

Printed in the United States of America. 10 9 8 7 6 5 4 3 2 1
1-59745-160-6 (e-book)

Library of Congress Cataloging-in-Publication Data

Wiart, Christophe.
Ethnopharmacology of medicinal plants : Asia and the Pacific /
Christophe Wiart.
p. cm.
Includes bibliographical references and index.
ISBN 1-58829-748-9 (alk. paper)
1. Materia medica, Vegetable--Asia. 2. Ethnopharmacology--Asia.
3. Materia medica, Vegetable--Pacific Area. 4.
Ethnopharmacology--Pacific Area. I. Title.
RS179.W528 2006
615'.321--dc22

2006015502

"Observation and experiment for gathering material, induction and deduction for elaborating it; these are our only good intellectual tools."

F. Bacon, 1561–1626

Preface

In 1860, Oliver Wendell Holmes pointedly expressed himself to the Massachusetts Medical Society: "I firmly believe that if the whole *Material Medica*, as now used, could be sunk to the bottom of the sea, it would be all the better for mankind, and all the worst for the fishes." Should one think the same about the current approach in drug discovery from plants? Probably yes. Despite the spending of billions of US dollars, and three decades of efforts, high-throughput screenings have only allowed the discovery of a couple of drugs. One could have reasonably expected the discovery of an arsenal of drugs from the millions of plant extracts randomly tested, but "hits" can be inactive in vitro or too toxic, some molecules need to be metabolized first to be active, and false-positive and false-negative results are common.

The bitter truth is that the robotic approach in discovering drugs from plants has proven, to date, its inability to excavate the hundreds of molecules that will contribute to the health progress of Man. However, one can reasonably see that the last patches of primary rainforest on earth hold still hundreds of spectacularly active drugs that await discovery. The successful isolation of these drugs will depend on rational and selective collection of plants, heightened powers of observation, creation of original concepts, and formulation of new hypotheses to attain the sudden insight of which will be born new theories to extend the frontier of knowledge. As is often the case, that new theory might first be rejected out-of-hand by the dominant conservative group of established scientific schools of thoughts, the proponent of the new theory often being considered a quack. Gradually, however, if that theory is refined, developed and proven and leads to the discovery of wonder drugs, the real therapeutic usefulness, will be identified as a result of serendipity. Perhaps the future will see this new "Hippocratic" way of direct observation and logical interpretation displacing "robotic theories."

At this point in time, ethnopharmacologists represent a little heteroclite community of scientists who assess the last traditional systems of medicine: Pacific Rim, Amazon, and Africa. For the research scientist who penetrates the unknown of medicinal plants alone, no guide books are possible because the territory they travel is uncharted. For the first time in the history of medicinal plant research, *Ethnopharmacology of Medicinal Plants: Asia and the Pacific* sheds some lights on the pharmacological potentials of one of the most exciting and enormously rich sources of potential drugs: the medicinal plants of the Pacific Rim, which encompasses more than 6000 species that are virtually unexplored for pharmacology.

Ethnopharmacology of Medicinal Plants: Asia and the Pacific is written for all who will participate in the field of drug discovery from plants and offers stimulating, thoughtful, and critical information that should contribute in some way to the scientific progress of ethnopharmacology and to the discovery of drugs. *Ethnopharmacology of Medicinal Plants:*

Asia and the Pacific emphasizes the fundamental importance of the precise observation of the use of each medicinal plant, combined with pharmacological experiments and its botanical classification, and provides the base for a new theory of ethnopharmacology.

Christophe Wiart
Pharm.D.

Contents

1 Anti-Inflammatory Plants

GENERAL CONCEPT

Inflammation is a dynamic process that is elicited in response to mechanical injuries, burns, microbial infections, and other noxious stimuli that may threaten the well-being of the host. This process involves changes in blood flow, increased vascular permeability, destruction of tissues via the activation and migration of leucocytes with synthesis of reactive oxygen derivatives (oxidative burst), and the synthesis of local inflammatory mediators, such as prostaglandins (PGs), leukotrienes, and platelet-activating factors induced by phospholipase A_2, cyclooxygenases (COXs), and lipoxygenases. Arachidonic acid is a key biological intermediate that is converted in to a large number of eicosanoids with potent biological activities. The two major pathways of arachidonic acid metabolism are the COX pathway, which results in the formation of both PGs and thromboxanes, and the 5-lipoxygenase pathway, which is responsible for the formation of leukotrienes and 5S-hydroxy-6E, 8Z, 11Z, 14Z-eicosatetraenoic acid (5-HETE). Classic examples of herbs traditionally used to treat inflammation in Western medicine are *Matricaria chamomilla* L. and *Arnica montana* L. (Asteraceae), *Salix alba* (Salicaceae), and *Glycyrrhiza glabra* (Fabaceae).

The dried capitula of *Matricaria chamomilla* L. (Asteraceae), or German chamomile, have been used as anti-inflammatory and antispasmodic remedies since very early times on account of its contents in bisabolol oxides the activity of which has been experimentally substantiated. The plant is listed in several European pharmacopeias, and is used in the form of tinctures, extracts, lotions, ointments, shampoos, and sunscreen products.

Arnica montana L. (Arnica) has been used for treating bruises and swelling in Western medicine on account of its ability to elaborate sesquiterpene lactones, such as helenalin and dihydrohelenalin, which are thought to inhibit the activation of transcription factor nuclear factor (NF)-κB, which is responsible for the transcription of genes involved in encoding mediators for the inflammatory process.

Many topical preparations containing arnica are commercially available. Arnica is most commonly prepared as a tincture that can also be used as the base for creams, ointments, compresses, and poultices. Arnica oil may also be used in topical preparations.

From: *Ethnopharmacology of Medicinal Plants: Asia and the Pacific*
Edited by: C. Wiart © Humana Press Inc., Totowa, NJ

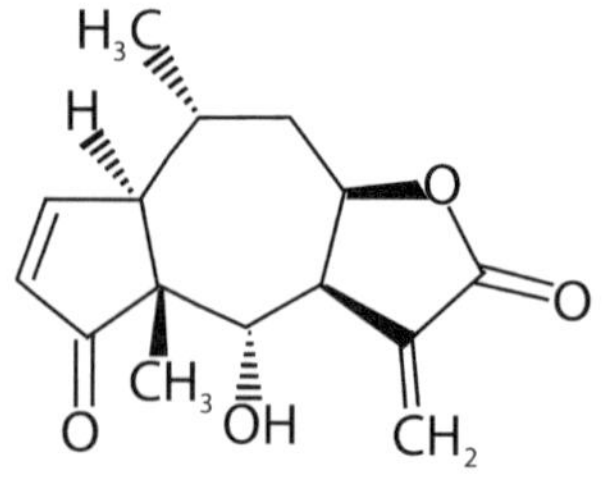

Helenanin

The effect of *Salix alba* L. (white willow) is largely owed to a glycoside, salicin. Salicin is antipyretic and analgesic and has been used in the treatment of rheumatic fever (salicilin tablets; *British Pharmaceutical Codex*, 1949). In 1893, Felix Hofmann, a chemist working for the Bayer chemical company in Germany, first synthesized acetylsalicylic acid, the acetylated form of salicin. Aspirin is one of the most commonly used pharmaceuticals containing salicin. Today, the main commercial sources of salicin are *Salix fragilis* and *Salix purpurea* (Salicaceae), which are native to Eurasia.

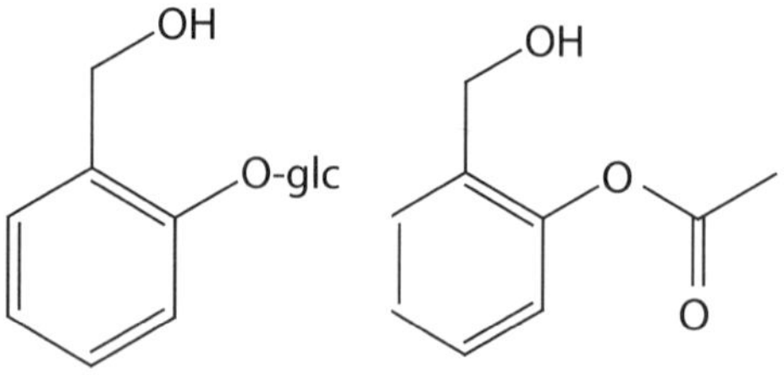

Salicin Acetylsalicylic acid

The mechanism by which aspirin elicits its anti-inflammatory activity is based on the fact that it irreversibly inactivates COX by covalent acetylation.

The roots of *Glycyrrhiza glabra* (liquorice) were known to Roman physicians as *Radixdulcis* and to Arab physicians as a remedy for cough, and the plant has been cultivated in Europe since the 18th century for its peculiar taste. *Glycyrrhiza glabra* is listed in the *British Pharmaceutical Codex* (1973 ed.) and contains triterpenes glycyrrhizin (6–13%) and glycyrrhizic acid, which have anti-inflammatory activity.

Glycyrrhizic acid is mainly absorbed after hydrolysis as glycyrrhetic acid, which is a potent inhibitor of 11-β-hydroxysteroid dehydrogenase an enzyme that catalyzes the conversion of cortisol to cortisone, hence mineralocorticoid action. A large amount of commercial teas, ointments, tobaccos, and suppositories are available on the market. In cosmetology, the drug is used for sunscreen and skin-care products. Other well-known plant products with anti-inflammatory activity are the distillate of *Hamamelis virginiana* (witch hazel; Hamamelidaceae), *Echinacea* species including *Echinacea angustifolia* (purple coneflower; Asteraceae), and *Ananas comosus* (pineapple; Bromeliaceae).

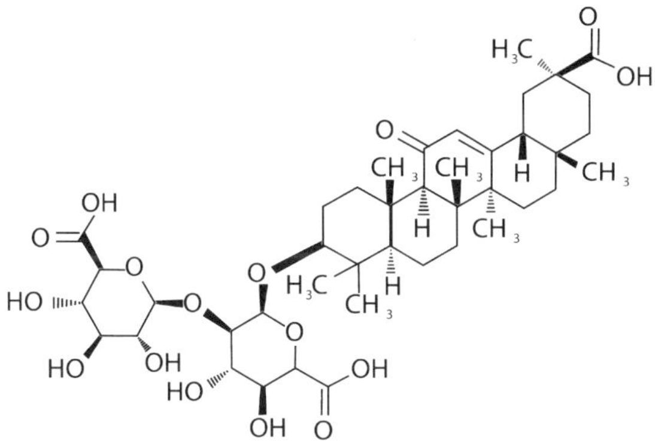

Glycyrrhizic acid

Common examples of Asian anti-inflammatory plants are *Curcuma domestica* Val. and *Curcuma longa* L. (turmeric), *Curcuma xanthorrhiza* Roxb. (temoe-lawaq), and *Zingiber officinale* Rosc. (Zingiberaceae). The rhizomes of C. *longa* L. (turmeric) from Java were introduced in Europe probably through Arab traders. Dioskurides mentions it as an Indian plant that looks like ginger but contains a yellow dye and has a bitter taste. The Indians and Chinese have been using *Curcuma longa* L. for centuries as a cosmetic and for the making of curry, and it was found in a list of medicinal plants sold in Frankfurt in 1450.

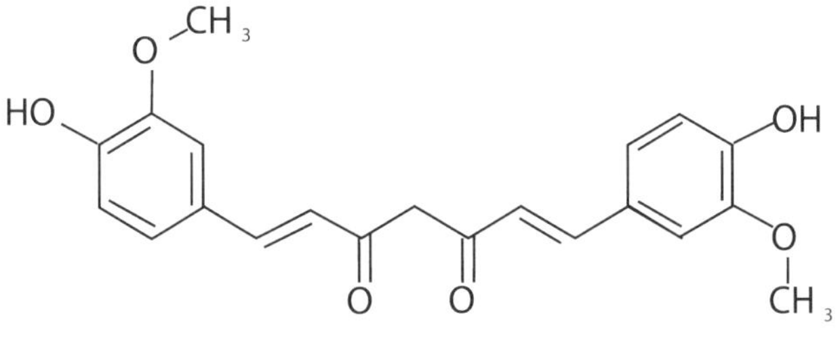

Curcumin

The yellow principle of *Curcuma longa* L. is a yellow pigment, curcumin. This dye inhibits the enzymatic activity of both COX and nitric oxide synthetase (NOS) and showed clinical potentials for the treatment of inflammation. *Zingiber officinale* L. (ginger) is native to Gingi area near Pontichery, India and the first European to have seen the whole living plant is said to be the Venetian Marco Polo around 1285. It was used to flavor food and beverages by the Greeks and Romans, who imported it via the Red Sea. During the Middle Ages, ginger was an important economical product controlled by the Venetians. Venetians had established houses of business at Constantinople and Sudak on the shore of the Black Sea, had the monopol of ginger, which was brought by caravannes following the Silk Road. The Venetian monopol survived until the late 15th century when Portuguese navigators were able to sail via the cape to Mozambique and then direct to India to Calicut. Ginger was brought in South America for cultivation by Francisco Mendoza and was exported to Spain as early as 1547. The plant contains arylalkalones, which inhibit the enzymatic activity of COX with potentials for the treatment of inflammation.

Encompassing approx 6000 medicinal plant species, the medicinal flora of Asia and the Pacific comprise a fantastic source of pharmacologically active products, and the number of plant species principally used for the treatment of inflammation can be estimated to be more that 380. This chapter will focus on the potentials of medicinal plants of Asia as a source of original anti-inflammatory drugs, with particular interest payed to inhibitors of phospholipase A_2, COX, lipoxygenases, elastase, and NOS.

INHIBITORS OF PHOSPHOLIPASE A_2

Phospholipase A_2 or phosphatide acylhydrolase 2, is an enzyme that catalyzes the hydrolysis of the acyl group attached to the 2-position of intracellular membrane phosphoglycerides. This hydrolysis release arachidonic acid from membrane phosphoglycerides. Arachidonic acid is the precursor of PGs, thromboxanes, and leukotrienes (Fig. 1). In regard to the possible mechanisms observed so far, the inhibition of phospholipase A_2 is mediated via lipocortine or by direct interaction with the enzyme itself. The former mechanism utilizes a protein known as lipocortine, the synthesis of which is commanded by steroidal hormones and steroid-like plants known as triterpenoids. Examples of lipocortine-mediated phospholipase A_2 inhibitors that are of therapeutic value and potent anti-inflammatory drugs are cortisone, prednisolone, and betamethasone. The other possible mechanism involves a direct binding with the enzyme itself, a mechanism thus far unused in therapeutics, but with promise. One such compound is also a triterpene: betulinic acid *(1)*. When looking for an inhibitor of phospholipase A_2 from medicinal plants, one could look into plant species that are traditionally used as snake-bite antidotes because hemolytic and myolytic phospholipases A_2 are often present in snake venom, which results in damage to cell membranes, endothelium, skeletal muscle, nerves, and erythrocytes.

Other medicinal features to consider when searching for plants with potential as phospholipases A_2 are abortifacient, analgesic, antipyretic, and hypoglycemic uses. Such features are present in the following plant species.

Medicinal Aristolochiaceae

The family Aristolochiaceae is a family of herbaceous plants often used in Asia and the Pacific to counteract snake poisoning, promote urination and menses, mitigate stomachache, and treat dropsy and skin diseases. During the past 20 years, members of this family, especially from the genus Aristolochia have attracted much interest and has been the subject of numerous chemical and pharmacological studies. The anti-inflammatory property of Aristolochia species is probably the result of a direct

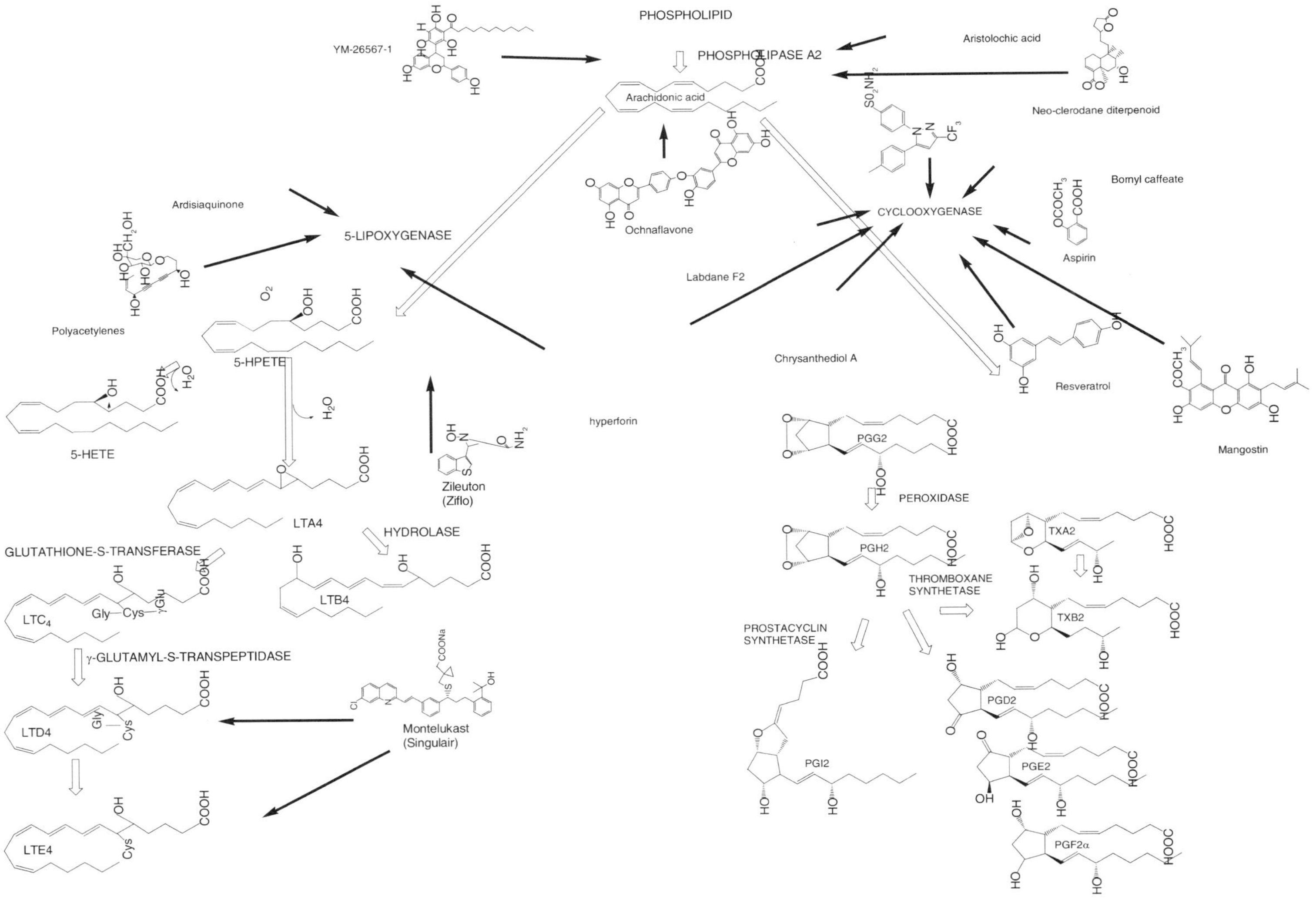

Fig. 1. Biosynthetic pathway of arachidonic acid metabolites.

interaction between aristolochic acid and derivatives of phospholipase A_2. *Aristolochia indica* L., *Aristolochia kaempferi*, and *Aristolochia recurvilabra* Hance are used for the treatment of inflammatory conditions.

A. *indica* L. Indian *Aristolochia*, also known as Indian birthwort, *ishvara* (Sanskrit), or *adagam* (Tamil), is a bitter climber native to India. The medicinal material consists of the rhizome, which is to resolve inflammation (India), counteract insect poison, and as an antipyretic (Philippines and Vietnam). The rhizome contains aristolochic acid, which inhibits in vitro and dose-dependent phospholipid hydrolysis by the human synovial fluid phospholipase A_2, snake venom phospholipase A_2, porcine pancreatic phospholipase A_2, and human platelet phospholipase A_2 *(2)*.

***Aristolochia kaempferi* Willd.** (*Aristolochia chrysops* [Stapf] E.H. Wilson ex Rehder, *Aristolochia dabieshanensis* C.Y. Cheng and W. Yu, *Aristolochia heterophylla* Hemsl., *Aristolochia kaempferi* f. *heterophylla* S. M. Hwang, *Aristolochia kaempferi* f. *mirabilis* S. M. Hwang, *Aristolochia neolongifolia* J.L. Wu and Z.L. Yang, *Aristolochia mollis* Dunn, *Aristolochia shimadae* Hayata, *Isotrema chrysops* Stapf, *Isotrema heterophyllum* [Hemsl.] Stapf, and *Isotrema iasiops* Stapf), or yellow mouth Dutchman's pipe, *ma tou ling, yi ye ma dou ling* (Chinese), is a perennial climber that grows to a height of 1 m in forests, thickets, and the mountain slopes of China, Taiwan, and Japan. The plant is herbaceous and develops small yellow flowers in the summer. The fruits are cylindrical or ovoid, 3–7- × 1.5–2-cm, dehiscing capsules. The drug consists of the fruit, which is shaped like human lungs, and is therefore recommended in China for all forms of pulmonary infections. Other diseases for which they are prescribed are hemorrhoids, ascite, and heartburn. The plant is known to contain phenanthrene alkaloid derivatives

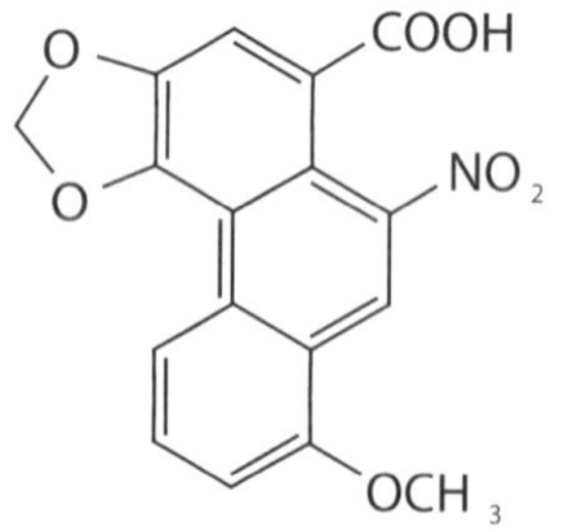

Aristolochic acid

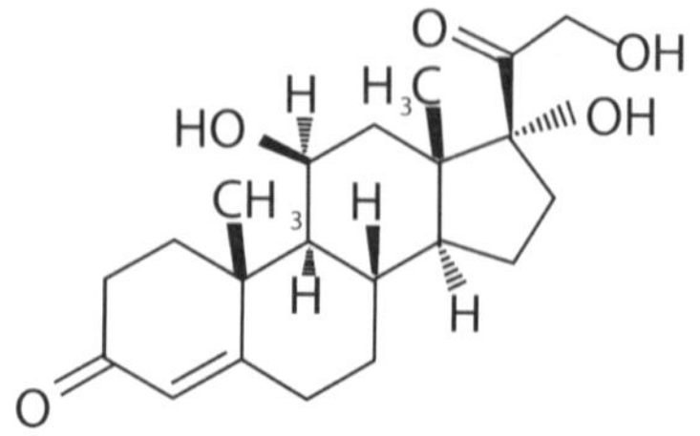

Cortisol

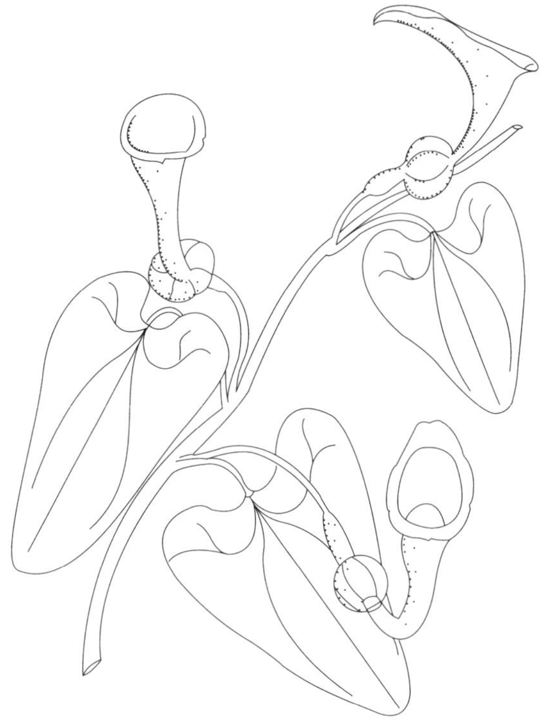

Fig. 2. *Aristolochiaceae recurvilabra.*

including aristoliukine-C, aristofolin A and E, aristolochic acid-Ia methyl ester, and aristolochic acid, as well as kaempferol-3-O-rutinoside and quercetin kaempferol-3-O-rutinoside *(3,4)*.

The plant is known elaborate a series of quite unusual phenanthrene alkaloid derivatives, of which aristoliukine-C, aristofolin A and E, aristolochic acid-Ia methyl ester, and aristolochic acid. Other chemical constituents found in this plant are flavonoid glycosides such as kaempferol-3-O-rutinoside and quercetin kaempferol-3-O-rutinoside *(3,4)*.

Exposure to Aristolochiaceae family is associated with the development of cancer in humans. A significant advance is the toxicological effects of aristolochic acid has been provided by the work of Pezzuto et al. They showed that aristolochic acid is a mutagen *(5)*.

Aristolochia recurvilabra Hance (*Aristolochia debilis* Sieb. et Zucc, *Aristolochia sinarum* Lindl., *Aristolochia longa* L.), or *ch'ing-mu-hsiang, pai-shu, ma dou ling, sam pai liang yin yao* (Chinese), is a climber that grows to a height of 1.5 m in thickets, mountain slopes, and moist valleys to 1500 m altitude in China, Taiwan, and Japan by roadsides, in thickets, and in meadows. The flowers are tubular and dark purple at the throat (Fig. 2). The drug consists of the rhizome. It is highly esteemed and was, at one time, worth 300 silver taels. The rhizome can be easily mistaken for ginger. It is used to treat digestive disorders, fluxes, diarrhea, dysentry, and snake bites. Levi et al. reported cases of hepatitis following ingestion of teas containing aristolochic acid *(6)*.

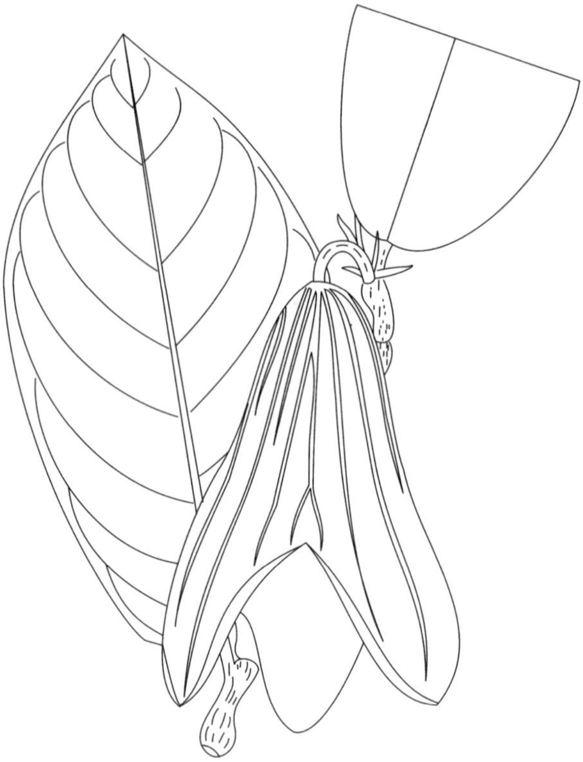

Fig. 3. *Thottea grandiflora* Rottb. From KL 1719. Phytochemical Survey of the Federation of Malaya. Geographical localization: Fort Iskandar, South Pahang, primary forest. Field collector: M. C. Wood, 3/2/1959. Botanical Identification: Ding Hou, November, 1984.

Hong et al. showed that a methanol extract of ***Aristolochia debilis*** is a potent inhibitor of COX-2 activity *(7)*.

***Thottea grandiflora* Rottb.** is a shrub that grows in the primary rainforests of Malaysia, Thailand, and Singapore. The stems are terete and hairy. The leaves are simple, alternate, thick, glossy, and glaucous underneath and grow up to 25 cm long. The flowers are axillary, 15 cm long, purple, membranaceous, and three-lobed. The fruits are linear follicles (Fig. 3). The roots are used to invigorate, break fevers, treat agues, and as a postpartum remedy. The pharmacological potential of this plant is unexplored.

Medicinal Myristicaceae

The Myristicaceae family has attracted a great deal of interest on account of its ability to produce series of unusual phenylacylphenols—of possible symbiotic origin—that might have some potential for the treatment of inflammation. One such compound is YM-26567-1 from *Horsfieldia amygdalinia* (Wall.) Warb. isolated by Mikaye et al. *(8)*

***Horsfieldia amygdalinia* (Wall.) Warb** (*Myristica amygdalina* Wall, *Horsfieldia tonkinensis* H. Lecomte, *Horsfieldia thorelii* H. Lecomte, *Horsfieldia tonkinensis* var. *multiracemosa* H. Lecomte, *Myristica glabra* auct. non Blume, *Horsfieldia glabra* auct. non (Blume)

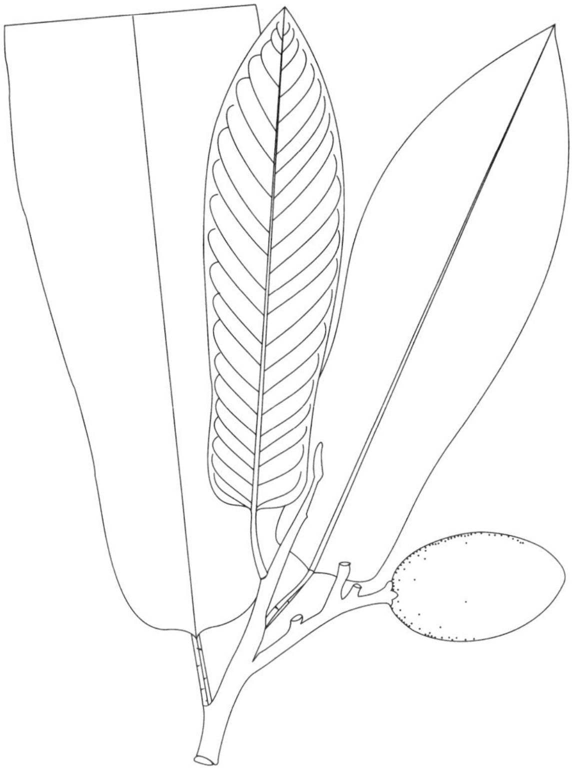

Fig. 4. *Horsfieldia valida*. From Forest department Brunei. Flora of Brunei. BRU 137. Geographical localization: B. Ingei. Primary forest seasonal swamp. 100 feet. Riverine alluvium. Field collector: Ashton, 7/7/1957. Botanical identification: J. Sinclair.

Warb, *Horsfieldia prunoides* C.Y. Wu), or *feng chui nan* (Chinese), is a timber tree that grows to a height of 25 m in hilly, sparse forests or dense forests of mountain slopes and groves in China, India, Laos, Burma, Pakistan, Thailand, Vietnam, Malaysia, and Indonesia. The bark is grayish-white and exudes sticky blood-like latex. The mature fruits are ovoid to elliptical drupes that are orange and to 2.5 cm long. The seeds are oily and completely enclosed in a crimson tunic (Fig. 4). The leaves and bark are used to make a tea to treat intestinal discomfort, and the bark is used to heal sores and pimples. The anti-inflammatory property of *Horsfieldia amygdalinia* (Wall.) Warb is confirmed in vitro. Mikaye et al. reported that YM-26567-1 from the fruit of this plant competitively inhibits the enzymatic activity of phospholipase A_2. In the course of further screening for YM-26567-1 derivatives, YM-26734 was selected, and inhibited phospholipase A_2 from rabbit platelets with an inhibition concentration 50% (IC_{50}) value of 0.085 mM (8).

Horsfieldia valida (Miq.) Warb. (*Myristica valida* Miq., *Endocomia macrocoma* [Miq.] de Wilde subsp. *prainii* [King] de Wilde; *Horsfieldia merrillii* Warb.; *Horsfieldia oblongata* Merr., *Horsfieldia prainii* [King] Warb., *Myristica prainii* King.), or *yunnan feng chui nan* (Chinese), is a buttressed tree that grows to a height of 25 m and a girth of 50 cm in the

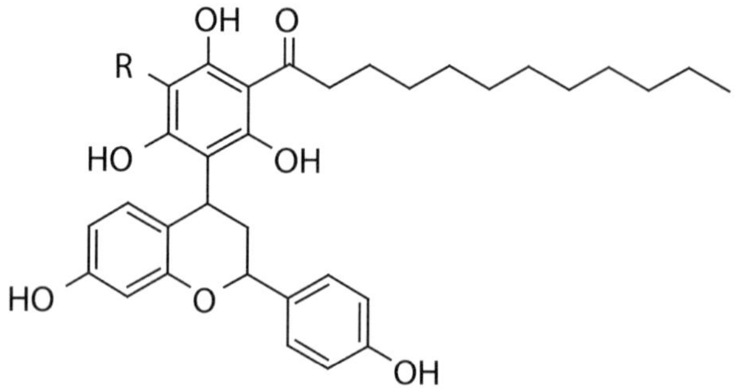

R= H, YM-26567-1

primary rainforests of Indonesia, Malaysia, and the Philippines. The bark is red-brown and minutely scaly. Red sap is present. The stems are terete, pubescent to puberulous, lenticelled, and longitudinally fissured. The leaves are simple, spiral, and exstipulate. The petiole is 2.3 cm × 3 mm, woody, and cracked. The blade is obovate-oblong, 19 cm long by 6 cm large, 24 cm long by 8 cm large, 24 cm long by 6 cm large, and shows 18–25 pairs of secondary nerves prominent on both surfaces. Male flowers are yellowish or subglobose, three- to five-lobed, and minute. The female flowers are ovoid-globose and 2.5–2.8 mm long. The fruits are red, ovoid, edible, and resinous in flavor, and 6 × 3.5 cm on a 5-mm-long pedicel. The seeds are 2–4 cm long and enclosed in a waxy, orange aril (Fig. 4). In Indonesia, the bark is used to treat sprue. Pharmacological properties are unexplored.

Medicinal Caprifoliaceae

The family Caprifoliaceae comprises approx 400 species, of which *Lonicera japonica* Thunb., *Lonicera affinis* Hook and Arn, *Lonicera confusa* DC, *Sambucus javanica* Reinw. ex. Bl, *Sambucus sieboldiana* (Miq.) Graebn, and *Weigela floribunda* (Sieb. and Zucc.) K. Koch. are used to treat inflammatory conditions in Asia and the Pacific. There is an expanding body of evidence to suggest that biflavonoids from this family might hold some potential as phospholipase A_2 inhibitors. One such compound is ochnaflavone from *Lonicera japonica* Thunb.

***Lonicera japonica* Thunb.** (*Lonicera chinensis* Wats, *Lonicera brachypoda* DC. var. *repens* Sieb.), or Chinese honeysuckle, *kim ngam, day nhan dong* (Vietnamese), *jen-tung* (Chinese), is a climbing shrub. The flowers are tubular, up to 4 cm long, and white when fresh but yellow when dry. In China, the flowers, stems, and leaves are used in medicine as febrifuge, correctives, and astringents and are used to treat infections and poisoning. The dried flowers are a common sight in the Chinese pharmacies of Malaysia, where they are prescribed as an antipyretic. In Vietnam, a decoction of stems or flowers is drunk to treat syphilis and rheumatism. The anti-inflammatory and antipyretic properties of *Lonicera japonica* Thunb. are confirmed and involve a biflavonoid, ochnaflavone, strongly inhibited the enzymatic activity of rat platelet phospholipase A_2 (IC_{50} approx 3 μM). This activity was strong and dependent of the pH, noncompetitive, and irreversible. In addition, the inhibitory activity of ochnaflavone is rather specific against group II phospholipase A_2 than group I phospholipase A_2 (IC_{50} approx 20 μM). These results indicate that the inhibition of phospholipase A_2 by ochnaflvone may result from direct interaction with the enzyme *(9)*.

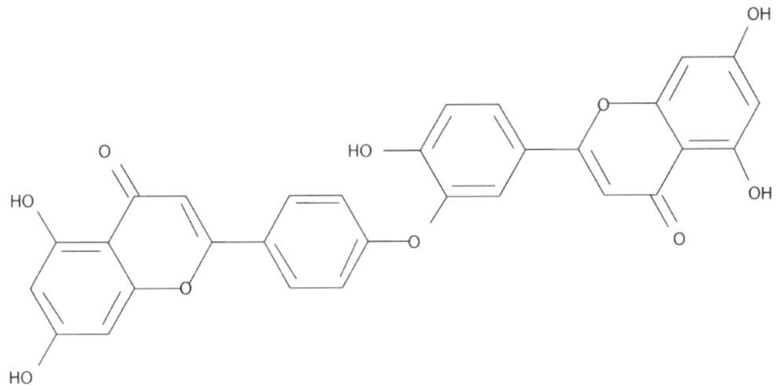

Ochnaflavone

Sambucus javanica **Reinw. ex Bl.** (*Sambucus hookeri* Rehd, *Sambucus thunbergiana* Bl.), or *so tiao, chieh ku ts'aois* (Chinese), or *kambiang beriak* (Indonesian), is a deciduous shrub of open spaces of land in town or countryside that are abandoned and where plants can grow freely, village outskirts, and wasteland. The flowers are white, starry, and small, and the fruits are red berries (Fig. 5). In Indonesia, the leaves and bark are used to cure itching. The plant is also used to treat rheumatism, assuage pain, reduce fever, and resolve swellings. The pharmacological potentials of this plant are unknown.

Weigela floribunda **(Sieb. & Zucc.) K. Koch.** (*Diervilla* versicolor Sieb. & Zucc.), crimson weigela, or Japanese wisteria, is a deciduous shrub that grows up to 2.5 m in Asia and was introduced as an ornamental shrub in the United States. The flower appears from May to June, and is large and purplish (Fig. 6). The plant is medicinal in China and Indonesia, where it is used to wash sores. The pharmacological potentials of the plant are unknown.

Medicinal Asteraceae

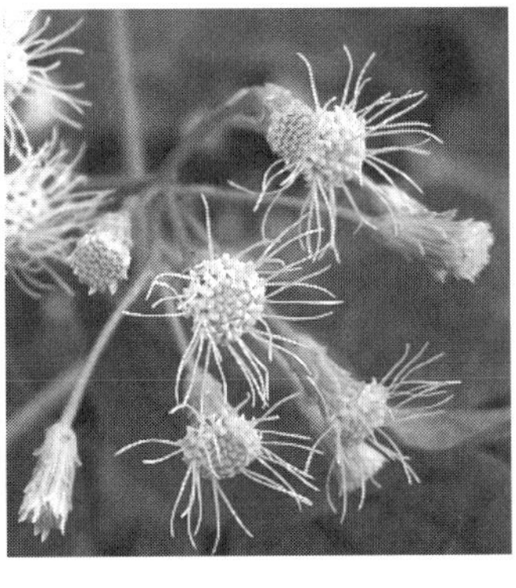

Classical examples of anti-inflammatory Asteraceae are *Arnica montana* and *Calendula officinalis*, both used in European medicine to treat bruises and contusions. There is an expanding body of evidences to suggest that Asteraceae could be a useful source of anti-inflammatories, such as sesquiterpene lactones and/or triterpene alcohols, the latter being known to inhibit 12-O-tetradecanoylphorbol-13-acetate (TPA)-induced inflammation in mice as efficiently as commercial indomethacine by possible inhibition of phospholipase A_2 *(10)*.

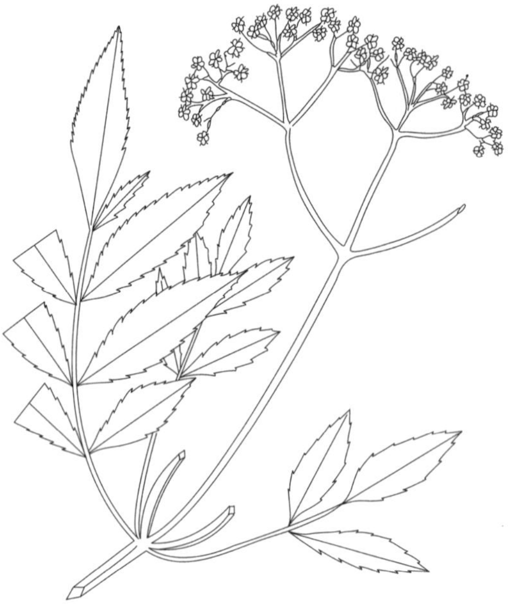

Fig. 5. *Sambucus javanica* Reinw. ex Bl. From Plants of Indonesia. Bali Timur, karangasem. On skirt of Gunung Agung, 1–3 km of Besakih. altitude: 1100 m, 8° 21′ S – 115° 26′ E. in secondary forest.

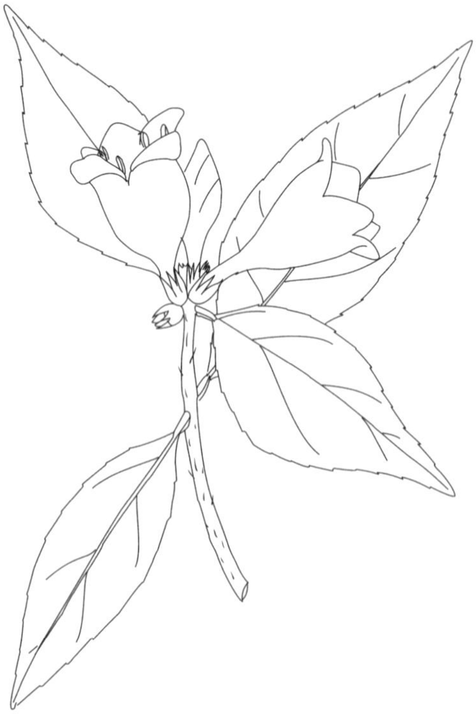

Fig. 6. *Weigela floribunda* (Sieb. & Zucc.) K. Koch.

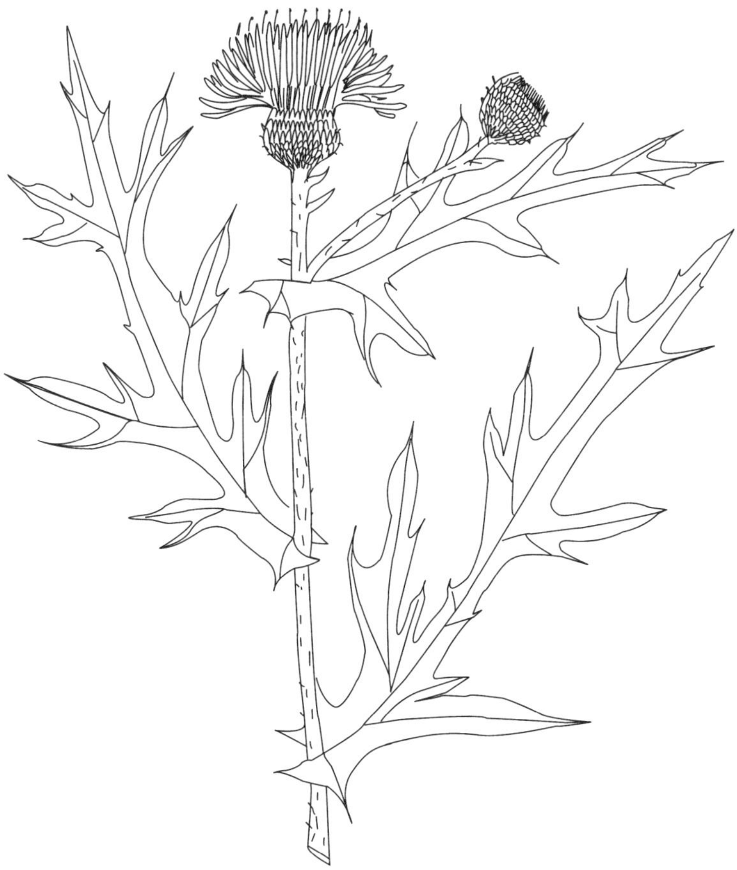

Fig. 7. *Cirsium japonicum* DC.

One of the most exiting findings in this area is perhaps the isolation of Bt-CD, a neoclerodane diterpenoid from *Baccharis trimera* (Less) DC or *carqueja* (Brazil) used to treat rheumatism and diabetes that shows anti-phospholipase A_2 activity *(11)*. Note also the anti-phospholipase A_2 and anti-inflammatory activity of *Santolina chamaecyparissus (12)*. *Cirsium japonicum* DC, *Crossotephium chinense* L. Makino, *Inula chinensis* Rupr. ex Maxim., and *Sigesbeckia orientalis* L. are used in Asia for the treatment of inflammatory conditions.

Cirsium japonicum DC (*Cnicus japonicum* Maxim, *Cnicus spicatus*), or Japanese thistle, *azami* (Japanese), *ta chi, hu chi, ma chi, tz'u chi, shan nin p'ang, chi hsiang ts'ao, yeh hung hua*, and *ch'ien chen ts'ao* (Chinese), is an herb that grows to 2 m in height. The plant is spiny and produces conspicuous purple capitula (Fig. 7). The drug consists of the root and is used to treat menstrual difficulties, irritable uterus, wounds, and snake bites. A decoction of the aerial part is used to stop bleeding from the nose. In Taiwan, the plant is used to heal burns. In Cambodia and Laos, the root is applied to ulcers and abscesses. The pharmacological properties of this herb are unknown.

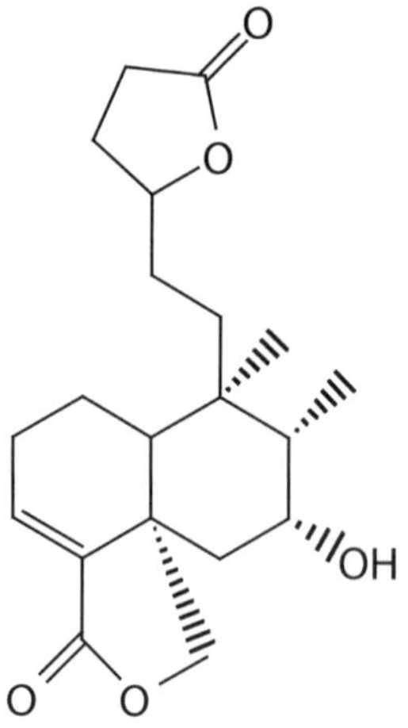

Neo-clerodane diterpenoid

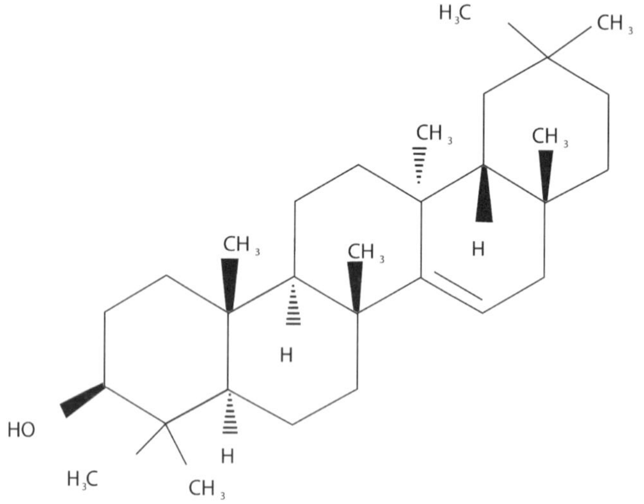

Taraxerol

Crossotephium chinense L. Makino (*Crossostephium artemisoides* Less, *Artemisia judaica* sensu Lour, *Artemisia loureiro* Kostel.) is a sub-shrub growing in crevices in the rocks in Japan and is cultivated in other Asian countries as pot ornamental. The plant is glaucous with dissected fleshy leaves (Fig. 8). In China, the leaves are used to calm itching. In Taiwan, the leaves are applied to contusions and wounds. In Vietnam, Cambodia, and Laos, an infusion of the plant is drunk to treat congestion. The plant is known to elaborate taraxerol, taraxeryl acetate, and taraxerol, which might participate in the medicinal uses (*13*). It would be interesting to know whether further studies on this herb discloses inhibitors of phospholipase A_2.

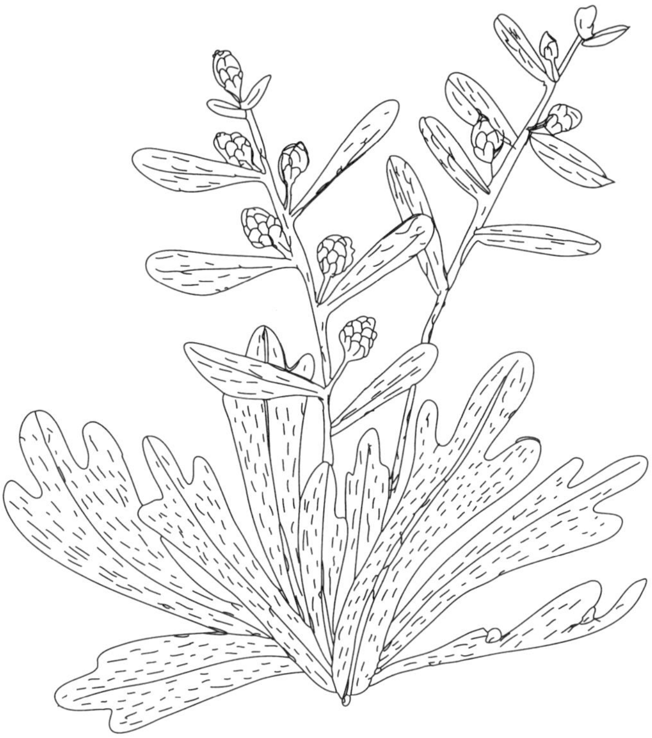

Fig. 8. *Crossotephium chinense.*

INHIBITORS OF COX

An example of a medicinal plant used for the treatment of inflammation based on its activity on COX is *Harpagophytum procumbens* DC (Pedaliaceae), or devil's claw, which has long been used in South Africa for the management of pain and inflammation. Two isoforms of COX, designated COX-1 and COX-2, are known to catalyze the synthesis of PGs from arachidonic acid (Fig. 1). A body of evidence suggests that PGs are involved in various physiopathological processes including carcinogenesis. COX-1 is present in most tissues, whereas COX-2 is inducible by carcinogens, cytokines, and tumor promoters, and therefore involved not only in inflammation, but also the growth of cells. Thus, compounds that inhibit the activity of COX-2 might also be an important target for cancer chemoprevention. Nonsteroidal anti-inflammatory drugs are widely used in the treatment of pain and inflammation associated with acute injury or chronic diseases, such as rheumatoid arthritis or osteoarthritis. Classic examples of COX inhibitors of therapeutic value are aspirin, paracetamol, ibuprofen, and recently introduced and withdrawn "coxibs" such as celecoxib (Celebrex®) and rofecoxib (Vioxx®). Coxibs abrogate the formation of cardioprotective PGI2, leading to a rise in blood pressure, atherogenesis, and heart attack by the rupture of an atherosclerotic plaque.

There is, therefore, a need for original coxibs, and one might think to look into the medicinal flora of Asia and the Pacific, as an increasing body of evidence suggests the families Apocynaceae, Clusiaceae, Asteraceae, Polygonaceae, Lamiaceae, and Convolvulaceae to elaborate ast sources of biomolecules which are able to inhibit the enzymatic activity of COX.

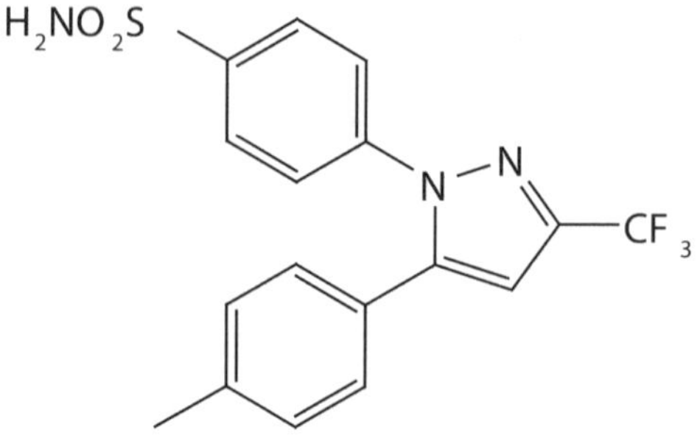

Celecoxib(Celebrex®)

Medicinal Apocynaceae

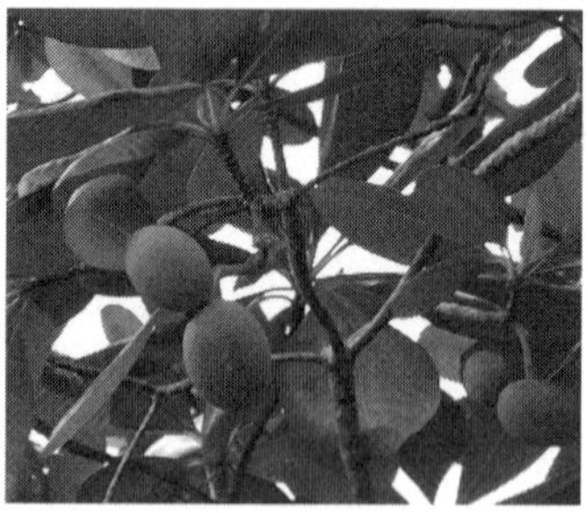

The family Apocynaceae consists of about 250 genera and 2000 species of tropical trees, shrubs, woody climbers, or herbs classically known to elaborate monoterpenoid indole alkaloids of therapeutic usefulness, such as vinblastine and vincristine characterized from the aerial part of *Catharanthus roseus* G. When looking for such principles, one might investigate members of the subfamily Plumerioideae, which includes the Plumerieae (*Alstonia*, *Aspidosperma*, *Catharanthus*), Tabernaemontaneae (*Crioceras*, *Tabernaemontana*, *Tabernanthe*, *Voacanga*), Rauvolfieae (*Ochrosia*, *Rauvolfia*, *Kopsia*, *Vallesia*), and Carissae (*Hunteria*, *Melodinus*, *Picralima*). About 80 species of plants classified within the family Apocynaceae are medicinal and are often used to treat gastrointestinal ailments, reduce fever and pains, and treat diabetes and infectious diseases. *Alstonia scholaris* (L.) R. Br, *Plumeria rubra* L. *sensu lato*, (*Plumeria acuminata* Ait, *Plumeria acutifolia* Por, *Plumeria alba* L.), *Ervatamia divaricata* (L.) Burk. (*Ervatamia coronaria* Stapf, *Tabernaemontana coronaria* Willd, *Tabernaemontana divaricata* R. Br.), *Trachelospermum jasminoides* (Lindl.) (*Rynchospermum jasminoides* Lindl.), and *Trachelospermum asiaticum* (Sieb. & Zucc.) Nak. are used in Asia to treat inflammation and have virtually been unstudied as a source of COX inhibitors.

***Trachelospermum asiaticum* (Sieb. & Zucc.) Nak.** (*Trachelospermum divaricatum* K. Schum), or Asian jasmine, is a climber native to Southeast Asia. The stems are smooth and reddish-brown and exude a milky liquid when cut. The small, leathery leaves are glossy, deep green, and arranged in opposite pairs along the stems. The flowers are light yellow and fragrant (Fig. 9). The plant is used in Korea to treat rheumatism, heal

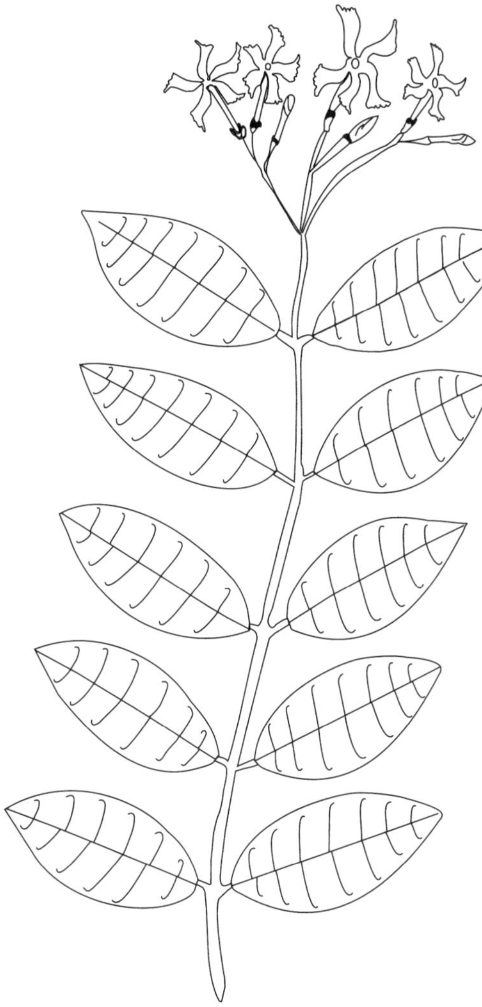

Fig. 9. *Trachelospermum asiaticum* (Sieb. & Zucc.) Nak.

abscesses and ulcers, and sooth laryngitis. To date, this anti-inflammatory property is not confirmed, and it will be interesting to learn whether it is be mediated via inhibition of the enzymatic activity of COX as measured with an ethanol extract of stem of *Trachelospermum jasminoides* (Lindl.) (*14*). If confirmed, this activity might involve alkaloids or lignans, such as arctigenin, and/or flavonoids or iridoids, which are known to occur in the plant (*15*).

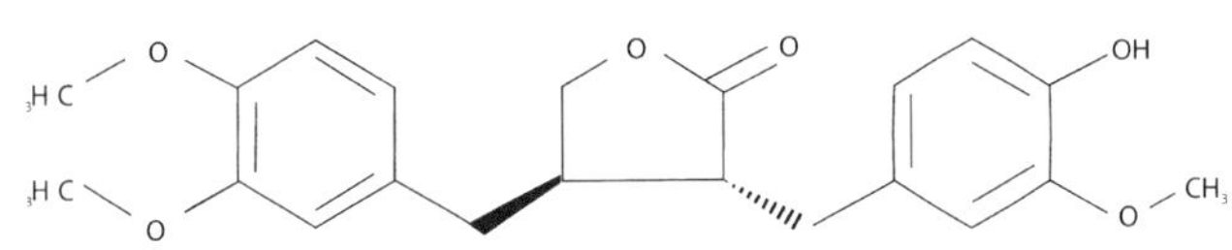

Arctigenin

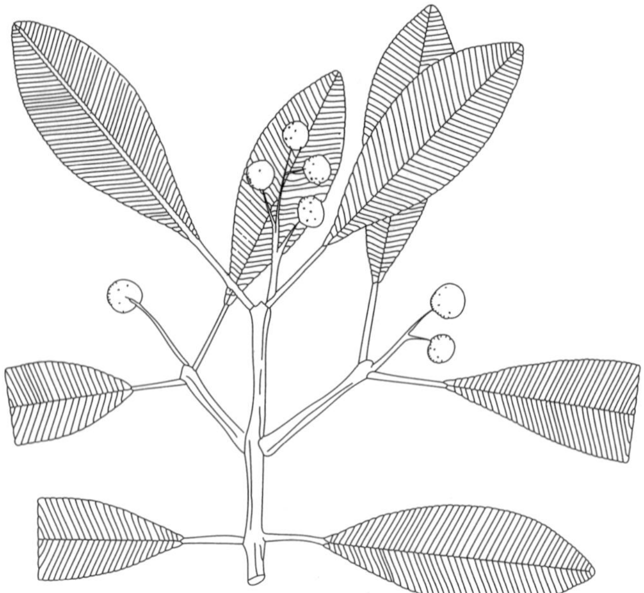

Fig. 10. *Calophyllum teysmanii* var. *inophylloides*. From Flora of Malaya. No FRI: 12776. Geographical localization: Terengganu, Gunong Padang, narrow ridge crest alt. 3300 feet. Date: 9/21/1969. T. C. Whitmore.

Medicinal Clusiaceae

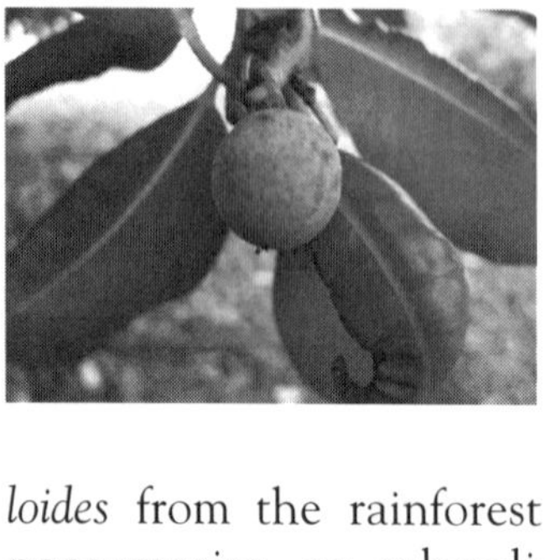

The family Clusiaceae, or Guttiferae, consists of 50 genera and 1200 species of tropical trees, climbers, or herbs. Regarding the chemical constituents of Clusiaceae, there is a massive body of evidences, which cleary demonstrate that neoflavonoids, prenylated xanthones, dipyranocoumarins, and quinones are common in member of thus family. Perhaps no other Clusiaceae has contributed antiviral research than *Calophyllum teysmanii* var. *inophylloides* from the rainforest of North Borneo. This tree produces series of dipyranocoumarins, or calanolides with anti-HIV potentials (Fig. 10). If the antiviral properties of Clusiaceae are being investigated, less work has been done in regard to the central nervous system properties of this family, although monoamine oxidase (MAO; of MAO A and, to a lesser extent, of MAO-B) activities have been measured experimentally, hence its potential to fight depression. An example of central nervous system-active Clusiaceae is *Hypericum perforatum* L. (St. John's Wort), the flowering tops of which can be found in several over-the-counter products, and the safety of which is controversial. One such compound is γ-mangostin from *Garcinia mangostana* L., which is found to directly inhibit activity of both COX isoforms in microsomal preparations *(16)*. The family Clusiaceae and the genera *Garcinia* therefore represent an interesting source of potential COX inhibitors.

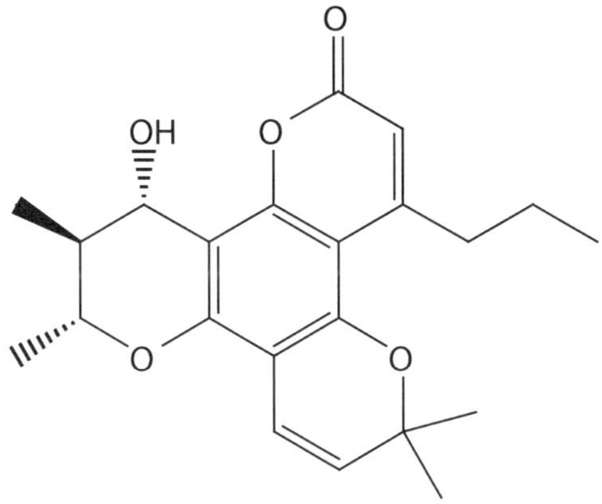

Calanolide

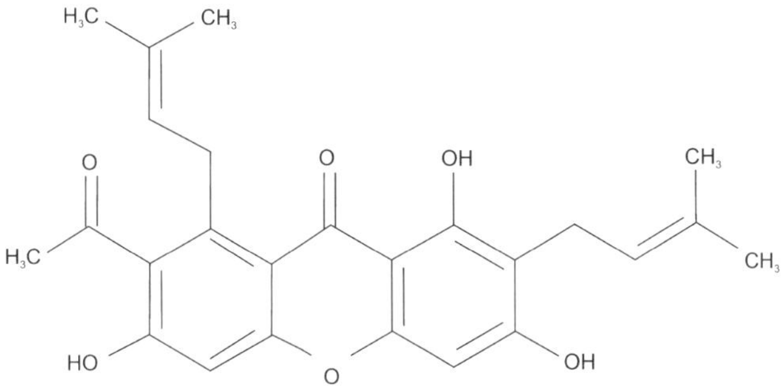

Hypericin

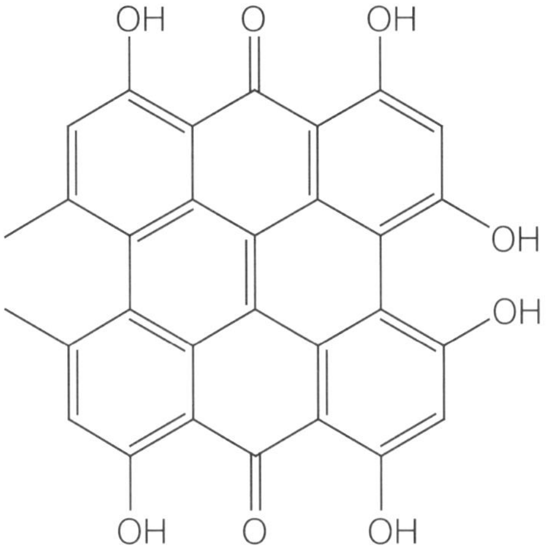

Hypericin

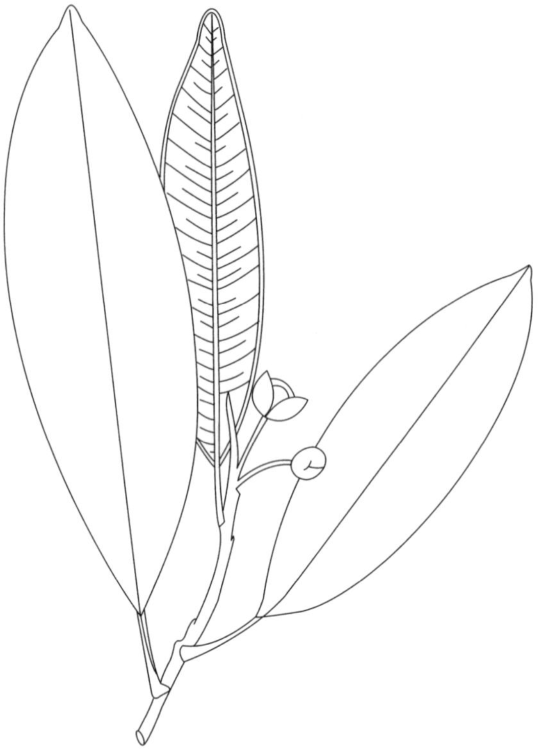

Fig. 11. *Garcinia atroviridis* Griff. From Flora of Malaya. FRI No: 13275. Geographical localization: Semangkok F.R. North Selangor, in primary forest, hillside, alt. 2700 feet.

***Garcinia atroviridis* Griff.**, or *asam geluggur* (Malay), *som khaek, som ma won* (Thai), is a tree that grows to a height of 15 m. The leaves are decussate and glossy, long (25 × 6.5 cm), and show about 18 pairs of secondary nerves. The flowers are dark red and the fruits are pumpkin-like berries that are edible and sour (Fig. 11). In Malaysia, a decoction of leaves and roots is used to mitigate earaches; the sap of the leaves is used as a postpartum remedy. One might give the hypothesis that the anti-inflammatory property of the plant involves atroviridine, a xanthone structurally related to mangostin. Is atroviridin an inhibitor of COX?

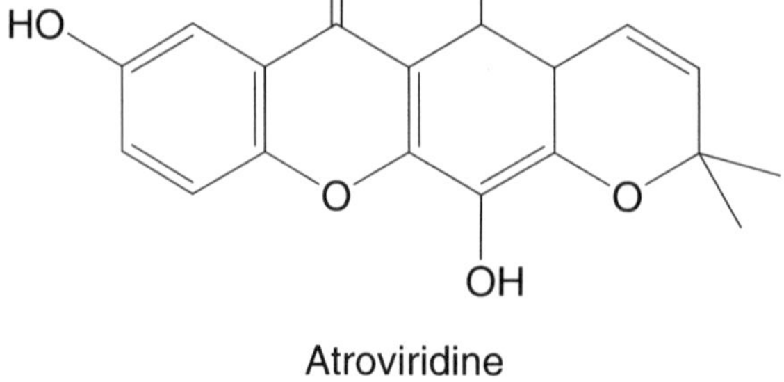

Atroviridine

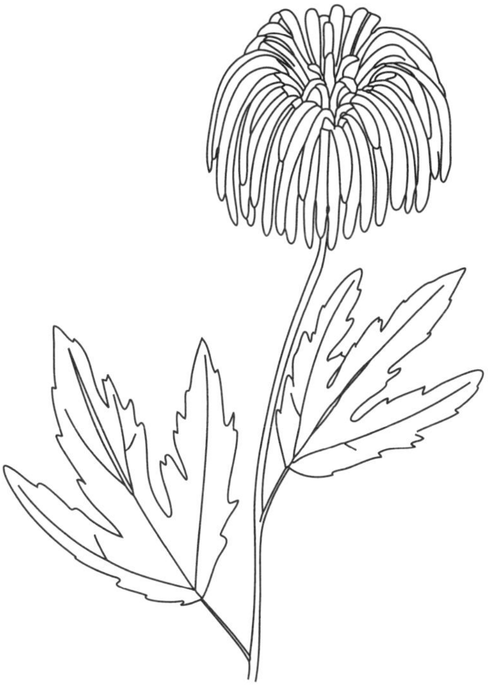

Fig. 12. *Chrysanthemum sinense* Sab.

Medicinal Asteraceae

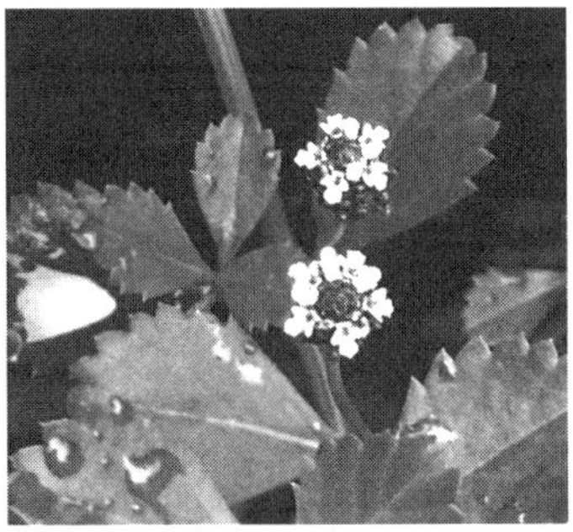

An example of Asteraceae reported to inhibit COX is *Cichorium intybus* L., or chicory *(17)*. In Asia, *Chrysanthemum sinense* Sab. (*Chrysanthemum morifolium* Ramat) and *Bidens bipinnata* L. are used as anti-inflammatories on account of their likely ability to inhibit COX.

***Chrysanthemum sinense* Sab.** (*Chrysanthemum morifolium* Ramat), or chrysanthemum or *chu-hua*. (Chinese), is a herb native to China and Japan that grows to a height of 30 cm. The plant is ornamental, aromatic, and a perennial herb. The leaves are pinnately lobed and toothed. The capitula are small, yellowish-pink, and globose (Fig. 12). The flowers are used to treat colds and headaches, to soothe inflamed eyes, and to prevent hair loss. A tincture of flowers is used to promote digestion and blood circulation, and to treat nervousness. A decoction of the whole plant is drunk to promote menses and applied externally to heal infected and cancerous sores. The medicinal properties mentioned here have not been confirmed experimentally; however, the plant is known to elaborate a series of sesquiterpenes, such as chrysanthediol A, which might have some level of activity against COXs, as demonstrated with *Chrysanthemum parthenium* (L.) Bernh. *(18,19)*. Note that the plant has antivenom properties, and this is not surprising because celecoxib, an inhibitor of COX-2, attenuates the action of venom phospholipase A_2 *(20)*.

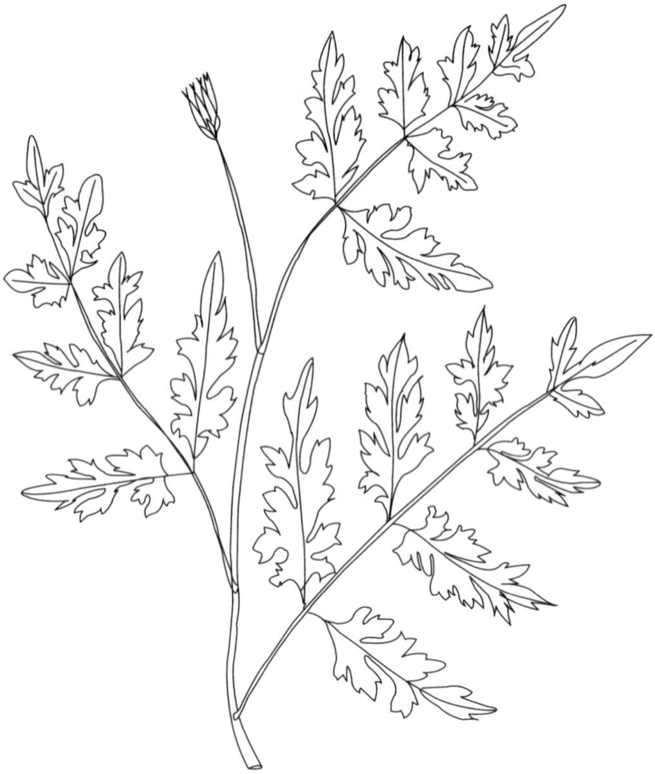

Fig. 13. *Bidens bipinnata* L.

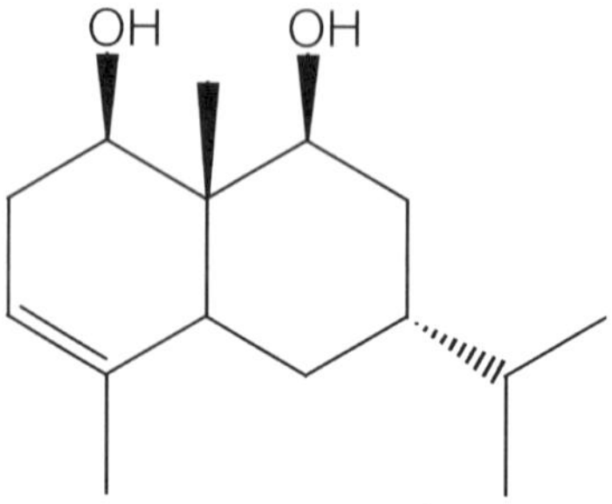

Chrysanthediol A

Bidens bipinnata L., or Spanish needles, is an herb that grows to a height of 80 cm. The plant is native to the United States and grows wild in tropical regions. The stems are quadrangular and dichotomously branching from tap roots. The leaves are deeply bipinnatifid. The capitula are yellow. The fruits are needle-like, hence the common name (Fig. 13). In China, the plant is used to counteract snake bites and insect stings. In Taiwan, a decoction of the plant is drunk to treat diarrhea. The antivenom property may involve inhibitors of phospholipase A_2 and possibly COXs because extracts of *Bidens pilosa* L. inhibit the enzymatic activity of COX in vitro *(21)*.

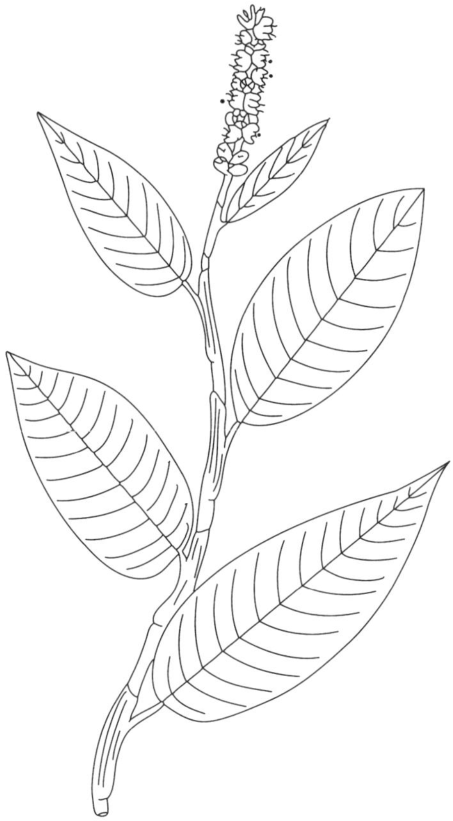

Fig. 14. *Polygonum amphibium* L.

Medicinal Polygonaceae

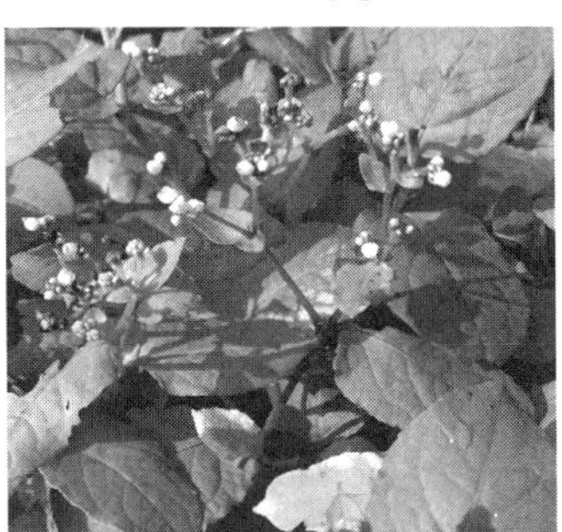

Polygonaceae are interesting because they elaborate a series of stilbene derivatives including resveratrol, which has displayed so far a broad array of pharmacological effects, including the inhibition of the enzymatic activity of rat polymorphonuclear leukocytes lipoxygenase and COX *(22)*. A classic example of anti-inflammatory Polygonaceae is *Polygonum amphibium* L.

***Polygonum amphibium* L.**, or water smartweed, water knotweed, or *t'ien liao* (Chinese), is a common temperate herb that grows in marshes and around ponds and lakes. The plant is erect, may be both branched or not, and grows up to 1 m in height. The leaves are dark green, glossy, are characterized by a conspicuous yellowish midrib and lanceolate, and the flowers are arranged in pinkish spikes (Fig. 14). In China, the juice expressed from the rhizomes and stems is used to heal infected sores and to treat rheumatism. To date, the pharmacological potential of this plant is unexplored, and it will be interesting to learn whether or not it holds any potential as a COX inhibitor.

Medicinal Laminiaceae

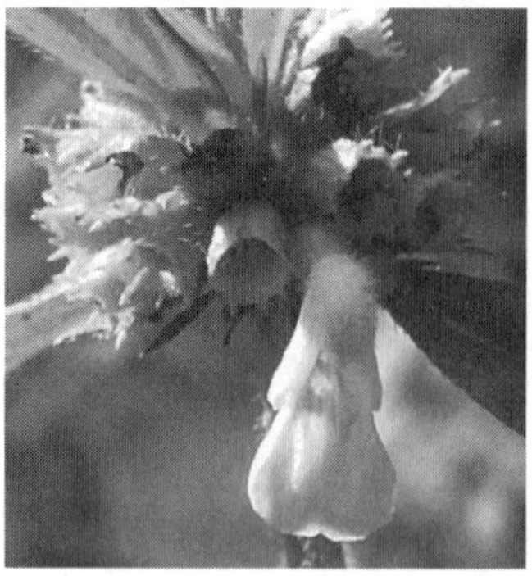

The family Lamiaceae comprises 200 genera and 3200 species of aromatic herbs including *Mentha piperita*, (peppermint, *British Pharmaceutical* Codex, 1954), *Lavendula officinalis* (lavender oil, *British Pharmaceutical Codex, 1963*), *Salvia officinalis* (sage, *British Pharmaceutical Codex*, 1934), and *Rosmarinus officinalis* L. (rosemary oil, *British Pharmaceutical Codex*, 1963). About 60 species of Lamiaceae are of medicinal value in Asia and the Pacific and, in regard to the potentials of Lamiaceae against COX, one might set the hypothesis that the stockhouse of diterpenes present in this family could be an interesting source of COX inhibitors. A signicant advance in that field of research has been provided by the work of Pang et al. Using ionophore-stimulated rat peritoneal leukocytes, they identified from *Sideritis javalambrensis*, a labdane called labdane F2, which inhibits the generation of COX and 5-lipoxygenase products of arachidonate metabolism *(23)*. An example of anti-inflammatory Lamiaceae where COX could be involved are *Ocimum basilicum* L. and *Glechoma brevituba* Kuprian which are described next.

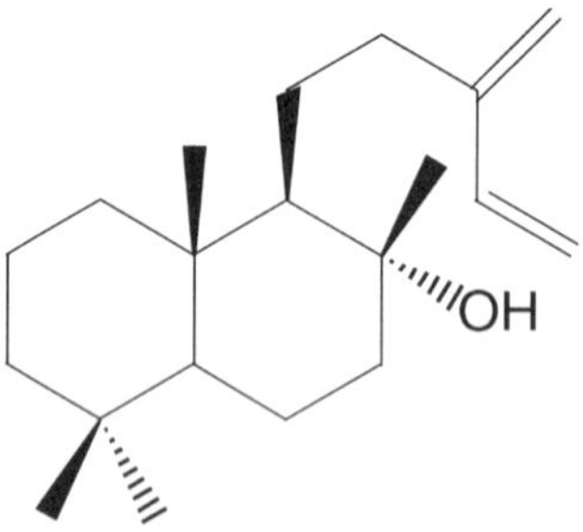

Labdane F2

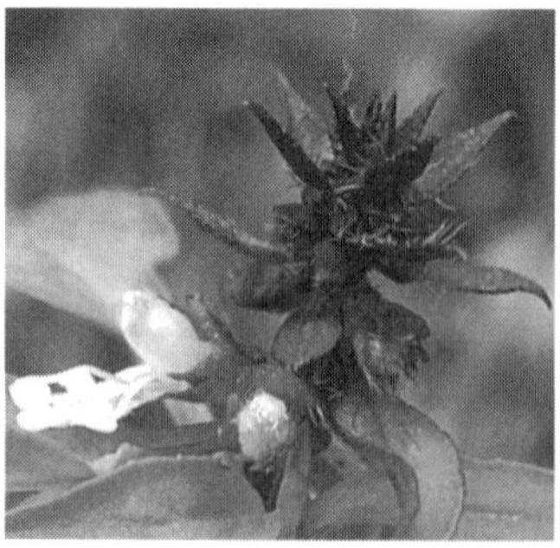

***Ocimum basilicum* L.**, or basil, *selaseh* (Malay), *telasih* (Javanese), *manglak luk* (Thai), *basilic* (French), *tirunitru* (Tamil), *babul* (Hindi), *barba* (Sanskrit), *badruj* (Arab), or *hsiang ts'ai* (Chinese), is an erect herb that grows to a height of 90 cm. The stem is purplish and the leaves are lanceolate, glossy, and fragrant. The flowers are tubular, bilabiate, purplish, and packed in whorled racemes (Fig. 15). In China, the seeds are used to soothe pain and inflammation. In India, the juice expressed from the leaves is used as nasal douche, and the plant is used to treat inflammation and assuage chronic pain in the joints. In Malaysia, the juice expressed from the leaves is drunk to calm cough, and the plant

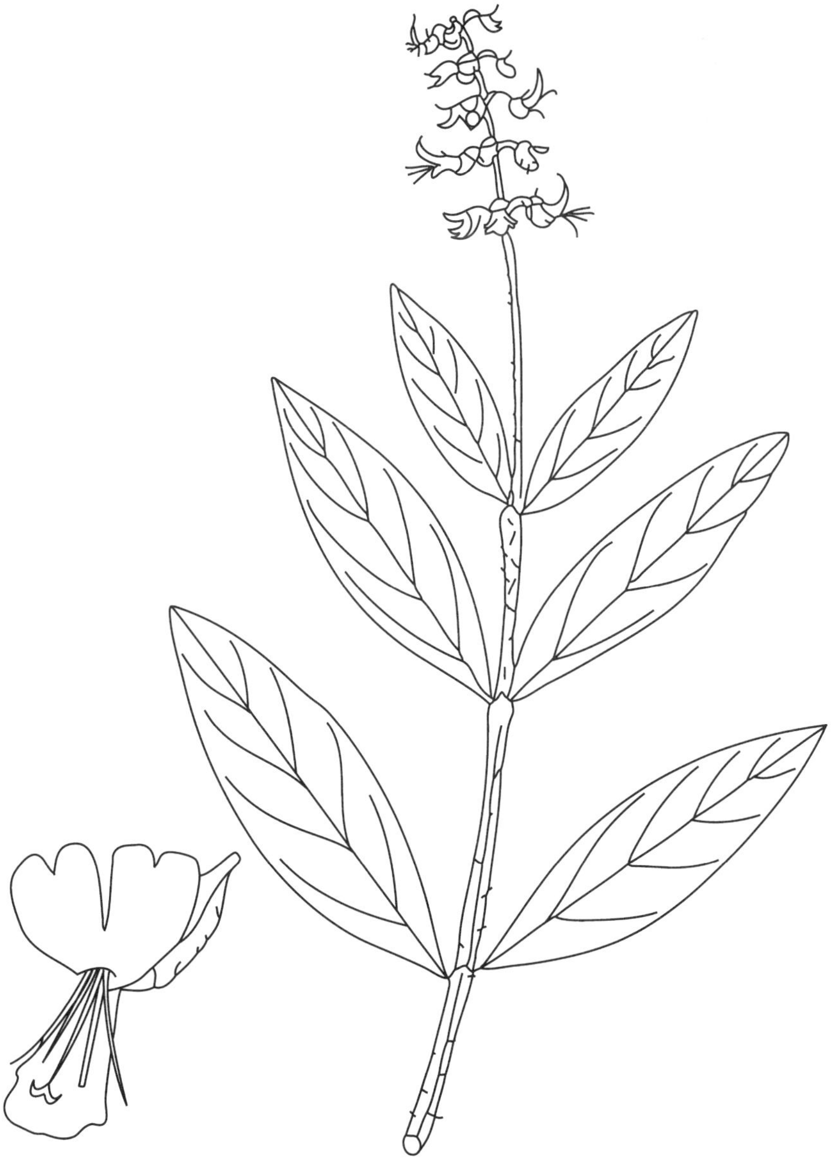

Fig. 15. *Ocimum basilicum* L.

is used to abrogate pregnancy. In Cambodia, Vietnam, and Laos, the leaves are used to break fever. The anti-inflammatory property of the plant is confirmed by Singh et al. They showed that the fixed oil inhibits carrageenan-induced and arachidonic acid- and leukotriene-induced paw edema, possibly by blockade of the enzymatic activity of both COX and lipoxygenaseas demonstrated for *Ocimum sanctum* L. and Holy basil *(24)*. Possible constituents responsible for COX inhibition might be phenolic compounds, such as phenylpropanes. Phenylpropanes are simple alkylated phenolic substances, which inhibit the PG synthesis. Such compounds are responsible for the anti-inflammatory properties of several medicinal plants in the family Convolvulaceae (*25,26*).

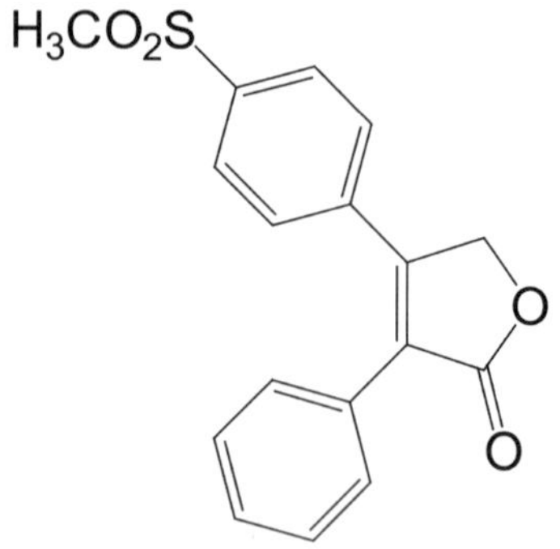

Rofecoxib

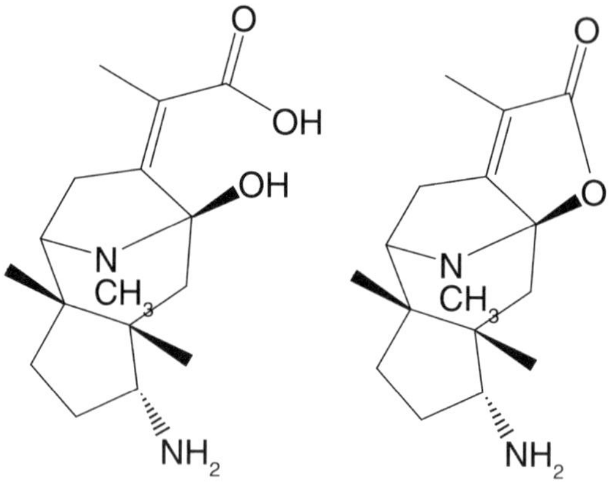

Hederacine A Hederacine B

***Glechoma brevituba* Kuprian.** is a stoloniferous, perennial, prostrate herb that grows in China. The leaves are simple, decussate and exstipulate. The petioles are long. The base of the blade is cordate. The flowers are tubular, dilated at apex, and bilobed. The fruits are dark brown, oblong-ovoid, smooth or impressed-punctuate, and glabrous. The plant is used in China to reduce fever, promote urination and the heart tone, and to cure colds and gravel. The pharmacological potential of *Glechoma brevituba* Kuprian. remains unexplored. An interesting feature of the *Glechoma* species is their ability to elaborate long-chain unsaturated fatty acids with anti-inflammatory, analgesic, antipyretic potentials. One such fatty acid is (9S,10E,12Z)-9-hydroxy-10,12-octadecadienoic acid, an antagonist of PGs E_1 and D_2 (*27,28*). Note also the the presence in the *Glechoma* species of a very unusual series of alkaloids (*29*), the structural features of which has some similarity to rofecoxib. Therefore, it would be interesting to learn whether these alkaloids hold any potential as a COX inhibitor or not.

INHIBITORS OF LIPOXYGENASES

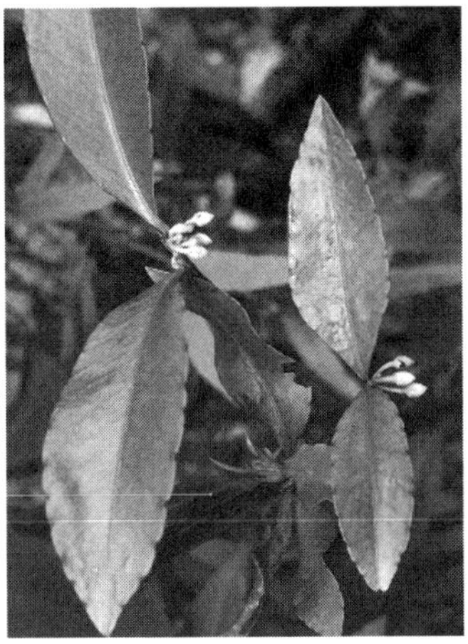

Lipoxygenases are present in leukocytes, tracheal cells, keratinocytes, and airway and stomach epithelium, and they catalyze the introduction of a molecule of oxygen to the 5-position of arachidonic acid to give the intermediate (5S)-hydroxy-(6E,8Z,11Z,14Z)-eicosatetraenoic acid or 5-HETE, which is immediately followed by the rearrangement of 5-HETE to leukotrienes. Another potential site of action for anti-inflammatory drugs is, therefore, at the level of lipoxygenases, thus inhibiting the biogenesis of leukotriene and 5-HETE. The search for specific inhibitors of lipoxygenase activity from medicinal plants results in the characterization of anti-inflammatory agents. Lipoxygenase inhibitors might hold some potential for the treatment of asthma, psoriasis, arthritis, allergic rhinitis, cancer, osteoporosis, and atherosclerosis. The evidence currently available suggests the families Myrsinaceae, Clusiaceae, and Asteraceae have potential as sources of lipoxygenase inhibitors.

Medicinal Myrsinaceae

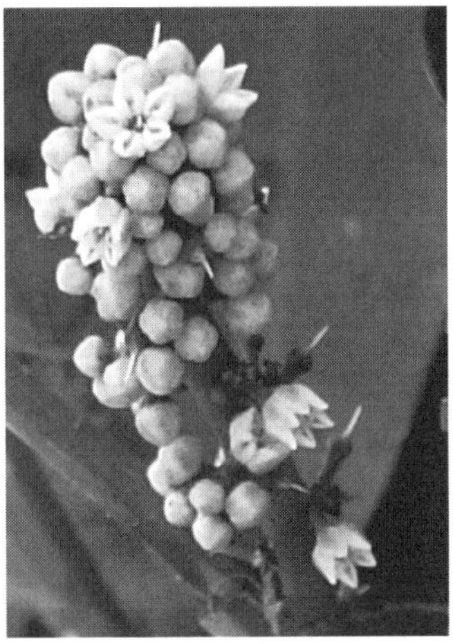

The family Myrsinaceae consists of 30 genera and about a 1000 species of tropical plants that have attracted a great deal of interest for their quinones and saponins, which have exhibited a large spectrum of pharmacological activities. About 40 species of plants classified within the family Myrsinaceae are medicinal in the Asia–Pacific region, particularly for the treatment of inflammatory conditions. One of these medicinal herbs is *Ardisia villosa* Roxb.

***Ardisia villosa* Roxb.**, or *xue xia hong* (Chinese), is a shrub that grows up to 3 m tall in the wild in China, Taiwan, Thailand, and Malaysia. The stems are stoloniferous, blackish, rusty villous, or hirsute almost throughout. The leaves are simple, spiral, and exstipulate. The blade is selliptic-lanceolate, somehow fleshy, light green, and marked with numerous blackih dots. The flowers are lavender or pink. The fruits are dark red or blackish with globose berries (Fig. 16). The plant is used in China to treat contusions and rheumatic and neuralgic pains. In Malaysia, a decoction of leaves is used as bath to treat dropsy; the roots are used to reduce fever and treat cough. An interesting feature of *Ardisia* species, and the Myrsinaceae family in general, is the production of a very unusual series of dimeric benzoquinones known as ardisiaquinones, which are known to inhibit the enzymatic activity of 5-lipoxygenases, a feature that could explain the frequent use of *Ardisia* species to treat inflammatory conditions. One such compound is ardisiaquinone G isolated from *Ardisia teysmanniana*, which is known to inhibit the enzymatic activity of lipoxygenase *(30,31)*.

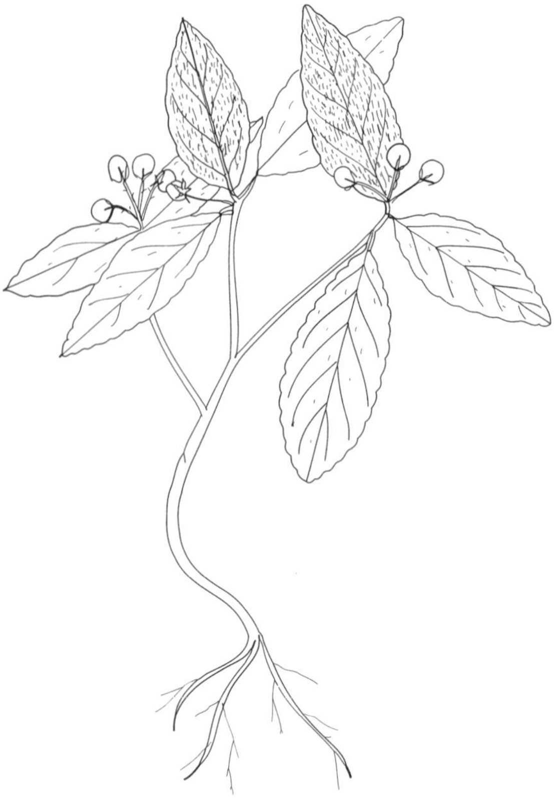

Fig. 16. *Ardisia villosa* Roxb.

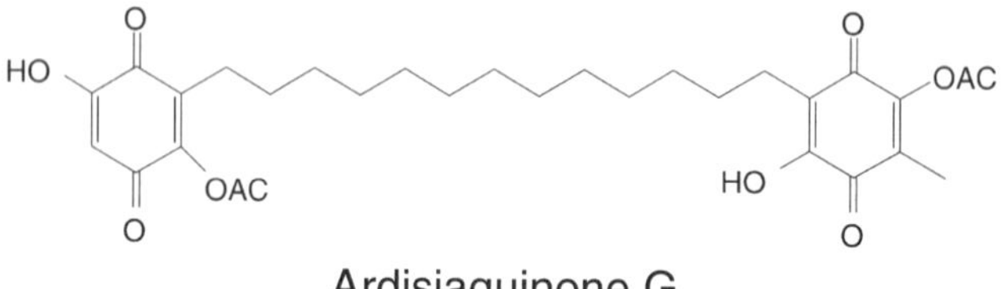

Ardisiaquinone G

Medicinal Clusiaceae

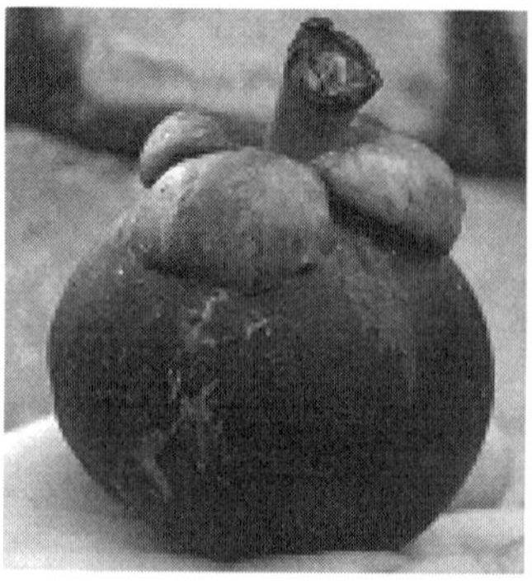

Hyperforin, the major constituent in *Hypericum perforatum* (St. John's Wort), inhibits the enzymatic activity of 5-lipoxygenase and COX-1 in platelets, acts as a dual inhibitor of 5-lipoxygenase and COX-1, and might have some potential in inflammatory and allergic diseases connected to eicosanoids *(32)*. Several *Hypericum* species are of medicinal value in Asia and the Pacific. One of these is *Hypericum erectum* Thunb., the potential of which as a source of 5-lipoxygenase is given here.

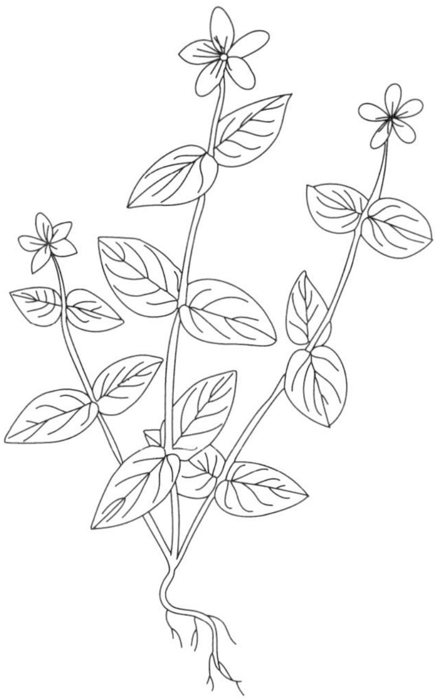

Fig. 17. *Hypericum erectum* Thunb.

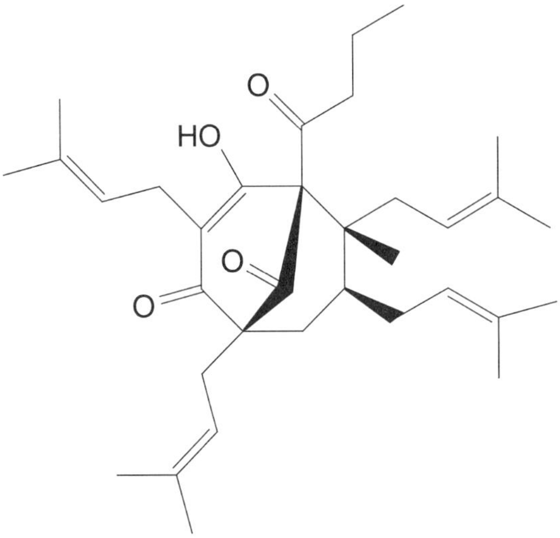

Hyperforin

***Hypericum erectum* Thunb.**, or *otogirisou* (Japanese), is an herb of grassy places and thin woods in the hills and mountains of Japan, Korea, and China. The plant is a lithe herb with decussate leaves and yellow flowers (Fig. 17). In Japan, the juice expressed from the leaves is used to heal cuts and sooth bruises. A decoction of the fruits is used to stop bleeding. In Vietnam and Cambodia, a paste of the aerial parts is applied to dog bites and bee stings, and is used internally for the treatment of malarial fever. *Hypericum erectum* Thunb. is an important herb in Chinese medicine as an anti-hemorrhagic agent, astringent, and antibiotic that is known to contain antiviral phloroglucinol derivatives, as well as the anti-hemorrhagic compounds otogirin and otogirone. Also, because the plant is known to elaborate a series of polyprenylated phloroglucinol derivatives including erectquione A, B, C, its potential as a lipoxygenase inhibitor would be worth assessing *(33)*.

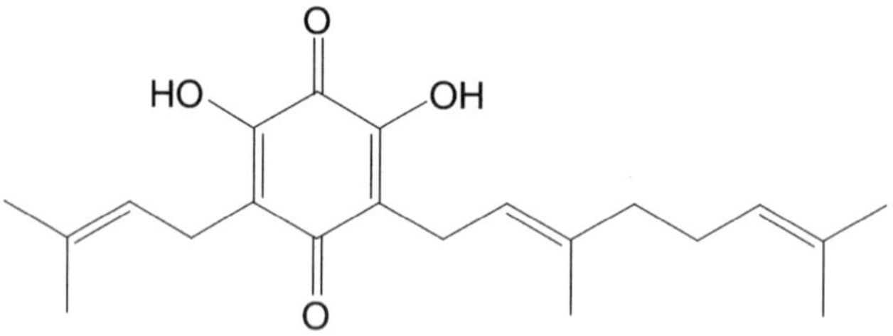

Erectquione A

Medicinal Asteraceae

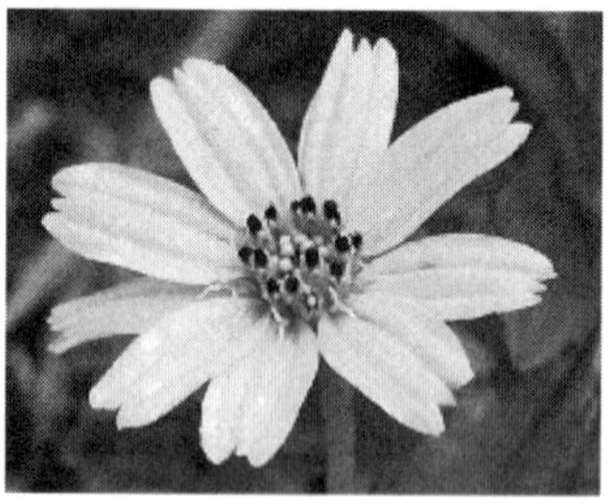

One of the richest sources of lipoxygenase inhibitors is perhaps the family Asteraceae, where three different types of principles have been characterized. The sesquiterpene lactone helenalin, which can be isolated from several plant species of the Asteraceae family, is a potent anti-inflammatory and antineoplastic agent. In human granulocyte, helenalin inhibited 5-lipoxygenase (IC_{50} 9 mM after 60 min preincubation) in a concentration- and time-dependent fashion *(34)*. Polyacetylenes from *Artemisia monosperma* showed some levels of activity against lipoxygenase (35). The third group of lipoxygenase inhibitors in this family are bornyl cinnamoyl derivatives from *Verbenisa* species, such as bornyl caffeate from the South American herb *Verbenisa turbacensis* Kunth.

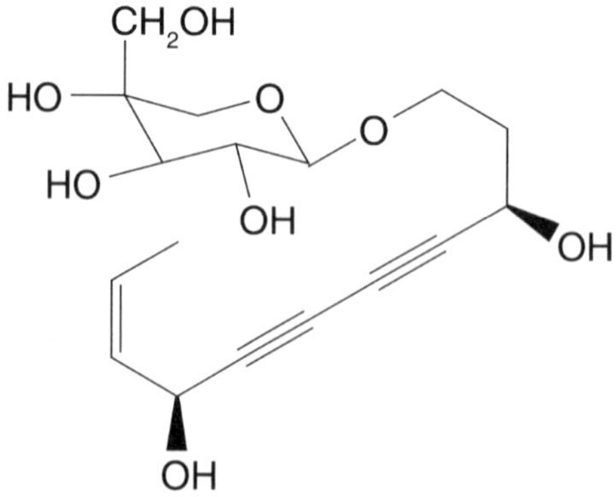

Polyacetylene

Medicinal Apiaceae

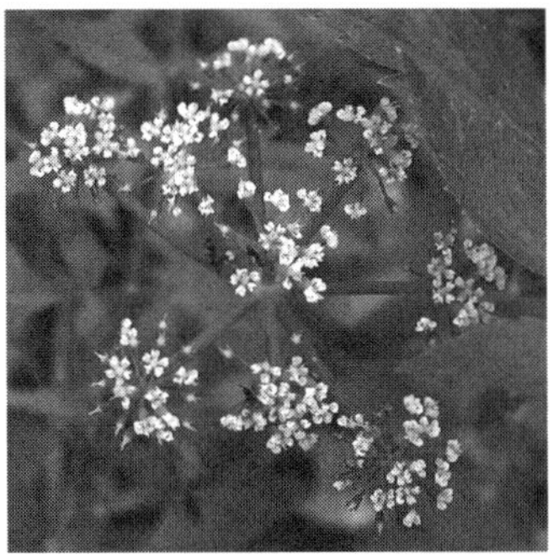

The family Apiaceae is a large group of flowering plants which comprises some 250 genera of herbs, mostly growing in temperate regions, the principal botanical hallmark of which is the presence of umbels, dissected leaves, pungent or aromatic smell, and hollowed and articulate stems. A large number of Apiaceae is of value in Western medicine, notably *Anethum graveolens L.* (dill, *British Pharmaceutical Codex*, 1954), *Foeniculum vulgare* (fennel, *British Pharmaceutical Codex*, 1963), *Apium graveolens* L. (celery, *British Pharmaceutical Codex*, 1949), *Carum carvi* L. (caraway, *British Pharmacopoeia*, 1963), *Coriandrum sativum* L. (coriander, *British Pharmacopoeia*, 1963), and *Pimpinella anisum* (anise, *British Pharmaceutical Codex*, 1954). A number of plants classified in this family are drastically toxic on account of coniine, such as *Conium maculatum* L. (hemlock leaf, *British Pharmaceutical Codex*, 1949).

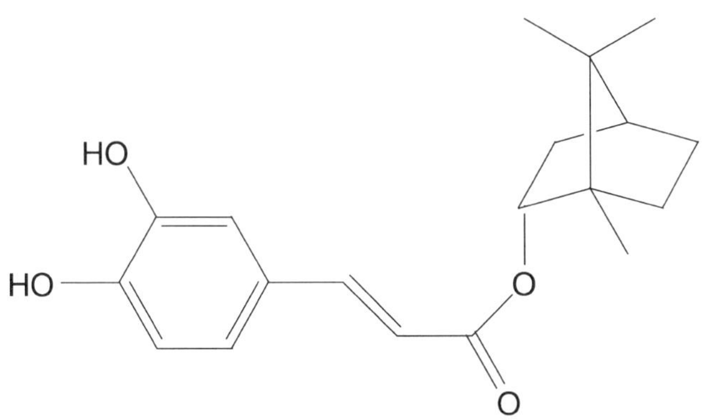

(-)-Bornyl caffeate

The traditional system of medicine of the Pacific Rim uses approx 80 species of Apiaceae, for instance, *Centella asiatica* (L.) Urban (*Hydrocotyle asiatica* L.; centella, *Indian Pharmaceutical Codex*, 1955). The plant has been used in India since early times for skin diseases and as a diuretic. It has long been a popular remedy in India for leprosy and syphilis. However, large doses are said to have narcotic action. The plant was used also by the surgeons of Napoleon's army.

***Bupleurum chinense* DC** (*Bupleurum falcatum* L. var *scorzoneraefolium* (Willd.) Ledeb, *Bupleurum octoradiatum* Bge. *Bupleurum chinense* Franch, *Bupleurum chinense* f. *vanheurckii* (Muel.- Arg) R. H. Shan & Yin Li, *Bupleurum falcatum* f. *ensifolium* H. Wolff, *Bupleurum togasii* Kitagawa, *Bupleurum vanheurckii* Muel- Arg), or *bei chai hu, tz' u hu, ch'ai hu* (Chinese), is a perennial herb that grows to a height of 90 cm in China, Mongolia, India, Korea, and Taiwan from a stout elongate, brown, and woody root.

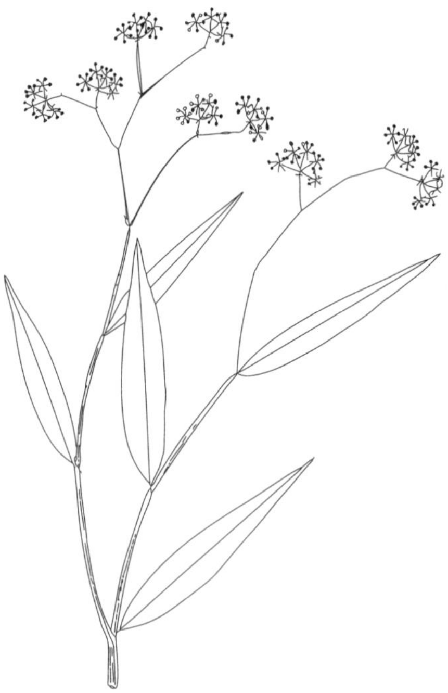

Fig. 18. *Bupleurum chinense* DC.

The leaves are simple, spiral and 4–7 cm × 5–8 mm. The blades of basal leaves are ellipticat and the cauline ones are linear-lanceolate. The inflorescence consists of numerous umbels spreading to form a large, loose panicle. The flowers are bright yellow. The achenes are oblong, brown, and prominently ribbed (Fig. 18).

In Asia, this plant is valued as a remedy for fever, rheumatism, gout, and inflammatory illnesses. In China, the roots are used as febrifuges, deobstruents, and carminatives, and are used to assuage muscle pains, thoracic and abdominal inflammations, puerperal fever, and diarrhea.

A significant advance in the understanding of the anti-inflammatory properties of *Bupleurum fruticescens* has been provided by Prieto et al. (36). The showed that a methanol extract from the aerial parts had a significant effect on 5-lipoxygenase activity, inhibiting both LTB_4 and 5(S)-HETE production, with IC_{50} values of 112 and 95 μg/mL, respectively. At concentrations of 200 μg/mL, the extract inhibited COX-1 (90%) and elastase activities (54%). What are the principles involved here, saponin?

INHIBITORS OF ELASTASE

The seeds and vegetative part of plants contain several sorts of inhibitors of insect, fungal, mammalian, and endogenous proteinases. These inhibitors may be involved in plant defense mechanisms against predators and participate in the development of the plant itself. Peptidic proteinase inhibitors are well studied in the families Fabaceae, Poaceae, Asteraceae, and Solanaceae (37). Non-proteinaceous inhibitors of serine protease are, in comparison, less known. Among serine proteinases are human neutrophils and macrophages, which digest degrade elastin, cartilage proteoglycans, fibronectin, and foreign materials ingested during phagocytosis.

In normal physiological conditions, it is inhibited by α-1-protease inhibitor of plasma. Damage to connective caused by leakage of elastases leads to damage associated with inflammatory diseases, such as pulmonary emphysema, adult respiratory distress syndrome, septic shock, cystic fibrosis, carcinogenesis, chronic bronchitis, and rheumatoid arthritis. Compounds that directly inhibit elastase or its release from human neutrophils are of enormous pharmaceutical and cosmetological interest in the development of new anti-inflammatory drugs. A possible source for elastase inhibitors are the medicinal Asteraceae and Droseraceae, particularly those used as traditional medicine in Asia.

Medicinal Asteraceae

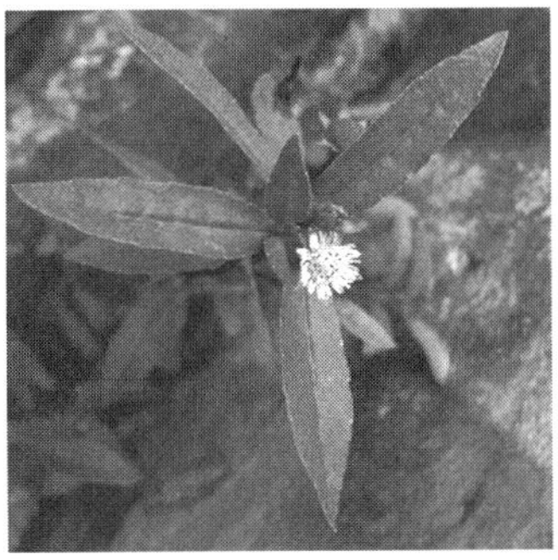

The family Asteraceae is a prolific source of sesquiterpene lactones, among which, melampolides have been shown to inhibit the enzymatic activity of elastases. Melampolides are a common member of the *Melampodiinae* subtribe. Examples of medicinal Asteraceae known to elaborate melampolides are *Sigesbeckia orientalis* L. and *Mikania cordata* (Burm.f.) B.L. Robinson.

***Sigesbeckia orientalis* L.**, or sigesbeckia, commonly known as St. Paul's wort, *sa phaan kon* (Thai), *hi lien*, *chu kao mu*, *hu kao*, *kou kao*, and *nien hu ts'ai* (Chinese), is an annual, branched herb that grows up to 1.2 m tall in Asia and the Pacific Islands. The capitula are bright yellow (Fig. 19). The plant has the reputation of "smelling like a pig" in China, where it is used to treat fever, snake bites, skin diseases, loss of appetite, chronic malaria, numbness of the extremities, and cancerous sores. In Taiwan, the plant is used to reduce swellings. In the Philippines, a decoction of the plant is used to heal wounds. A patent showed the ability of the plant to stimulate wound healing, to promote healing, and to restore elasticity to damaged skin. The dermis is thick, supple, and sturdy layer of connective tissue that encompasses a dense meshwork of collagen and elastin fibers, which are responsible for elasticity, tone, and texture. When the coils of collagen and elastin suffer cuts and crosslinking damage and the skin losses much of its strength and elasticity, wrinkles appear. This initial research led to an investigation of *Sigesbeckia orientalis* L.'s ability to restore normal quantities of collagen and elastin fibers in abnormal stretching of the dermis (pregnancy, change in weight) from a linear scar or from some endocrine disorders. Are melanpolides involved here? (38,39; Fig. 20).

***Sigesbeckia glabrescens* Mak.**, or *hi chum* (Korean; Fig. 21), is used in Korea to treat liver and kidney diseases, asthma, allergic disorders, costiveness, deafness, and blindness. In China, the plant is prescribed for rheumatic pain, numbness, weak bones, and to wash boils. The anti-inflammatory property of *Sigesbeckia glabrescens* Mak. is

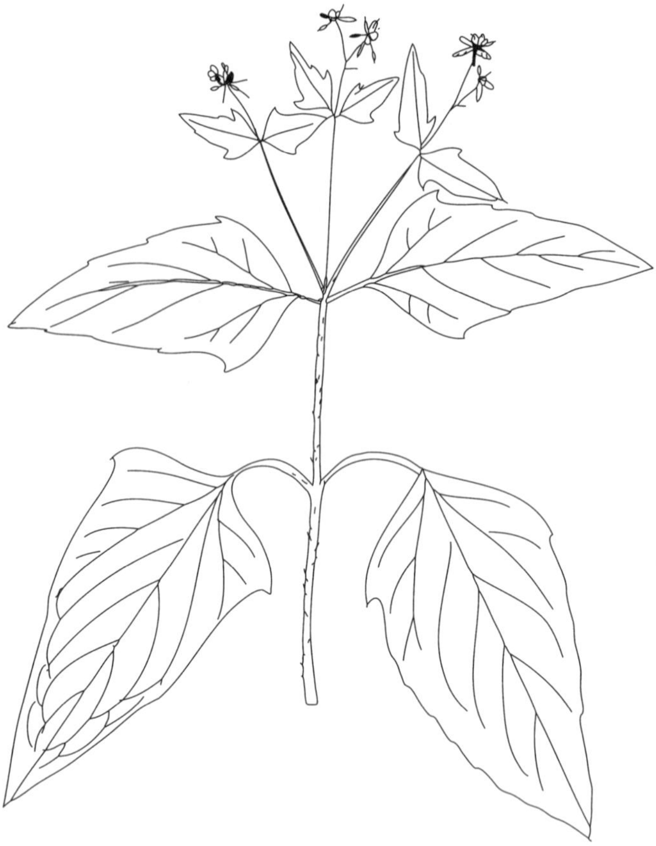

Fig. 19. *Sigesbeckia orientalis.*

confirmed experimentally, as an intraperitoneal injection of an aqueous extract of the plant inhibited compound 48/80 induced systemic anaphylaxis in mice. The extract dose-dependently inhibited the release of histamine from peritoneal mast cells by compound 48/80. The plant has a strong antianaphylactic activity by inhibition of histamine release from mast cells *(40)*. The extract dose-dependently inhibited the active systemic anaphylaxis and serum IgE production induced by immunization with ovalbumin and interleukin (IL)-4-dependent IgE production by lipopolysaccharide (LPS)-stimulated murine whole spleen cells *(41)*. Note that serine protease enzymes induces the release of significant amounts of histamine from mast cells, and that the antihistaminic effect described earlier could result from a possible inhibition of elastase by melampolides, but this remains to be confirmed *(42)*.

Note that darutoside, a diterpene including isolated from *Siegesbeckia glabrescens* Mak. abrogated early pregnancies in experimental rats at a dosage of 20–40 mg/kg *(43)*.

Mikania cordata (Burm.f.) B.L. Robinson (*Mickania scandens* [L.] Willd, *Eupatorium caudatum* Burm.f, *Eupatoirum volubile* Vahl, *Mikania volubilis* [Vahl] Willd, *Mikania chenopodifolia* Willd), or river vine, heartleaf hem vine, or climbing hemp vine, is a climber native to tropical America. The plant grows throughout Southeast Asia to the

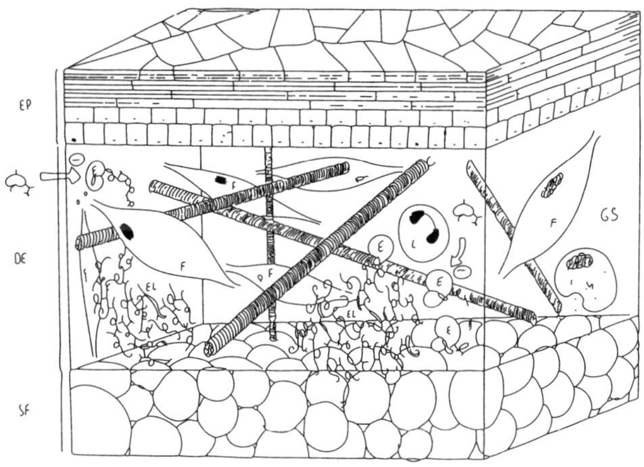

Fig. 20. Hypothetical mode of action of melampolides on skin. C, collagen; F, fibroblast; GS, ground substance; EL, elastine.

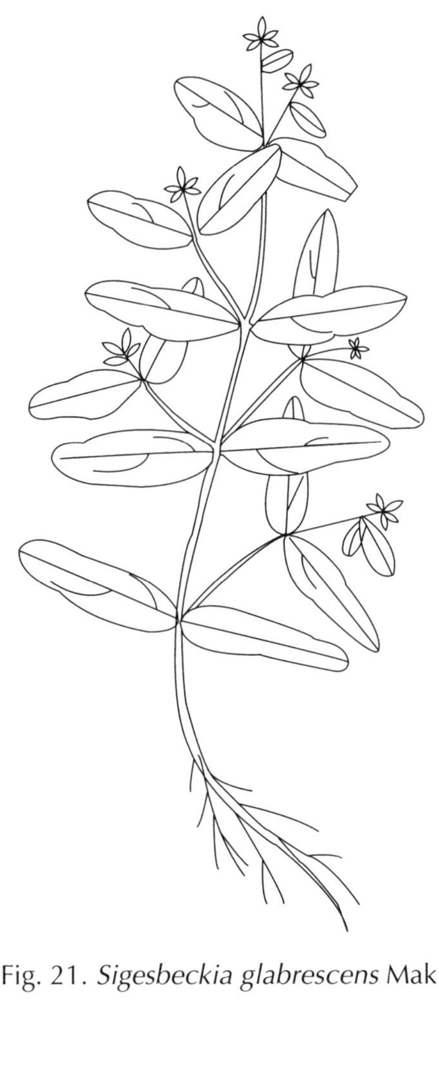

Fig. 21. *Sigesbeckia glabrescens* Mak.

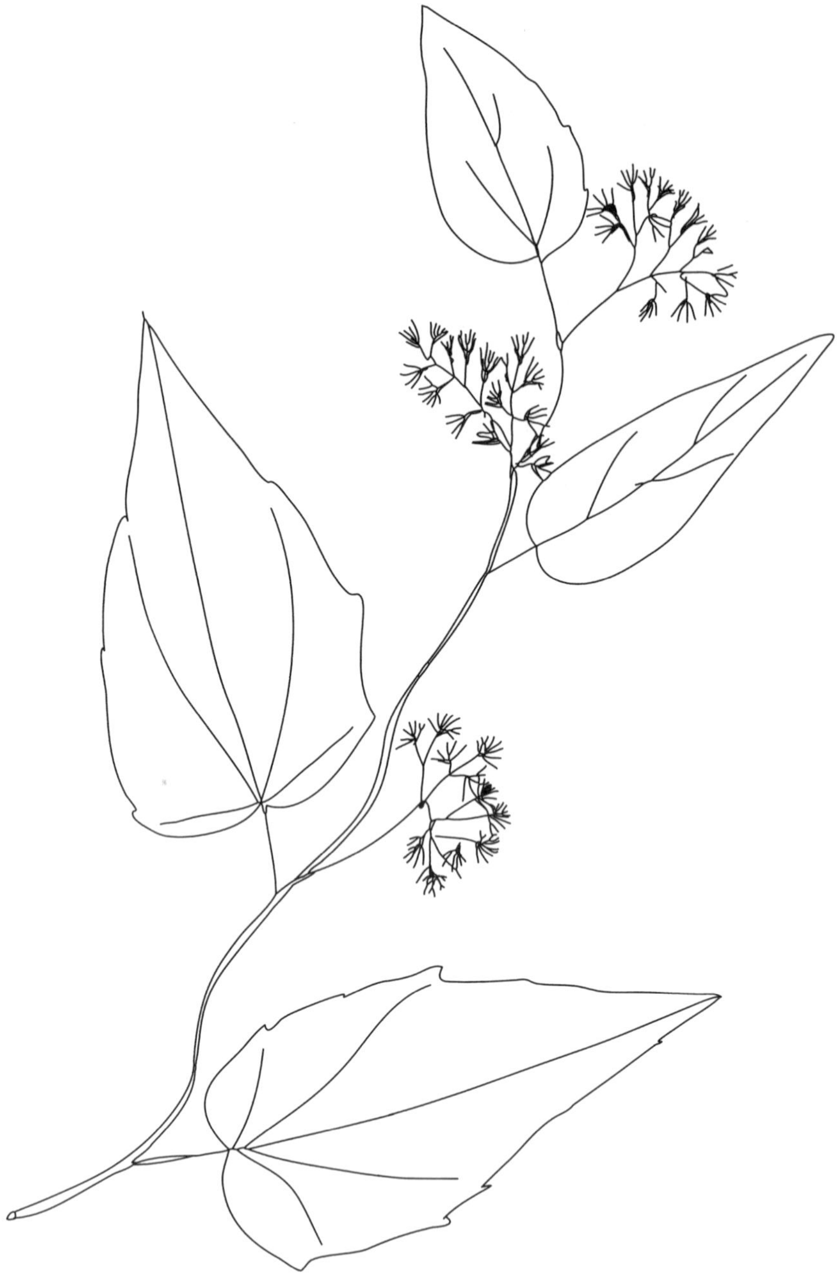

Fig. 22. *Mikania cordata* (Burm.f.) B.L. Robinson.

Bismarck Archipelago. The leaves are cordate, and the capitula are grouped in panicles (Fig. 22). In Taiwan, the plant is used to resolve swellings. In Malaysia, it is used to calm itches, and in Indonesia it is used to heal wounds.

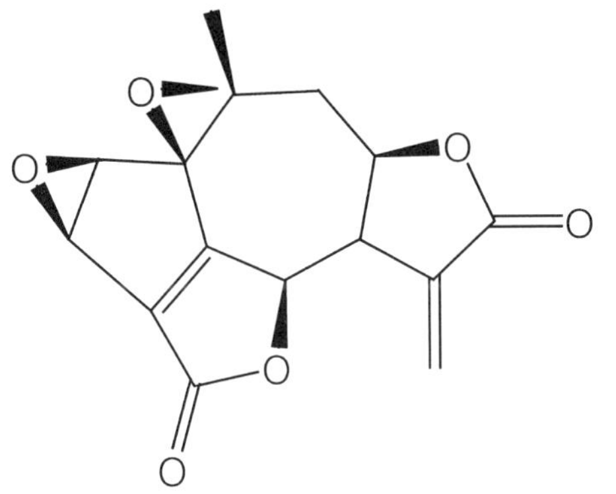

Mikanolide

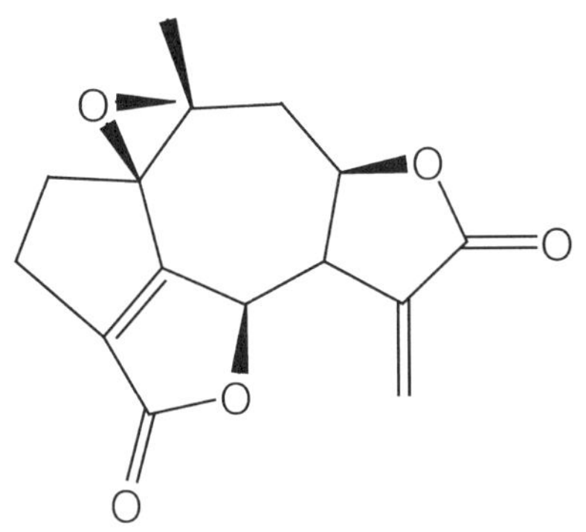

Deoxymikanolide

Mikania cordata is known to elaborate a series of sesquiterpene lactones, among which deoxymikanolide significantly inhibits acetic acid-induced writhing in mice *(44,45)*. The plant also contains a series of melampolides that inhibit the enzymatic activity of elastase *(46)*.

Medicinal Droseraceae

The family Droseraceae consists of four genera and about 100 species of perennial herbs, of which *Drosera burmannii* Vahl, *Drosera rotundifolia* L, *Drosera indica* L., and *Drosera peltata* Sm. are used in Asia for the treatment of cough. Naphthoquinones and flavonoids, which occur in this family, have not been fully studied for pharmacology, and it appears that flavonoids inhibit human neutrophil elastase, hence the potential for the treatment of inflammation.

***Drosera rotundifolia* L.**, or round leaf sundew, is a little perennial herb that can reach 35 cm in height. The plant is found in temperate bogs and swampy areas. The leaves are simple, fleshy, broadly ovate and arranged into rosettes. The leaves are covered with sticky, shiney, red tentacles. The flowers are pink (Fig. 23).

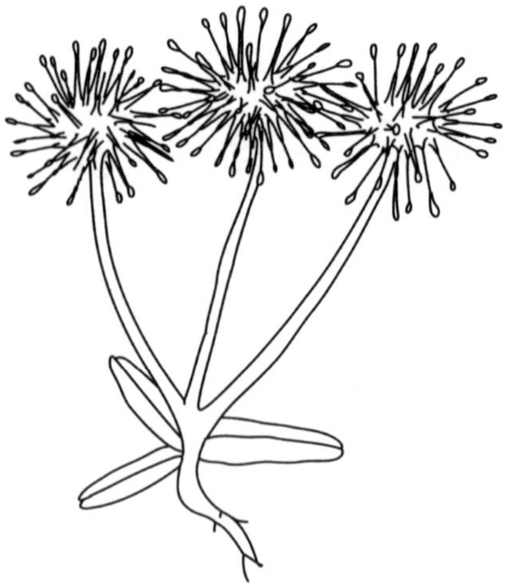

Fig. 23. *Drosera rotundifolia* L.

The plant has been traditionally used in Europe to treat chronic bronchitis, asthma, and whooping cough, and the entire air-dried plant, or *Drosera*, was listed in the *French Pharmacopoeia* in 1965 (tincture, 1 in 5; dose 0.5–2 mL), and in 1880, Murray described its uses in the Royal Hospital for whooping cough. In Japan, a decoction of the plant is used to treat cough. This effect is probably mediated by flavonoids such as hyperoside, quercetin, and isoquercitrin, which are known to abound in the plant *(47)*. Quercetin from *Drosera madagascariensis* inhibits human neutrophil elastase with an IC_{50} value of 0.8 μg/mL, as well as hyperoside (IC_{50} 0.15 μg/mL) and isoquercitrin (IC_{50} 0.7 μg/mL *[48]*).

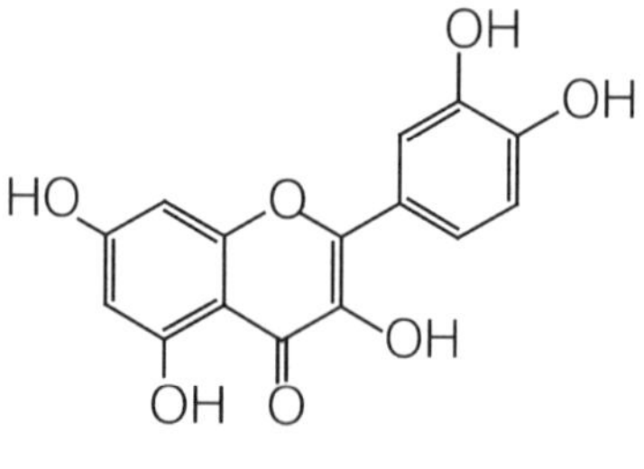

Quercetin

INHIBITORS OF NITRIC OXIDE SYNTHETASE

NOS is an important enzyme involved in the regulation of inflammation, vascular tone, neurotransmission, and cancer. NO is generated via oxidation of the terminal guanidine nitrogen atom from L-arginine by NOS. NO is a very toxic free radical that can cause substantial tissue damage in high concentrations, especially in the brain. In stroke, for example, large amounts of NO are released from nerve cells to cause damage to surrounding tissues including neurones and myocytes. NO is also released during inflammation and is involved in the growth of tumors; it is understood that endogenously formed NO induces the malignant transformation of mouse fibroblasts. Among NOSs, inducible NOS is involved in the overproduction of NO and is expressed in response to IL-1β, tumor necrosis factor-α, and LPS, the genetic expression of which is notably commanded by the NF-κB macrophages. Molecules capable of inhibiting inducible NOS and/or induction of NF-κB activation may be of therapeutic benefit in various types of inflammation. Such molecules could be of sesquiterpenic nature as discussed under the following subeadings.

Medicinal Asteraceae

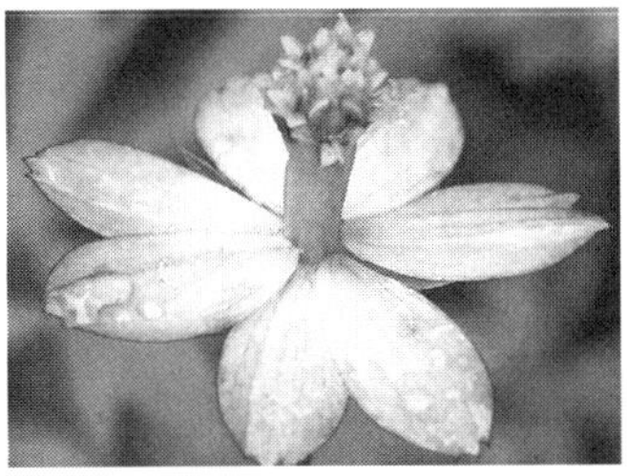

There is an expanding body of evidence to suggest that sesquiterpene lactones inhibit the synthesis NO synthetase. One such compound is an ambrosanolides-type sesquiterpene known as cumanin characterized from *Ambrosia psilostachya*. This sesquiterpene inhibit the enzymatic activity of NO synthetase with an IC_{50} value of 9.38 μM *(49)*. Another example is the well-known artemisinin, a sesquiterpene used as an alternative drug in the treatment of severe and multidrug-resistant malaria, which inhibits NO synthesis in cytokine-stimulated human astrocytoma T67 cells *(50)*.

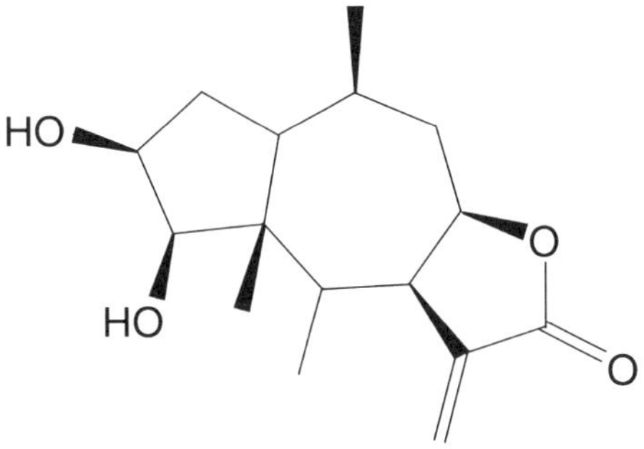

Cumanin

Other sorts of NO inhibitors are triterpenes, such as ursolic acid and 2-α-hydroxy ursolic acid and 2-α-hydroxy ursolic acid from *Prunella vulgaris* L., inhibit the production of NO by murine leukaemic monocyte macrophage cells, RAW 264.7, cultured in vitro. The IC_{50} values were 17 μM for ursolic acid and 27 μM for 2-α-hydroxy ursolic *(51)*.

***Inula chinensis* Rupr. ex Maxim.** (*Inula japonica* Thunb., *Inula britannica* L.), or *hsuan fu hua*, is indigenous of northern China, Mongolia, Korea, and Japan (Fig. 24). It is a perennial herb that grows to a height of 60 cm. The drug consists of the flowers dried in the sun, are used in China as analgesic, to treat swellings, sore throat, cough, vomiting, fullness of chest and as a deobstruent and laxative, diuretic, depurative, tonic, and carminative. Hernandez et al. characterized from

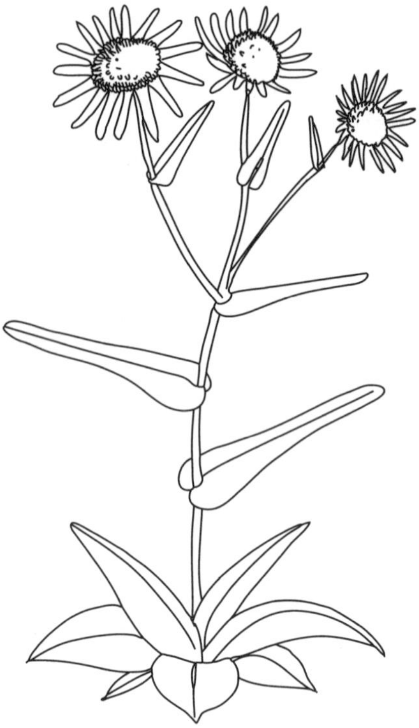

Fig. 24. *Inula chinensis* Rupr. ex Maxim.

Inula viscosa a sesquiterpene lactone, inuviscolide, which reduces the phospholipase A_2-induced edema with an inhibitory dose at which half of the phospholipase A_2-induced edema was reduced, ID_{50}, value of 98 mmol/kg *(52)*. Han et al., studied the mechanism of action of 1-O-acetyl-4R,6S-britannilactone, a sesquiterpene isolated from the flowers of *Inula britannica* and showed that this substance suppressed NO and PGE2 synthesis in RAW 264.7 macrophages through the inhibition of iNOS and COX-2 gene expressionvia a blocking the binding of NF-κB to the promoter in the target genes *(53,54)*. Other sesquiterpenes able to inhibit the enzymatic activity of inducible nitric oxide synthase from the genus *Inula* are bigelovin, 2,3-dihydro-aromaticin and ergolide, which potently inhibits the activity on LPS-induced NOS in murine macrophage RAW 264.7 cells with an IC_{50} value of 0.46 mM, 1.05 and 0.69 μM, respectively *(55)*.

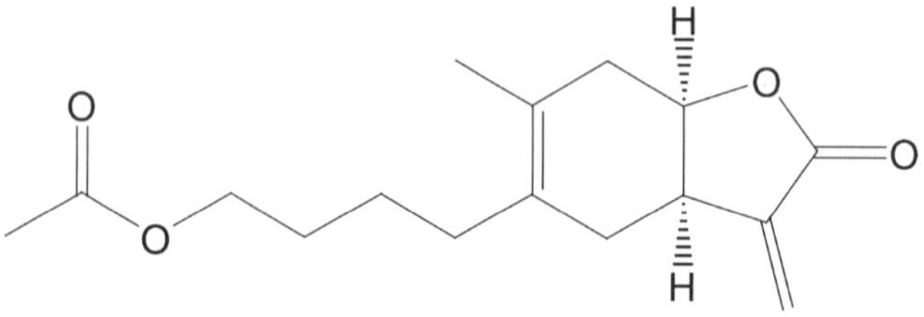

1-O-acetylbritannilatone

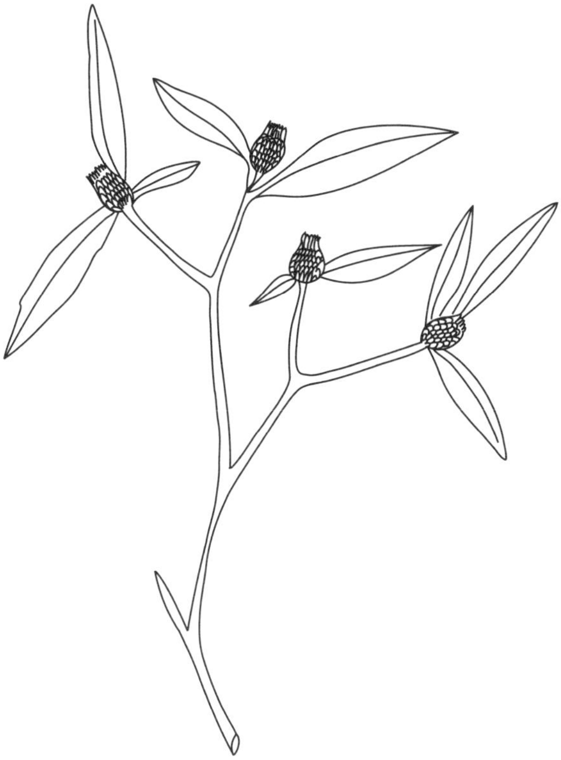

Fig. 25. *Carpesium divaricatum* Sieb. et Zucc.

***Carpesium divaricatum* Sieb. et Zucc.**, or *gankubisou* (Japanese), is an herb that grows to a height of 1 m in shady and damp waste places, roadsides, and hillsides in China, Japan, and Korea. The leaves are lanceolate, and the inflorescences consist of yellow, cylindrical capitula (Fig. 25).

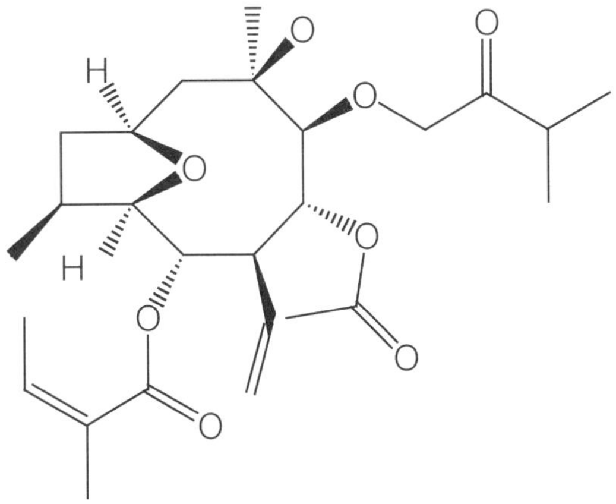

2β, 5-epoxy-5, 10-dihydroxy -6α-angeloyloxy -9β-isobutyloxy -germacran -8α, 12-olid

The plant has been used in traditional Korean herbal medicine for its antipyretic, analgesic, and anti-inflammatory properties vermifuge.
The active principle involved in the antipyretic, analgesic, and anti-inflammatory traditional uses is a sesquiterpene known as 2β,5-epoxy-5,10-dihydroxy-6α-angeloyloxy-9β-isobutyloxy-germacran-8α,12-olide. This sesquiterpene lowers the production of NO by LPS/IFN-γ-stimulated RAW 264.7 cells in a concentration-dependent manner, with an IC_{50} value of approx 2.16 mM. This carence in NO is not owed to inhibition of the enzymatic activity. In addition, Kim et al., showed that the cells exposed to the sesquiterpene had lower level in iNOS protein and mRNA suggesting inhibition of nuclear factor-kappaB (NF-kappaB) activation through a mechanism involving the inhibition of iNOS gene expression via inhibition of NF-κB DNA binding *(56,57)*.

Medicinal Lauraceae

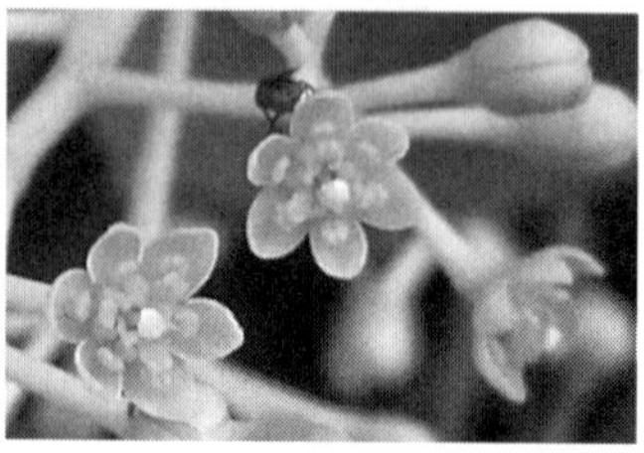

The family Lauraceae consists of 50 genera and 2000 species of trees, shrubs, and herbs, of which 70 are of medicinal value in the Asia–Pacific region. Lauraceae are well-known for elaborating isoquinoline alkaloids and sesquiterpenes, the latter most likely representing a vast source of material for the search for NOS. Examples of such compounds are costunolide and dehydrocostunolide found in the leaves of *Laurus nobilis* (bay leaf, laurel), the leaves of which are widely used as a spice, antiseptic, stomachic, and to treat rheumatism in traditional European medicine *(58)*. The potential of *Neolitsea zeylanica* Nees (Merr.) as a potential source of NOS inhibitor is discussed here.

***Neolitsea zeylanica* Nees (Merr.)** (*Tetradenia zeylanica* Nees, *Litsea zeylanica* Nees) or shore laurel, *tejur* (Malay), Or *nan ya xin mu jiang zi* (Chinese), is a tree that grows up to 20 m tall in forests and thickets from sea level up to 1000 m in Burma, Malaysia, Sri Lanka, Borneo, the Philippines, India, China, and Australia. The young stems are glabrous. The leaves are simple, alternate, or crowded at apex of stems. The blades are ovate-oblong or oblong and glaucous beneath. The flowers are small and arranged in axillary, subsessile, four- to five-flowered umbels. The fruits are subglobose, 8 mm–1.5 cm in diameter, and seated on a disc-shaped, wavy, marginated perianth.

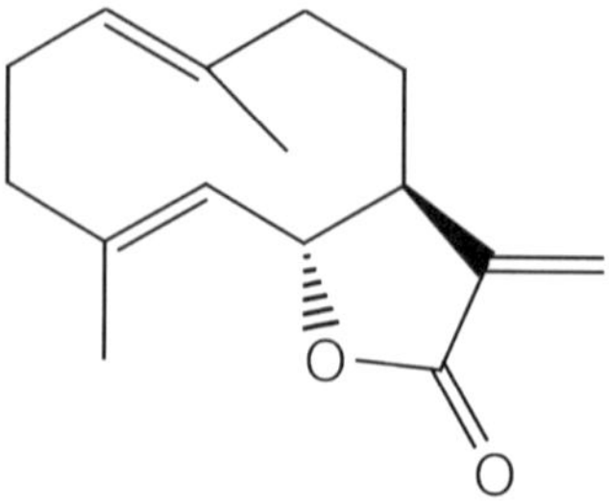

Costunolide

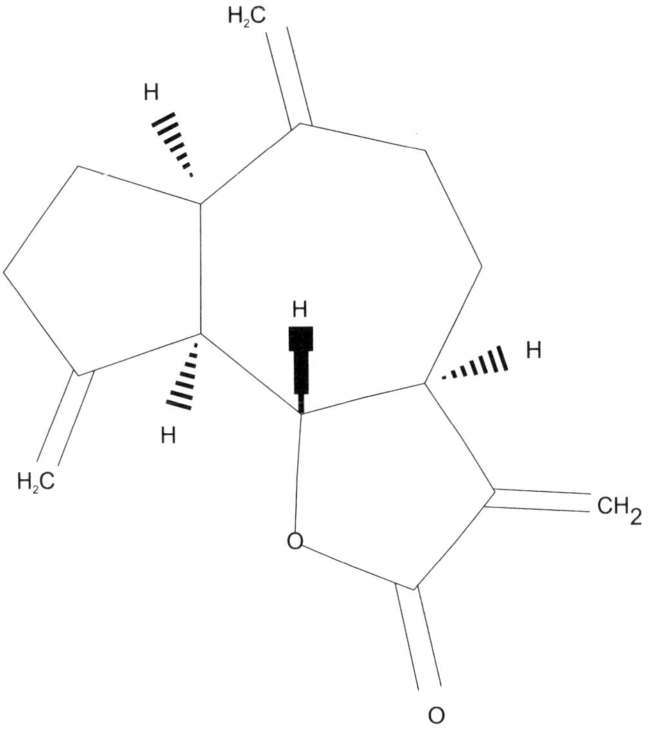

Dehydrocostus lactone

In Malaysia, a paste of the roots is applied to fingers to treat eruptions. The plant is known contain some sesquiterpene lactones including neolinderane, zeylanine, zeylanicine and zeylanidine *(59–61)*, the potential of which as an inhibitor of NOS would be worth investigation because pseudoneolinderane and linderalactone inhibited the production of superoxide anion generation by human neutrophils in response to fMLP/CB. The IC_{50} values for pseudoneolinderane and linderalactonewere 3.21 and 8.48 μg/mL, respectively *(62)*.

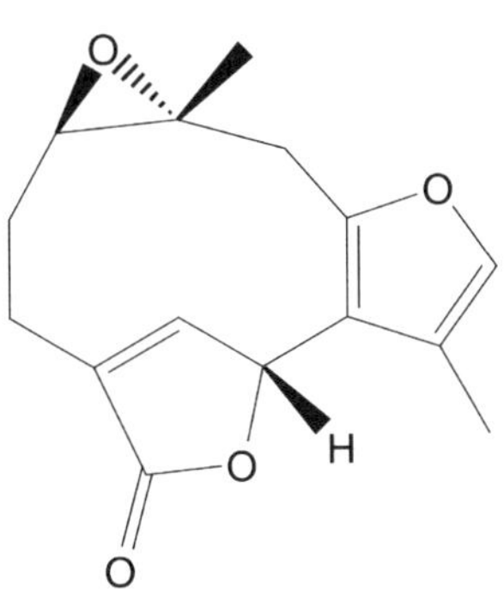

pseudoneolinderane

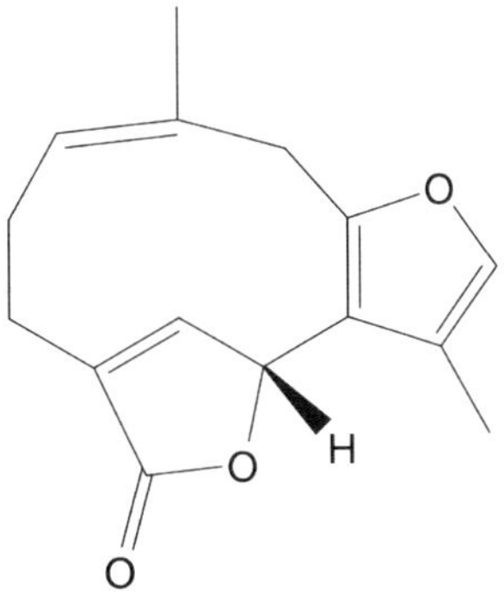

linderalactone

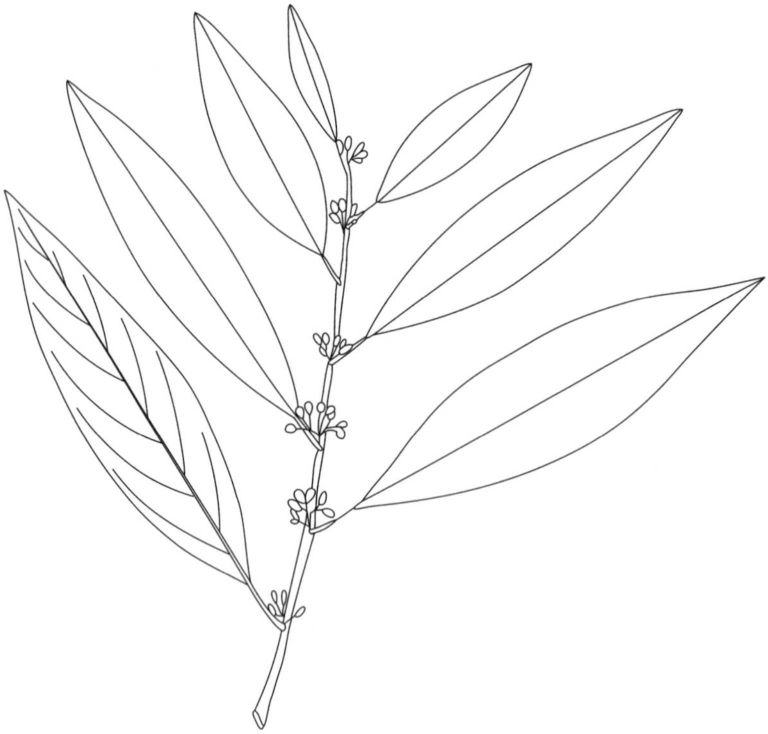

Fig. 26. *Litsea cubeba*. Flora of Malay peninsula. Geographical localization: Bukiy Kutu, Kudla Kubu. Date: 12/25/1930. No 23848. Field collector: Cooman. Botanical identification: F.S.P. Ng, 11/27/2001.

Litsea cubeba (Lour.) Pers. (*Litsea citrata* Bl., *Laurus cubeba* Lour., *Daphnidium cubeba*), or *pokok myuniak kayah puteh* (Malay, Indonesian), is a shrub which grows wild in China, Korea, Vietnam, and Indonesia. The stems are smooth; the leaves are aromatic, simple, and exstipulate. The petiole is about 1 cm long. The blade is lanceolate, thinly coriaceous, 12–4 cm × 3–1 cm and shows six to eight pairs of secondary nerves. The fruits are globose and 3 mm in diameter (Fig. 26).

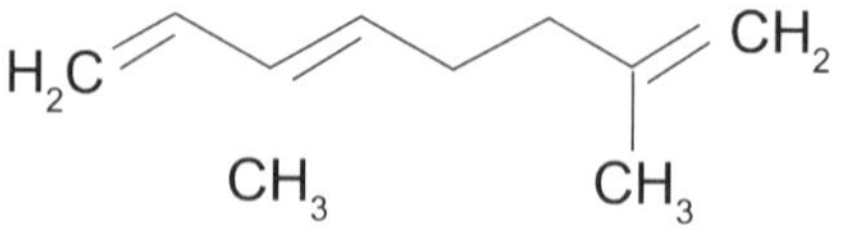

*cis*α–ocimene

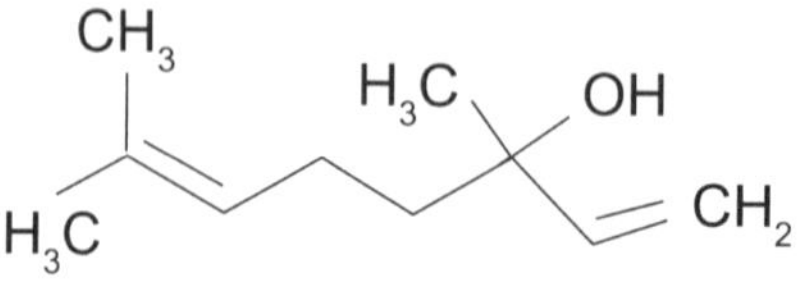

3,7-dimethyl-1,6-octadien-3-ol

In China, the seeds are eaten to promote digestion and treat cough and bronchitis. In Vietnam, Cambodia, and Laos, a decoction of the plant is used to treat mental disorders such as hysteria and forgetfulness. In Taiwan, the plant is used to treat athlete's foot and other skin diseases.

The plant is strongly aromatic on account of an essential oil which comprises *cis*-α-ocimene (25.11%), 3,7-dimethyl-1,6-octadien-3-ol (16.85%), and *trans*-nerolidol (13.89%), hence the use of the plant in aromatherapy. A methanolic extract of bark of *Litsea cubeba* (Lour.) Pers. and its fractions (0.01 mg/mL) from bark inhibit NO and PGE_2 production in LPS-activated RAW 264.7 macrophages without significant cytotoxicity at less than 0.01 mg/mL concentration. The methanol extract decreased the enzymatic activity of myeloperoxidase (0.05 mg/mL). These findings suggest that *L. cubeba* is beneficial for inflammatory conditions and may contain compound(s) with anti-inflammatory properties (63). Can we expect the vasorelaxant laurotetanine (64) isolated from the plant to exert such activity?

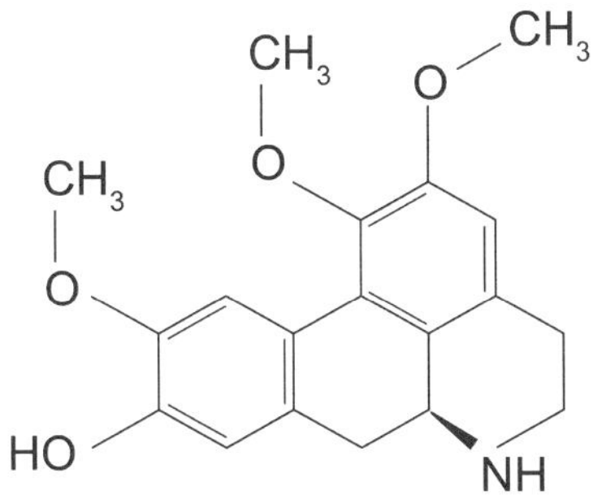

Laurotetanine

Litsea odorifera Val., or *medang pawas* (Indonesian), is a tree that grows in Indonesia and eastward to Papua New Guinea. The stem is slightly lenticelled. The leaves are simple, exstipulate, and glossy. The blade is broadly lanceolate, 7.5 × 5 cm, and shows four to five pairs of secondary nerves. The fruits are to 1 cm long, dark green with white spots, glossy, and ovoid (Fig. 27). The plant is used to treat biliousness, to promote lactation, and to heal boils and furuncles. The pharmacological potential of this plant is unexplored, and it would be interesting to know whether further study reveals evidence of nitric oxidase inhibition.

Medicinal Solanaceae

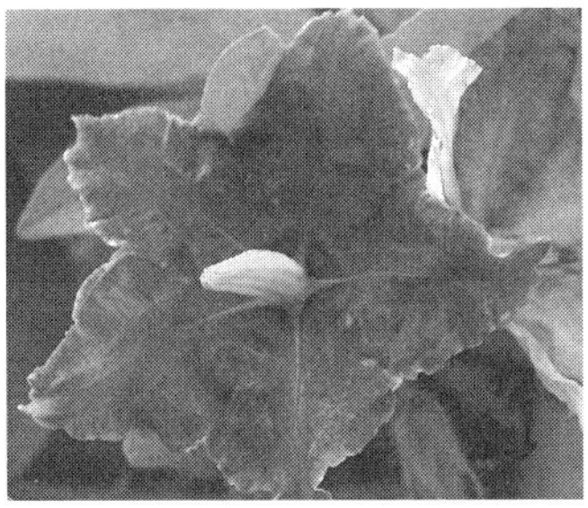

The family Solanaceae consists of about 85 genera and 2800 species of plants, of which, 80 are of medicinal value in the Asia–Pacific region. Solanaceaeare well known for their parasympatholytic tropane alkaloids, such as hyoscyamine. Classic examples are *Atropa belladonna* L. (belladona herb, *British Pharmacopoeia* 1963), *Datura stramonium* L. (stramonium, *British Pharmacopoeia*, 1963), and the dried leaves and flowering tops of *Hyoscyamus*

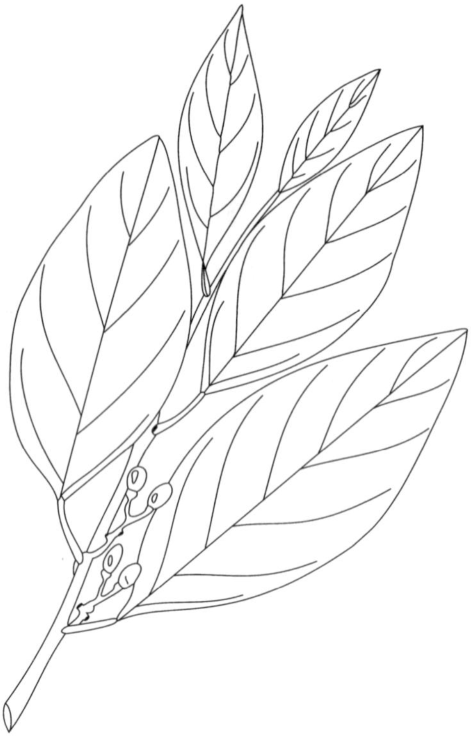

Fig. 27. *Litsea odorifera* Val. BOSWESEN. Nederlands New Guinea (Forestry Division Neth. New Guinea) Field collector: F. Schram No B 1737. Date: 3/9/1955. Geographical localization: New Guinea, Res. Manokawaii, Sidei, altitude: 7 m.

niger L. (hyoscyamus, *British Pharmacopoeia*, 1963), which have been used as antispasmodic drugs. In the family, the genus *Physalis* is known to produce 16,24-cyclo-13,14-secosteroidal terpenes called physalins, which might be of interest as inhibitors of NOS. An example of medicinal *Physalis* is *Physalis alkekengi*, a medicinal plant of the Asia–Pacific region.

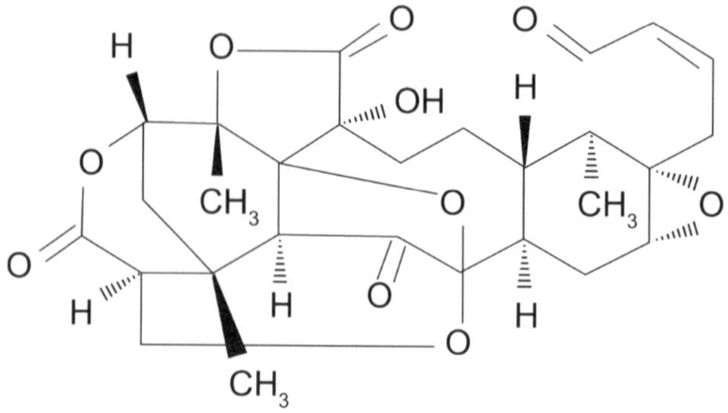

Physalin F

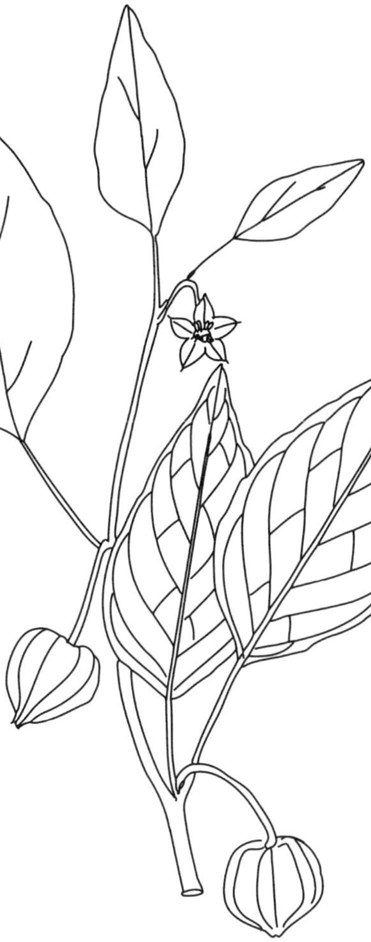

Fig. 28. *Physalis alkekengi.*

Physalis alkekengi, or Chinese lantern, alkekengi, bladder cherry, ground cherry, strawberry tomato, winter cherry, *suan chiang*, or *teng leng ts'ao*, is an ornamental perennial herb that grows to a height of 80 cm in Eurasia. The leaf blade is narrowly to broadly ovate. The flowers are mostly white, with a greenish or yellowish eye, and are rotate or campanulate. The fruits are shiny, orange-red, globose, 1–1.5 cm in diameter. The berries are enclosed in an inflated calyx that resembles a little lantern (Figs. 28 and 29). The plant is used in China to break fever, promote urination, and treat cough. The seeds are used to promote labor. *Physalis alkekengi* is known to elaborate a series of 16,24-cyclo-13,14-secosteroidals known as physalins, such as physalins N and O. Physalins B, F, and G from *Physalis angulata* L. lower NO, tumor necrosis factor-α, IL-6, and IL-12 release by macrophages stimulated with LPS and IFN-γ *(65)*. It would be interesting to learn whether further studies on Solanaceae, and *Physalis* species in general, disclose any molecule of therapeutic value in treating inflammation.

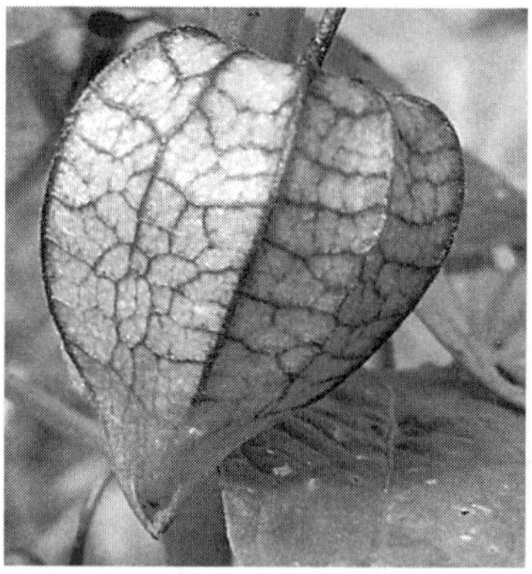

Fig. 29. Lantern-like fruits of *Physalis alkekengi*.

CONCLUSION AND FUTURE PROSPECTS

In summary, most of the evidence that has emerged from the investigation of medicinal plants of Asia and the Pacific for anti-inflammatory principles shows a clear predominance of sesquiterpene lactones from Asteraceae, which are able to inhibit the enzymatic activity of lipo-oxygenase, COX, NOS, and elastase, and we can reasonably expect the isolation of original anti-inflammatory drugs from this large family. Some evidence has already been presented that indicates that a large number of flowering plants owe their anti-inflammatory properties to flavonoids which inhibit a broad spectrum of enzymes and scavenge free radicals.

Such plants might be found in the Asteridae, particularly in the order Lamiales (Boraginaceae, Verbenaceae), Solanales (Convolvulaceae), Scrophulariales (Acanthaceae), Dipsacales (Caprifoliaceae), and Rubiales (Rubiaceae). *Cordia verbenacea* DC, *Cordia francisci*, *Cordia myxa*, and *Cordia serratifolia* in the Boraginaceae exhibit significant analgesic, anti-inflammatory, and antiarthritic properties in vivo *(66)*. Another example of Boraginaceae is *Carmona microphylla* (Lamk.) Don, which is known to produce quinones, ehretianone, and microphyllone, and which has exhibited anti-inflammatory potencies in vivo and in vitro *(67)*.

The family Convolvulaceae consists of 50 genera and 1500 species of vines is of substantial interest in the search for COX inhibitors because it is known that the phenolic compounds it elaborates, such as eugenol and *N-trans-* and *N-cis-*feruloyltyramines, inhibit the synthesis of PG. Note that the closely related Solanaceae are known to elaborate feruloyltyramines and could be also considered as a source of COX inhibitors. One of these, *Argyreia speciosa*, at the doses of 50, 100, and 200 mg/kg dose-dependently potentiates the delayed-type hypersensitivity reaction induced both by sheep red blood cells and oxazolone in rodents *(68)*. *Vitex negundo* L. (Verbenaceae) abrogates carrageenan- and formaldehyde-induced paw edema, inhibits antihistamine and PG synthesis, and stabilizes membrane and fight oxidation *(69,70)*. An ethanolic extract of the leaves of *Graptophyllum pictum* (L.) Griffith (Acanthaceae) given orally to rodents is anti-inflammatory *(71)*. *Acanthus* *ebracteatus* reduces the production of eicosanoid *(72)* and abrogates the edema induced by carrageenan in rats. In the Rubiaceae, extracts of *Paederia foetida* L. inhibit significantly the formation of granulation in cotton-pellet-implanted rats *(73)*. Note that anthocyanins and hydrolysable tannins (Rosidae, Hamamelidae) are anti-inflammatory because of their ability to scavenge free radicals, as in the case of aqueous extract of *Bridelia ferruginea*, which inhibits paw edema induced by carrageenan, with an ID_{50} value of 36 mg/kg *(74)*. Triterpene as anti-inflammatory principles are to be found particularly in the subclass Dilleniidae and especially in the Ebenaceae (*Diospyros* species) and Capparaceae (*Crateva* species), and are known to elaborate a series of pentacyclic triterpenes including betulin, betulinic acid, and ursolic acid.

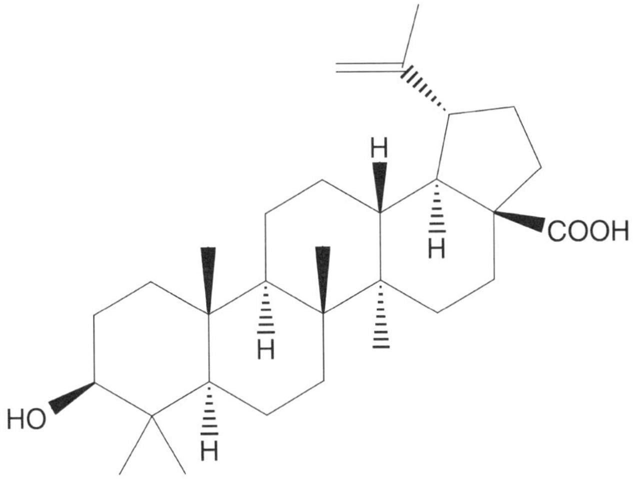

Betulinic acid

Lupeol, isolated from the stem bark of *Crataeva magna* (Lour.) DC. (Capparaceae), reduces the foot-pad thickness and complement activity in arthritic rats *(75)*. Oleanolic acid saponins isolated from the roots of *Momordica cochinchinensis* (Lour.) Spreng. is anti-pruritic in rodent *(76)*.

In comparison to the Asteraceae, Dilleniidae, and Rosidae, evidence available regarding the anti-inflammatory effects of Caryophyllaceae seems vestigial, hence the urgent need to assess this subclass for its anti-inflammatory potentials.

Caryophyllidae are an interesting source of oligosaccharides and peptides with potential anti-inflammatory and/or immunomodulating effect. These polar compounds might for instance explain the fact that the fresh juice expressed from *Aerva lanata* (L.) Juss. (Amaranthaceae) inhibits carrageenan-induced edema in rodent. Note that the seeds of *Gomphrena* species inhibit the formation of IL-6 by osteoblastic cells (MC3T3-E10) without cytotoxicity in vitro. Such property could be useful for the treatment of chronic rheumatoid arthritis, infection, and cancer. In the Lauraceae, *trans*-cinnamaldehyde from *Cinnamomum cassia* (Lauraceae, order Laurales) inhibits in vitro the activity of NOS. African medicinal plants *Cinnamomum latifolia* Sonder, *Cinnamomum myrtifolia* Stapf., *Cinnamomum transvaalensis* Burtt. Davy, *Cinnamomum woodii* Engl., and *Cinnamomum wyliei* Stapf., exhibited in vitro potent inhibition of COX-2 *(77)*.

Hong et al. *(7)* evaluated approx 170 methanol extracts of natural products, including Korean herbal medicines, for the inhibition of PGE_2 production (for COX-2 inhibitors) and NO formation (for iNOS inhibitors) in LPS-induced mouse macrophage RAW 264.7 cells. As a result, several extracts, such as *Aristolochia debilis* (Aristolochiaceae), *Cinnamomum cassia* and *Cinnamomum loureiroi* (Lauraceae), *Curcuma zedoaria* (Zingiberaceae), *Eugenia caryophyllata* (Myrtaceae), *Pterocarpus santalius* (Fabaceae), *Rehmania glutinosa* (Scrophulariaceae), and *Tribulus terrestris* (Zygophyllaceae), showed potent inhibition of COX-2 activity (>80% inhibition at the test concentration of 10 μg/mL). In addition, the extracts of *Aristolochiaceae debilis*, *Caesalpinia sappan*, *Curcuma longa*, *Curcuma zedoaria*, *Daphne genkwa* (Thymeleaceae), and *Morus alba* (Moraceae) were also considered as potential inhibitors of iNOS activity (>70% inhibition at the test concentration of 10 mg/mL). Investigation of these active extracts mediating COX-2 and NOS inhibitory activities are warranted for further elucidation of active principles for development of new cancer chemopreventive and/or anti-inflammatory agents.

REFERENCES

1. Bernard P, Scior T, Didier B, Hibert M, Berthon JY. Ethnopharmacology and bioinformatic combination for leads discovery: application to phospholipase A(2) inhibitors. Phytochemistry 2001;58:865–874.
2. Vishwanath BS, Fawzy AA, Franson R, et al. Edema-inducing activity of phospholipase A2 purified from human synovial fluid and inhibition by aristolochic acid. Inflammation 1988;12:549–561.
3. Wu TS, Leu YL, Chan YY. Aristofolin-A, a denitro-aristolochic acid glycoside and other constituents from aristolochia kaempferi. Phytochemistry 1998;49:2509–2510.
4. Wu TS, Leu YL, Chan YY. Constituents from the stem and root of *Aristolochia kaempferi*. Biol Pharm Bull 2000;23:1216–1219.
5. Pezzuto JM, Swanson SM, Mar W, Che CT, Cordell GA, Fong HH Evaluation of the mutagenic and cytostatic potential of aristolochic acid (3,4-methylenedioxy-8-methoxy-10-nitrophenanthrene-1-carboxylic acid) and several of its derivatives. Mutat Res 1988;206:447–454.
6. Levi M, Guchelaar HJ, Woerdenbag HJ, Zhu YP. Acute hepatitis in a patient using a Chinese herbal tea—a case report. Pharm World Sci 1998;20:43–44.
7. Hong CH, Sun KH, Jin O, Sun SK, Kyung AN, Sang KL. Evaluation of natural products on inhibition of inducible cyclooxygenase (COX-2) and nitric oxide synthase (iNOS) in cultured mouse macrophage cells. J Ethnopharmacol 2002;83:153–159.
8. Mikaye A, Yamamoto H, Takebayashi Y, Imai H, Honda K. The novel natural product YM-26567-1: a competitive inhibitor of group II phospholipase A2. J Pharmacol Exp Ther 1992;263:1302–1307.

9. Chang HW, Baek SH, Chung KW, Son KH, Kim HP, Kang SS. Inactivation of phospholipase A_2 by naturally occurring biflavonoid, ochnaflavone. Biochem Biophys Res Commun 1994;205:843–849.
10. Akihisa T, Ken Y, Hirotoshi O, Yoshimasa K. Triterpene alcohols from the flowers of Compositae and their anti-inflammatory effects. Phytochemistry 1996;43:1255–1260.
11. Januário AH, Simone LS, Silvana M, et al. Neo-clerodane diterpenoid, a new metalloprotease snake venom inhibitor from *Baccharis trimera* (Asteraceae): anti-proteolytic and anti-hemorrhagic properties. Chem Biol Interact 2002;150:243–251.
12. Sala AM, Carmen R, Giner M, Máñez SR. Anti-phospholipase A2 and anti-inflammatory activity of *Santolina chamaecyparissus*. Life Sci 2000;66:35–40.
13. Sasaki S, Aoyagi S, Hsu HY. The isolation of taraxerol, taraxeryl acetate, and taraxerone from *Crossostephium chinense* Makino (Compositae). Chem Pharm Bull (Tokyo) 1965;J13:87–88.
14. Li RW, David Lin G, Myers SP, Leach DN. Anti-inflammatory activity of Chinese medicinal vine plants. J Ethnopharmacol 2003;85:61–67.
15. Inagaki I, Sakushima A, Sueo N, Sansei H. Flavones and flavone glucosides from the leaves of *Trachelospermum asiaticum*. Phytochemistry 1973;12:1498.
16. Nakatani K, Norimichi N, Tsutomu A, Hideyuki Y, Yasushi O. Inhibition of cyclooxygenase and prostaglandin E_2 synthesis by γ-mangostin, a xanthone derivative in mangosteen, in C6 rat glioma cells. Biochem Pharmacol 2002;63:73–79.
17. Cavin C, Delannoy M, Malnoe A, et al. Inhibition of the expression and activity of cyclooxygenase-2 by chicory extract. Biochem Biophys Res Commun 2005;327:742–749.
18. Hu L, Zhongliang CH. Sesquiterpenoid alcohols from *Chrysanthemum morifolium*. Phytochemistry 1997;44:1287–1290.
19. Sumner H, Umit S, Knight DW, Hoult JRS. *Chrysanthemum parthenium* (L.); Bernh. Inhibition of 5-lipoxygenase and cyclooxygenase in leukocytes by feverfew: Involvement of sesquiterpene lactones and other components. Biochem Pharmacol 1992;43:2313–2320.
20. Chacur M, Gutierrez JM, Milligan ED, et al. Snake venom components enhance pain upon subcutaneous injection: an initial examination of spinal cord mediators. Pain 2004:111:65–76.
21. Jäger AK, Hutchings A, van Staden J. Screening of Zulu medicinal plants for prostaglandin-synthesis inhibitors. J Ethnopharmacol 1996;52:95–100.
22. Kimura Y, Hiromichi O, Shigeru A. Effects of stilbenes on arachidonate metabolism in leukocytes. Biochim Biophysica Acta 1985;834:275–278.
23. Pang L, de las Heras B, Hoult JR. A novel diterpenoid labdane from *Sideritis javalambrensis* inhibits eicosanoid generation from stimulated macrophages but enhances arachidonate release. Biochem Pharmacol 1996;51:863–868.
24. Singh S, Majumdar DK, Rehan HMS. Evaluation of anti-inflammatory potential of fixed oil of *Ocimum sanctum* (Holy basil) and its possible mechanism of action. J Ethnopharmacol 1996;54:19–26.

25. Pongprayoon U, Baeckstrom P, Jacobsson U, Lindstrom M, Bohlin L. Compounds inhibiting prostaglandin synthesis isolated from *Ipomoea pescaprae*. Planta Med 1991;57:515–518.
26. Dewhirst FE. Structure/activity relationship for inhibition of prostaglandin cyclooxygenase by phenolic compounds. Prostaglandins 1980;20:209–222.
27. Kuhn H, Wiesner R, Alder L, Schewe T. Occurrence of free and esterified lipoxygenase products in leaves of *Glechoma hederacea* L. and other Labiatae. Eur J Biochem 1989; 186:155–162.
28. Henry DY, Gueritte-Voegelein F, Insel PA, Ferry N, Bouguet J, Potier P, Hanoune J. Isolation and characterization of 9-hydroxy-10-*trans*,12-*cis*-octadecadienoic acid, a novel regulator of platelet adenylate cyclase from *Glechoma hederacea* L. Labiatae. Eur J Biochem 1987;170:389–394.
29. Yashodharan K, Cox PJ, Jaspars M, Lutfun N, Satyajit DS. Isolation, structure elucidation and biological activity of hederacine A and B, two unique alkaloids from *Glechoma hederaceae*. Tetrahedron 2003;59:6403–6407.
30. Yang LK, Khoo-Beattie C, Goh KL, et al. Ardisiaquinones from *Ardisia teysmanniana*. Phytochemistry 2001;58:1235–1238.
31. Fukuishi N, Takada T, Fukuyama Y, Akagi M. Antiallergic effect of ardisiaquinone A, a potent 5-lipoxygenase inhibitor. Phytomedicine 2001;8:460–464.
32. Dana A, Ilse Z, Dingermann T, Müller WE, Steinhilber D, Werz O. Hyperforin is a dual inhibitor of cyclooxygenase-1 and 5-lipoxygenase. Biochem Pharmacol 2002;64: 1767–1775.
33. An TY, Ming DS, Hu LH, Liu SJ, Chen ZL. Polyprenylated phloroglucinol derivatives from *Hypericum erectum*. Phytochemistry 2002;59:395–398.
34. Tornhamre S, Schmidt TJ, Näsman-Glaser B, Ericsson I, Ake L. Inhibitory effects of helenalin and related compounds on 5-lipoxygenase and leukotriene C_4 synthase in human blood cells. Biochem Pharmacol 2001;62:903–911.
35. Stavri M, Ford CH, Bucar F, et al. Bioactive constituents of Artemisia monosperma. Phytochemistry 2005;66:233–239.
36. Prieto JM, Giner RM, Recio MC, Manez S, Rios JL. Dual inhibition of cyclooxygenase-1 and 5-lipoxygenase by aerial part of Bupleurum fruticescens methanol extract. Fitoterapia 2004;75:179–186.
37. Konarev AV, Anisimova IN, Gavrilova VA, et al. Serine proteinase inhibitors in the Compositae: distribution, polymorphism and properties. *Phytochemistry* 2002;59: 279–291.
38. Barua RN, Ram PS, Gopalakrishna T, Werner H, Serengolam VG. New melampolides and darutigenol from *Sigesbeckia orientalis*. Phytochemistry 1980;19:323–325.
39. Zdero CF, Bohlmann RMK, Robinson H. Sesquiterpene lactones and other constituents from *Siegesbeckia orientalis* and *Guizotia scabra*. Phytochemistry 1991;30: 1579–1584.
40. Kang BK, Lee EH, Kim HM. Inhibitory effects of Korean folk medicine "Hi-Chum" on histamine release from mast cells *in vivo* and *in vitro*. J Ethnopharmacol 1997;57:73–79.

41. Kim HM, Lee JH, Won JH, Park et al. Inhibitory effect on immunoglobulin E production *in vivo* and *in vitro* by *Siegesbeckia glabrescens*. Phytother Res 2001;15:572–576.
42. He SH, Xie H, Zhang XJ, Wang XJ. Inhibition of histamine release from human mast cells by natural chymase inhibitors. Acta Pharmacol Sin. 2004;25:822–826.
43. Dong XY, Chen M, Jin W, Huang DX, Shen SM, Li HT. Studies on antifertility constituents of *Siegesbeckia glabrescens* Mak. Yao Xue Xue Bao 1989;24:833–836.
44. Ahmed M, Rahman MT. Alimuzzaman M, Shilpi JA. Analgesic sesquiterpene dilactone from *Mikania cordata*. Fitoterapia 2001;72:919–921.
45. Herz W, Subramaniam PS, Santhanam PS, Aota K, Hall AL. Structure elucidation of sesquiterpene dilactones from *Mikania scandens* (L.) Willd. J Org Chem 1970;35: 1453–1464.
46. Gutiérrez AB, Oberti JC, Sosa VE, Herz W. Melampolides from *Mikania cordifolia*. Phytochemistry 1987;26:2315–2320.
47. Krenn L, Beyer G, Pertz HH, et al. *In vitro* antispasmodic and anti-inflammatory effects of *Drosera rotundifolia*. Arzneimittelforschung 2004;54:402–405.
48. Melzig MF, Pertz HH, Krenn L. Anti-inflammatory and spasmolytic activity of extracts from *Droserae herba*. Phytomedicine 2001;8:225–229.
49. Lastra AL, Ramírez TO, Salazar L, Martínez M, Trujillo-Ferrara J. The ambrosanolide cumanin inhibits macrophage nitric oxide synthesis: some structural considerations. J Ethnopharmacol 2004;95:221–227.
50. Aldieri E, Atragene D, Bergandi L, et al. Artemisinin inhibits inducible nitric oxide synthase and nuclear factor NF-κB activation. FEBS Lett 2003;552(2–3):141–144.
51. Ryu SY, Oak MH, Yoon SK, et al. Anti-allergic and anti-inflammatory triterpenes from the herb of *Prunella vulgaris* Planta Med 2000;66:358–360.
52. Hernandez V, del Carmen Recio M, Manez S, Prieto JM, Giner RM, Rios JL. A mechanistic approach to the *in vivo* anti-inflammatory activity of sesquiterpenoid compounds isolated from *Inula viscosa*. Planta Med 2001:67;726–731.
53. Je KH, Han AR, Lee HT, Mar W, Seo EK. The inhibitory principle of lipopolysaccharide-induced nitric oxide production from *Inula britannica* var. chinensis. Arch Pharm Res 2005;27:83–85.
54. Han M, Wen JK, Zheng B, Zhang DQ. Acetylbritannilatone suppresses NO and PGE2 synthesis in RAW 264.7 macrophages through the inhibition of iNOS and COX-2 gene expression. Life Sci 2004;75:675–684.
55. Lee HT, Yang SW, Kim KH, Seo EK, Mar W. Pseudoguaianolides isolated from *Inula britannica* var. chinenis as inhibitory constituents against inducible nitric oxide synthase. Arch Pharm Res 2002;25:151–153.
56. Kim EJ, Hye KJ, Yong KK, et al. Suppression by a sesquiterpene lactone from *Carpesium divaricatum* of inducible nitric oxide synthase by inhibiting nuclear factor-κB activation. Biochem Pharmacol 2001;61:903–910.
57. Kim DK, Baek NI, Choi SU, Lee CO, Lee KR, Zee OP. Four new cytotoxic germacranolides from Carpesium divaricatum. J Nat Prod. 1997;60:1199–1202.
58. Matsuda H, Tadashi K, Iwao T, Hiroki U, Toshio M, Masayuki Y. Inhibitory effects of sesquiterpenes from bay leaf on nitric oxide production in lipopolysaccharide-activated

macrophages: structure requirement and role of heat shock protein induction. Life Sci 2000;66:2151–2157.

59. Joshi BS, Kamat VN, Govindachari TR. Sesquiterpenes of *Neolitsea zeylanica* merr. I: isolation of some constituents. Tetrahedron 1967;23:261–265.
60. Joshi BS, Kamat VN, Govindachari TR. Sesquiterpenes of *Neolitsea zeylanica* merr. II: structure of neolinderane. Tetrahedron 1967;23:267–271.
61. Joshi BS, Kamat VN, Govindachari TR. Sesquiterpenes of *Neolitsea zeylanica* Merr. III: structure of zeylanine, zeylanicine and zeylanidine. Tetrahedron 1967;23:273–277.
62. Chen KS, Hsieh PW, Hwang TL, Chang FR, Wu YC. Anti-inflammatory furanogermacrane sesquiterpenes from *Neolitsea parvigemma*. Nat Prod Res 2005;19:283–286.
63. Choi EM, Hwang JK. Effects of methanolic extract and fractions from Litsea cubeba bark on the production of inflammatory mediators in RAW264.7 cells. Fitoterapia 2004;75:141–148.
64. Chen WY, Ko FN, Wu YC, Lu ST, Teng CM. Vasorelaxing effect in rat thoracic aorta caused by laurotetanine isolated from *Litsea cubeba* Persoon. J Pharm Pharmacol 1994;46:380–382.
65. Soares MB, Bellintani MC, Ribeiro IM, Tomassini TC, Ribeiro dos Santos R. Inhibition of macrophage activation and lipopolysaccaride-induced death by seco-steroids purified from *Physalis angulata* L. Eur J Pharmacol 2003;459:107–112.
66. Ficarra R, Ficarra P, Tommasini S, et al. Leaf extracts of some *Cordia* species: analgesic and anti-inflammatory activities as well as their chromatographic analysis. Farmaco 1995;50:245–256.
67. Selvanayagam ZE, Gnanavendhan SG, Balakrishna K, et al. Ehretianone, a novel quinonoid xanthene from *Ehretia buxifolia* with anti-snake venom activity. J Nat Prod 1996;59:664–667.
68. Gokhale AB, Damre AS, Saraf MN. Investigations into the immunomodulatory activity of *Argyreia speciosa*. J Ethnopharmacol 2003;84:109–114.
69. Dharmasiri MG, Jayakody JR, Galhena G, Liyanage SS, Ratnasooriya W. Anti-inflammatory and analgesic activities of mature fresh leaves of *Vitex negundo*. J Ethnopharmacol 2003;87:199–206.
70. Alam MI, Gomes A. Snake venom neutralization by Indian medicinal plants (*Vitex negundo* and *Emblica officinalis*) root extracts. J Ethnopharmacol 2003;86: 75–80.
71. Ozaki Y, Sekita S, Soedigdo S, Harada M. Antiinflammatory effect of *Graptophyllum pictum* (L.) Griff. Chem Pharm Bull (Tokyo) 1989;37:2799–2802.
72. Laupattarakasem P, Houghton PJ, Hoult JR, Itharat. An evaluation of the activity related to inflammation of four plants used in Thailand to treat arthritis. J Ethnopharmacol 2003;85:207–215.
73. De S, Ravishankar B, Bhavsar GC. Investigation of the anti-inflammatory effects of *Paederia foetida*. J Ethnopharmacol 1994;43:31–38.
74. Olajide OA, Okpako DT, Makinde JM. Anti-inflammatory properties of *Bridelia ferruginea* stem bark. Inhibition of lipopolysaccaride-induced septic shock and vascular permeability. J Ethnopharmacol 1999;88:221–224.

75. Geetha T, Varalakshmi P. Anticomplement activity of triterpenes from *Crataeva nurvala* stem bark in adjuvant arthritis in rats. Gen Pharmacol 1999;32:495–497.
76. Matsuda H, Dai Y, Ido Y, et al. Studies on *Kochiae fructus*. V. Antipruritic effects of oleanolic acid glycosides and the structure-requirement. Biol Pharm Bull 1998;21:1231–1233.
77. Zschocke S, van Staden J. Cryptocarya-species substitute plants for *Ocotea bullata*? A pharmacological investigation in terms of cyclooxygenase-1 and -2 inhibition. J Ethnopharmacol 2000;71:473–478.

2 Plants Affecting the Central Nervous System

GENERAL CONCEPT

The use of plants to influence brain function has long been essential to medical practice, and one could say that the intake of new plant species by early hominids resulting from a change in the climate might have triggered the Mind's Big Bang 50,000 years ago which allowed us to prevail over the Neanderthals, who co-existed with us for tens of thousands of years.

With the arrival of *Homo sapiens* about 35,000 years ago, the first healers or shamans ingested or smoked mushrooms and plants in order to get into a trance and would mentally "fly" to another level of reality, in which they could communicate with animal spirits tell the hunters where preys were likely to be found.

Our early ancestors cultivated Valeriana (*Valeriana officinalis* L., Valerianaceae), hemp (*Cannabis sativa* L., Cannabinaceae), and opium (*Papaver somniferum* L.), the vestiges of which have been found in Croc-Magnon caves. Hippocrates mentions in the *Corpus Hippocraticum* three Solanaceae: *Hyoscyamus niger* (henbane), *Atropa belladona* L. (belladona), and *Mandragora officinarum* L. (mandrake), which were used later by witches to enter into delirium. The root of *Mandragora officinarum* L., with its human shape, played a prominent role in the European pharmacopeia of the Middle Ages, and had the reputation of being an aphrodisiac.

From earliest times, curious beliefs about the Human-shaped roots grew up. The Greeks considered the roots as human dwarfs. Theophrastus mentioned that at his time, the collection of Mandrake was following curious rituals including dances and recitation of formulas. During the Middle Ages it was believed that when being pulled from the ground, the plant would let out such a horrible scream that whoever heard the noise might die at once or become unsane. Eventually, only black dogs were employed to extract the root, after which, according to belief, the animal usually died. In Central America, *Lophophora williamsii* (*Echinocactus williamsii* [Lem. ex Salm-Dick] Coult.), or peyote, peyotl, anhalonium, or mescal button, has been used to cause hallucination. Peyote contains mescaline, the clinical properties of which are similar to those of lysergic acid diethylamide (LSD).

Classical examples of Asian medicinal plants are *Papaver somniferum* (opium, Papaveraceae), *Cannabis sativa* L. (cannabis, Cannabinaceae), and *Myristica fragrans*

From: *Ethnopharmacology of Medicinal Plants: Asia and the Pacific*
Edited by: C. Wiart © Humana Press Inc., Totowa, NJ

(nutmeg, Myristicaceae). *Papaver somniferum* was native to the Middle East and is possibly the oldest known narcotic; as early as 4000 BCE the Sumerians referred to it as the "joy plant." Opium was known by the Greeks for its constipating effect and sleep-inducing properties, and Celse mention it his *De re Medica* in about 30 BCE. The plant was brought to India and China by the Arabs, and Barbosa mentions the cultivation of opium in India in 1511. The medicinal use of opium was well established, and control of the opium trade was a central issue during the wars in China in 1839. Opium (*British Pharmacopoeia*, 1963), or the dried latex obtained by incision from the ripe capsules containing not less than 9.5% of anhydrous morphine, has been used as an analgesic and narcotic, and morphine, the active constituent, is used for the abrogation of pain.

Cannabis sativa L. (cannabis, *British Pharmaceutical Codex*, 1949) consists of the dried flowering or fruiting tops of the male *Cannabis sativa* L. It was used by the Chinese and Indians 3500 years ago to induce narcosis. According to Herodotus, hemp was brought by the Scythians in the Mediterranean when they invaded in about 1500 BCE, before the battle of Troy. Herodotus mentions in 600 BCE that the Scythians burned its seeds to produce a narcotic smoke. Dioskurides mentions that if the seeds of cannabis are eaten too freely, they destroy the virile powers, and that the juice is used to relieve earache. Galen asserts that in his time (Middle Ages), it was customary to give hemp seeds to the guests at banquets in order to promote hilarity and enjoyment *(1)*. The British physicians of the army of India *(2)* and Bonaparte's expedition to Egypt were responsible for its introduction into Europe in the 19th century. There it was consumed in intellectual circles, and the illicit use of cannabis spreaded rapidly. By 1972, at least 2 million Americans used marijuana daily. Cannabis (*British Pharmaceutical Codex*, 1949) has been used in Western medicine to treat mania and nervous disorders, as a cerebral sedative, and as an analgesic for migraine, headaches, and even herpes zoster. The active principle is a phenolic substance known as Δ-9-tetrahydrocannabinol (THC), which binds to the anandamide receptor, which might have potential in the treatment of various symptoms associated with disorders ranging from multiple sclerosis to AIDS to terminal cancer.

The dried kernels of the seeds of *Myristica fragrans* (nutmeg, *British Pharmaceutical Codex*, 1963) are aromatic and carminative. It was not known by the ancient Greeks and Romans, but was used by Indians and Arabs as early as 700 BCE. It was later introduced into Europe by Arab traders and, subsequently, by Portuguese and Dutch merchants. Reports on nutmeg intoxication date back to the Middle Ages, when William Cullen wrote about a patient in his treatise on the *Materia medica* in 1789: "About one hour after he had taken it (nutmeg), he was sized with a drowsiness, which gradually increased to a complete stupor and insensibility, waking from time to time he was quite delirious; and he thus continued alternately sleeping and delirious for several hours." The active principle in nutmeg is myristicin, a catecholamine-like phenylpropanoid.

The most fascinating aspect of the mechanism by which medicinal plants affect the brain function is their ability to elaborate molecules that are able to cross the hemato-encephalic barrier and infiltrate the brain where binding to protein receptors occurs.

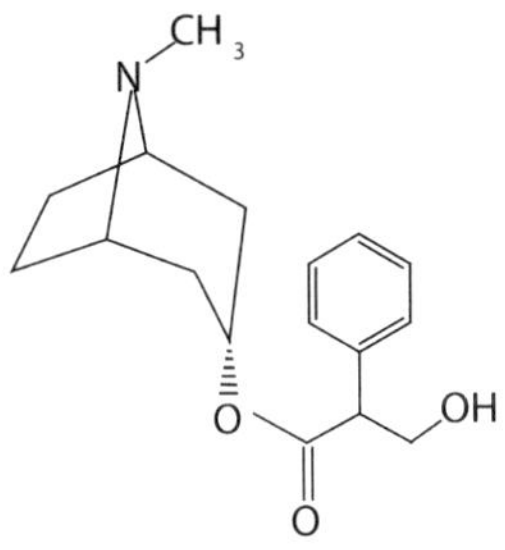

Atropine

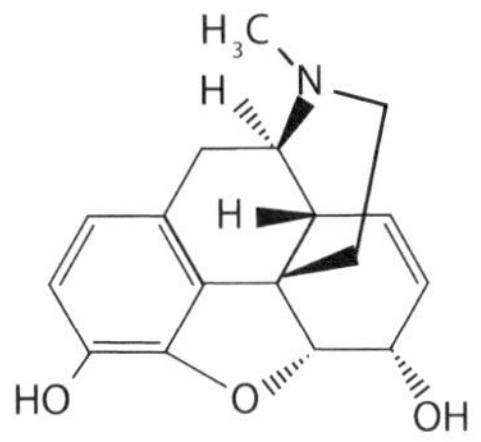

Morphine

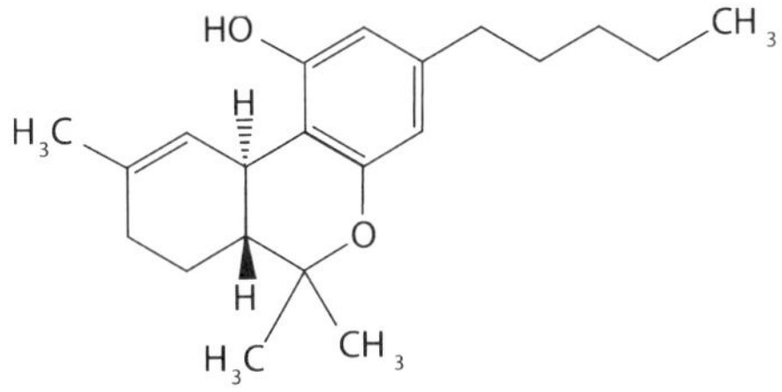

Tetrahydrocannabinol

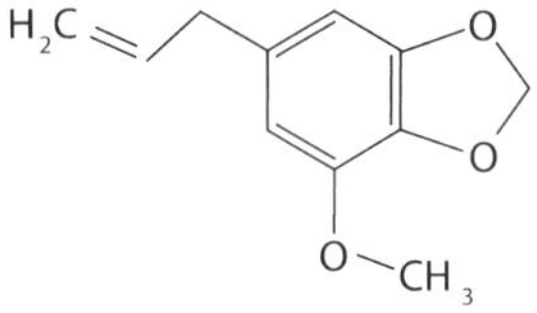

Myristicin

Fig. 30. Examples of natural products affecting the central nervous system.

One might set the hypothesis that the medicinal flora of Asia and the Pacific might hold a number of original molecules with potential for the treatment of central nervous disorders. The purpose of this chapter is to bring light onto some families and species of plants with such potentials, and to provide a basis for understanding the many mechanisms by which these herbs influence brain function, including their effects on the serotoninergic, γ-aminobutyric acid (GABA)ergic, glycinergic, and dopaminergic systems and opiate receptors.

PLANTS AFFECTING SEROTONINERGIC NEUROTRANSMISSION

5-Hydroxytryptamine, or serotonin, is a neurotransmitter in the central nervous system (CNS). The nerve-cell bodies of the major serotoninergic neurones are in the midline raphe nuclei of the rostral pons, and ascending fibers innervate the basal ganglia, hypothalamus, thalamus, hippocampus, limbic forebrain, and areas of the cerebral cortex. The serotoninergic system plays an important role in the control of mood and behavior, motor activity, hunger, thermoregulation, sleep, certain hallucinatory states, and some neuro-endocrine mechanisms.

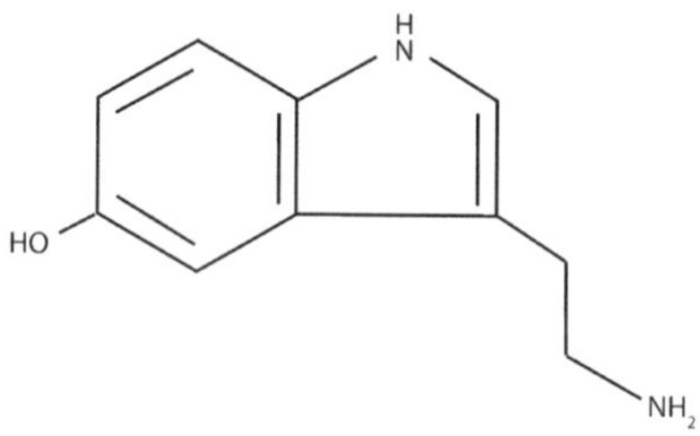

Serotonin

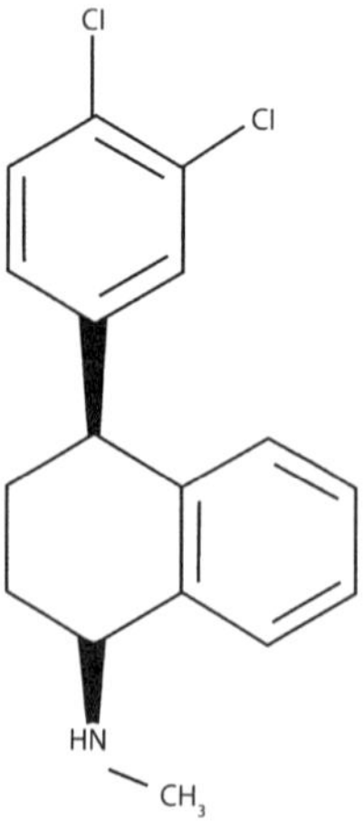

Sertraline (Zoloft®)

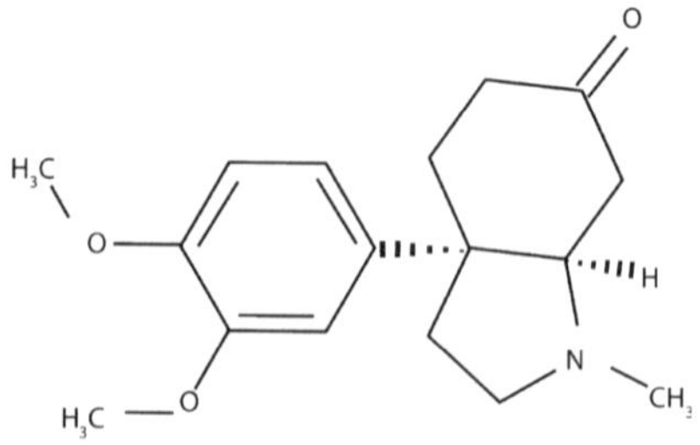

Mesembrine

5-Hydroxytryptaminergic ($5HT_{1A}$) receptors mediate in the CNS the autonomic control of hypothermia, hyperphagia, analgesia, blood pressure, venereal disease, anxiety, and several behavioral paradigms. It has been hypothesized that the anxiolytic property of buspirone is the result of a blockade of $5HT_{1A}$ receptors. Methysergide, a partial $5HT_1$ agonist, and sumatriptan, a $5HT_{1D}$ agonist, are drugs used to assuage headache.

Plants affecting the serotoninergic neurotransmission are therefore interesting because of their potentials for the treatment of depression, which is the eighth leading cause of death in the United States. It is generally agreed that there is a correlation between diminished serotonin neurotransmission and episodes of major depression, and a number or inhibitors of serotonin-uptake inhibitors are available on the market, such as sertraline (Zoloft®).

This type of action is found in kanna, or *Sceletium expansum* and *Sceletium tortuosum* (Aizoaceae), which have been used by South African shamans from prehistoric times to "enhance animal spirits, sparkle the eyes, and to stimulate gaiety." The active constituent of kanna is a serotonin-like alkaloid called mesembrine, which is a potent serotonin re-uptake inhibitor—hence, some potential for the treatment of anxiety and depression; however, careful clinical trials must be performed.

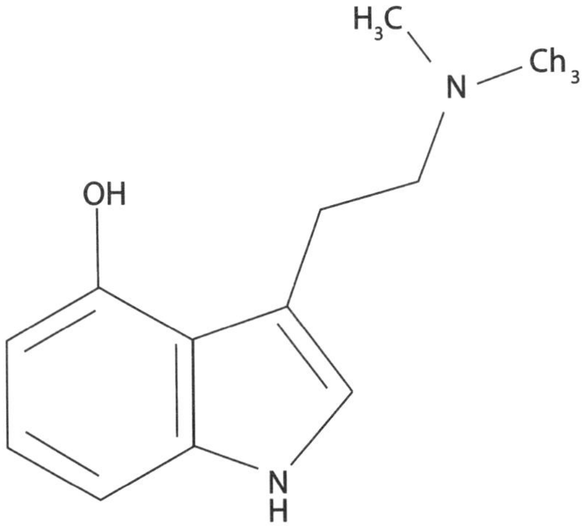

When looking for plants affecting serotoninergic neurotransmission, one might look into species that produce indole alkaloids, such alkaloids beingknown to impart to the plant's hallucinogenic properties.

Such alkaloids can be found particularly in the Myristicaceae, Malpighiaceae, Rutaceae, Apocynaceae, Rubiaceae, Loganiaceae, and Convolvulaceae. Such compounds are also found in mushrooms from the genera *Conocybe*, *Panaeolus*, *Psilocybe*, and *Stropharia* (Agaricaceae), which where used by the Aztecs of pre-Columbian America for their psilocin.

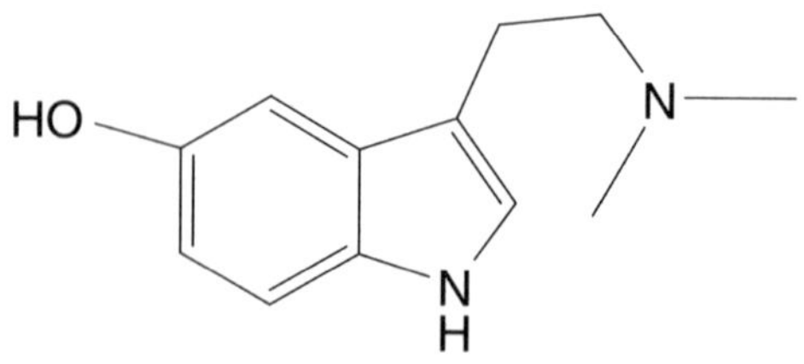

Bufotenine

Another example is bufotenine from Mimosaceae, *Anadenanthera peregrina* (L.) Spreg. (*Piptadenia peregrina* Benth.), a plant known as *yopo*, and a constituent of hallucinogenic snuffs in the Orinoco basin. *Banisteria caapi*, *Banisteria inebrians*, *Banisteria quitensis*, *Banisteria rusbyana*, and *Tetrapteris methystica* from the family Malpighiaceae are used to make a narcotic drink known as *caapi* in Brazil, *yage* in Columbia, and *ayahuasca* in Ecuador, Peru, and Bolivia that is an important tool of Amazonian religious ceremonies. The hallucinogenic and telepathic principles are a series of β-carboline derivatives, including harmine (banisterine, telepathine) and harmaline, the chemical structure of which is very much like serotonin and acts as a 5HT receptor agonist (Fig. 31). These alkaloids cause nausea, dizziness, and general malaise, together with pareasthesia of the hands, feet, and face, followed by numbness, dreams involving the stimulation of midbrain reticular formation, leading to such phenomena as double contours and persistence of after-images. Because of the growing interest in looking for serotoninergic agents, we shall consider the pharmacological potentials of the medicinal flora of Asia and the Pacific, and examine the molecules through which they are thought to act.

Medicinal Annonaceae

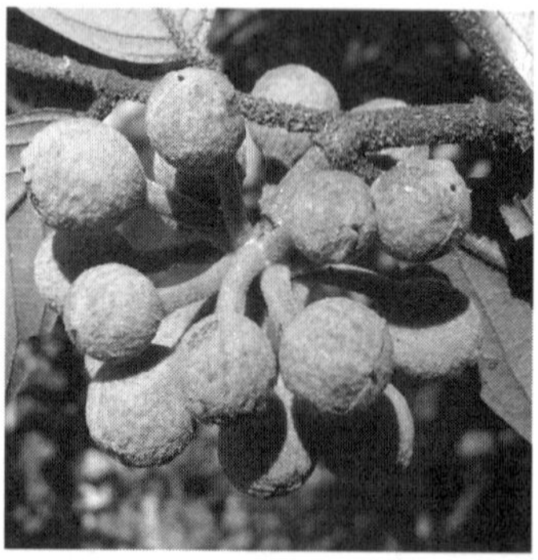

The family Annonaceae consists of about 120 genera and more than 2000 species of tropical trees, shrubs, or climbers, about 60 species of which are used for traditional medicine in Asia and the Pacific. Annonaceae have attracted a great deal of interest on account of their ability to elaborate isoquinoline alkaloids, which bind to the receptors of serotonin. Anonaine, nornuciferine, and asimilobine from *Annona muricata* L. block $5HT_{1A}$ receptors *(3)*. Such a property is not surprising because the molecular structures of anonaine, nornuciferine, and asimilobine are similar to the chemical structure of serotonin. For instance, anonaine, nornuciferine, and asimilobine from *A. muricata* L. block $5HT_{1A}$ receptors, thereby substantiating the anxiolytic use of the plant. Among the medicinal Annonaceae used in Asia, two possible candidates for the characterization of serotoninergic alkaloids are *Fissistigma lanuginosum* (Hook.f. & Thoms.) Merr. and *Cyathostemma micranthum* (A. DC.) J. Sinclair.

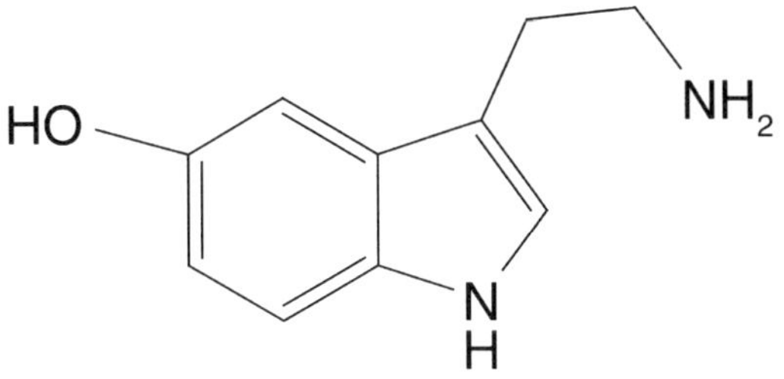

Serotonin

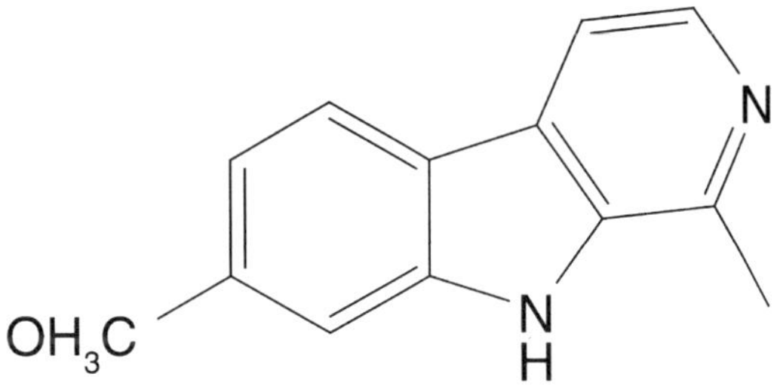

Harmine

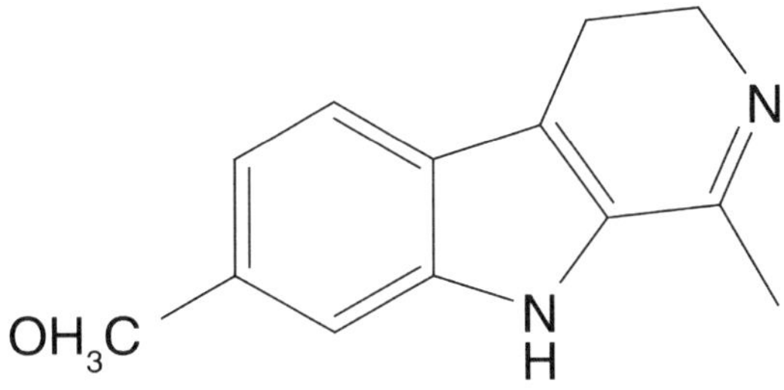

Harmaline

Fig. 31. Example of neuroactive indole alkaloids from plants. Note the similitude of chemical structure of harmine, harmaline, and serotonin.

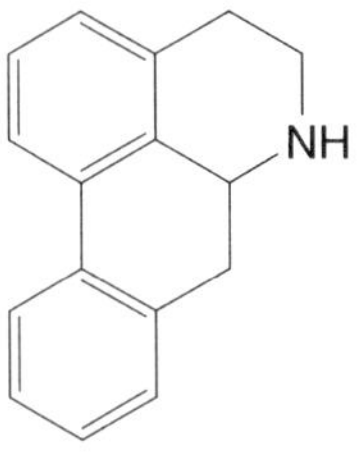

Nornuciferine

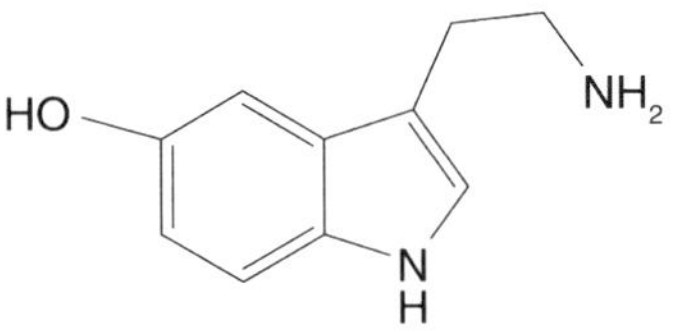

Serotonin

Fissistigma lanuginosum (Hook.f. & Thoms.) Merr. (*Uvaria tomentosa* Wall., *Melodorum lanuginosum* Hk f. et Th.) is a climber of the rainforests of Malaysia, Vietnam, Cambodia, Laos, and Thailand. The young stems are rusty tomentose. The leaves are simple, exstipulate, alternate, glossy, dark green, thick, and oblong. The fruits are velvety and globose to and grow up to 2 cm in diameter (Fig. 32).

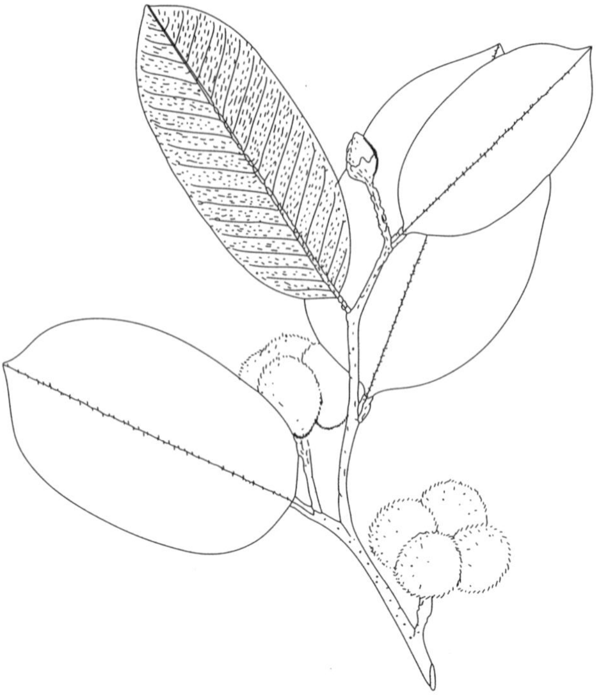

Fig. 32. *Fissistigma lanuginosum* (Hook. f. & Thoms.) Merr. From FRI Herbarium 023427. Flora of Malaya. Geographical localization: National Park, altitude: 700 feet in primary forest.

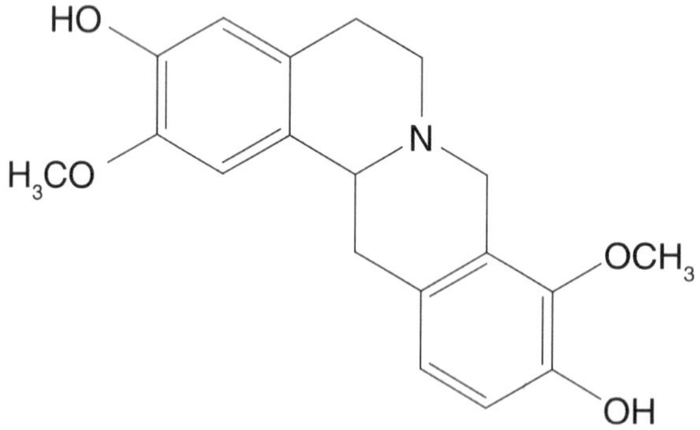

Discretamine

In Malaysia, a decoction of the roots is drunk to assuage stomachaches. The potential of this climber as a source of molecules affecting the serotoninergic neurotransmission would be worth investigating because (-)-discretamine characterized from *Fissistigma glaucescens* blocks α_1- and α_2-adrenoceptor and exerts a 5-hydroxytryptamine-antagonist activity. Note discretamine is spasmolytic, hence the use of the plant receptors (*4*).

Cyathostemma micranthum (A. DC.) J. Sinclair. (*Guatteria micrantha* A. DC, *Uvaria micrantha* Hk. f. et Th.), *Uvaria sumatrana Kurz*, *Anaxagorea sumatrana* Miq, *Cyathostemma sumatrana* Boerl, *Polyalthia fruticans* A. DC, *Popowia nitida* King), or *subang hitam* (Malay), is a climber that grows in the primary rainforest of Thailand, Burma, Malaysia, and east to Papua New Guinea. The roots have a very pleasant ginger-like fragrance. The stems are fissured and dark colored. The leaves are simple, oblong-lanceolate. The fruits are 1-cm-in-diameter ripe carpels with irregular bulges owing to the seeds (Fig. 33).

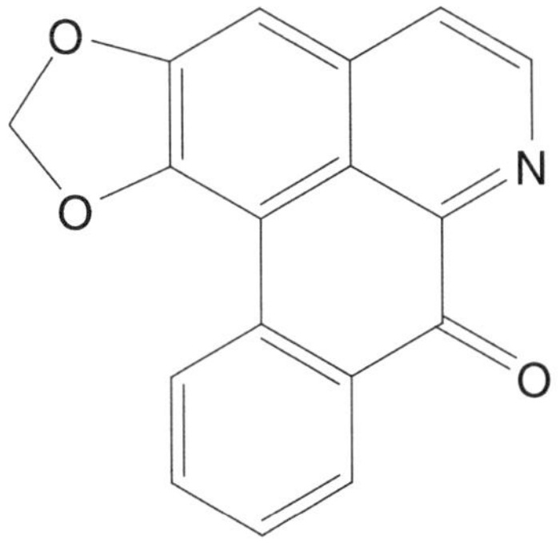

Liriodenine

In Malaysia, a decoction of the leaves or roots is drunk as a protective remedy after childbirth, and the plant is used to stimulate sexual desire and to invigorate. It is also used to promote sweating and to treat cough. The plant has not been yet investigated for pharmacology but one could suggest that the aphrodisiac and tonic properties might result from a mood elevation via inhibition of serotonin re-uptake. Note that the root of *Cyathostemma argenteum* contains liriodenine and discretamine (*5*). Liriodenine is known to block muscarinic receptors, but knowledge on its effects on the serotoninergic system is quite vestigial (*6*).

Medicinal Myristicaceae

The family Myristicaceae has about 16 genera and 380 species of tropical lowland rainforest trees that are easily recognizable in field collection because of their blood-like sap, conical crown, and nutmeg-like fruits. A very interesting feature of Myristicaceae species are their ability to elaborate series of neuroactive indole alkaloids, because it produces neuroactive indole alkaloids, which might hold potential for the treatment of anxiety, mood disorders, and other psychological disturbances.

Such alkaloids are *N*, *N*-dimethyl tryptamine, 5-methoxy-*N*, *N*-dimethyl tryptamine, and 2-methyl-1, 2, 3, 4-tetrahydro-β-carboline, which have been characterized from the resins of several *Virola* species, which is used by the witch doctors of several

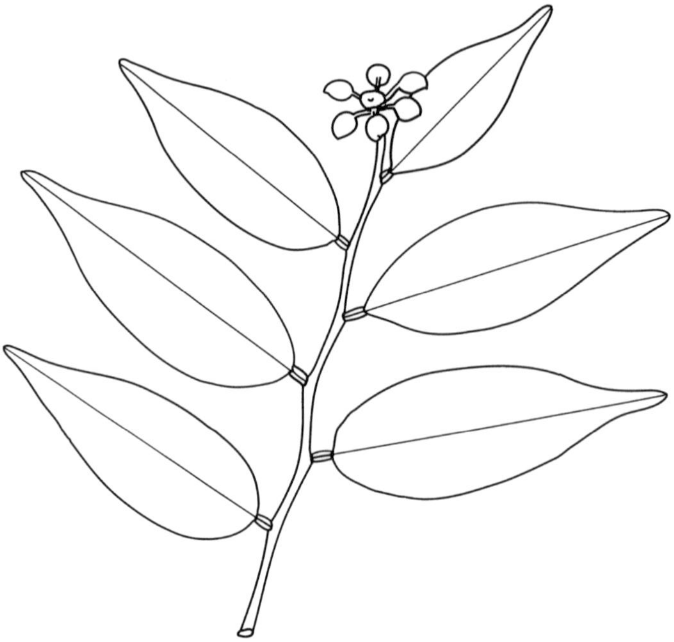

Fig. 33. *Cyathostemma micranthum* (A. DC.) J. Sinclair. From Herb. Hort. Bot. Singap. Field Collector: Burkill & Haniff, 11/24/1924. Geographical localization: Jerantut, Malaysia. Botanical Identification: J. Sinclair, 12/17/1948.

tribes in the Colombian Amazon to make a particularly intoxicating snuff known as *yakee*.

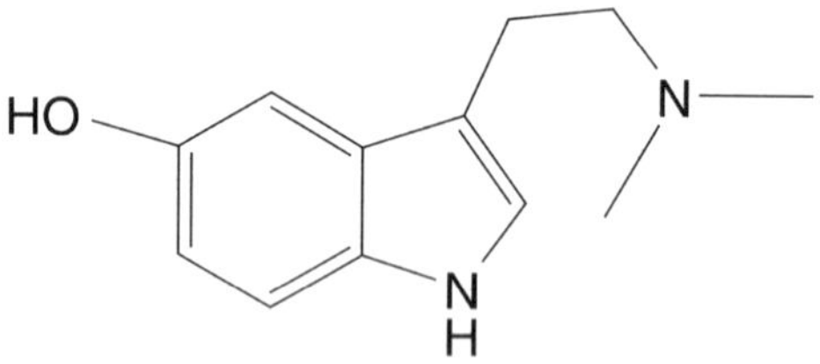

5-Hydroxy-*N*, *N*-dimethyl tryptamine

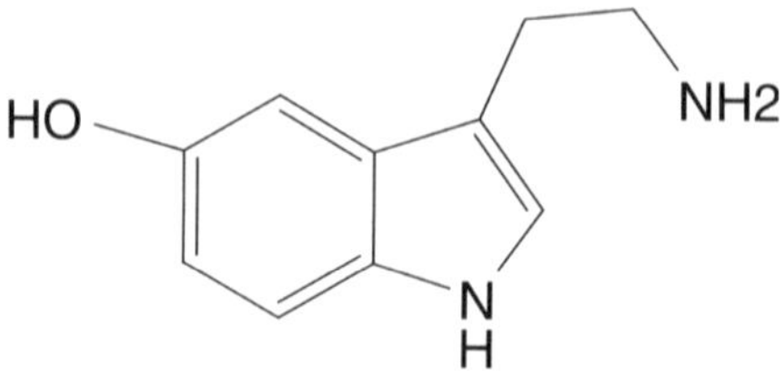

Serotonin

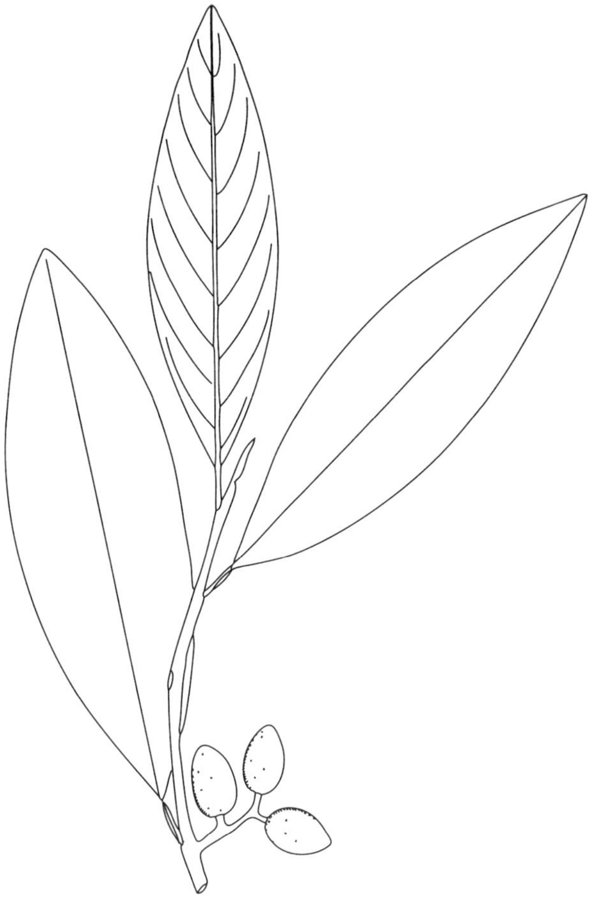

Fig. 34. *Horsfieldia glabra* (Bl.) Warb. Plants of Indonesia. East Bali, Karangasem, South slope of Gunung Agung, 1–2 km Southwest of Basket. Altitude: 750 m. 8° 21′, South–115° 26′ East in disturbed forest in ravine canopy.

According to Schultes, snuffing *yakee* produces scarily true hallucinations and an exhilarating euphoria. The subject performs prodigious feats of magic and strength because of a superhuman quality *(7)*. About 20 species of plants classified in the family Myristicaceae are medicinal, including *Myristica fragrans* Houtt. (mentioned earlier), as well as a few *Horsfieldia* species, including *Horsfieldia glabra* (Bl.) Warb.

***Horsfieldia glabra* (Bl.) Warb.**, or *feng chui nan* (Chinese), *kayu anak* (Indonesia), is a tree of up to 25 m tall that grows in Thailand, Malaysia, Indonesia, and China. The leaves are oblong-lanceolate, 13.8 × 3.8 – 15 × 4.9 cm, and show 7 to 10 pairs of secondary nerves. The fruits are ovoid to elliptical, 1.5–2.5 cm, orange color, aril orange color, and completely enclose seeds. In Indonesia, the bark and leaves are used to treat intestinal disturbances. The bark is also used to heal sores and boils on probable account of arylalkanones *(8)*.

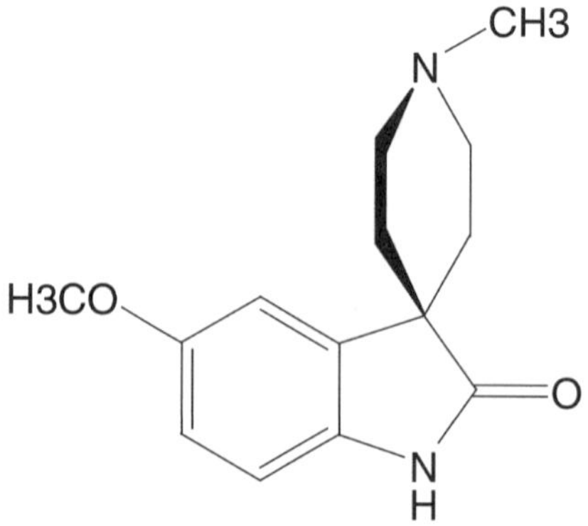

Horsfiline

One might set the hypothesis that intestinal disturbances, which are a common symptom in depression, could be the result of a serotonin-like mechanism because the *Horsfieldia* species, including *Horsfieldia superba* (Hk. f. et. Th.) Warb., are known to elaborate unusual series' of oxindole alkaloids, such as horsfiline (9).

Medicinal Convolvulaceae

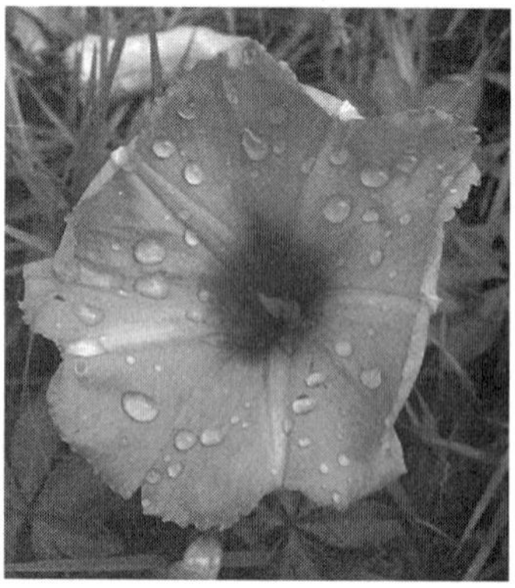

An interesting feature of the Convolvulaceae is their ability to elaborate LSD-like indole alkaloids. Both *Rivea corymbosa* (L.) Hall and *Ipomoea violacea* L., from which the Mexican magical drugs *ololiuqui* and *bado negro*, respectively, are prepared, contain a number of indoles related to the ergot alkaloids. D-Lysergic acid amide (ergine) is the major constituent of the seeds of both *Rivea corymbosa* and *Ipomoea violacea.* The seeds contain also small amounts of isowergine, chanoclavine, and elymoclavine.

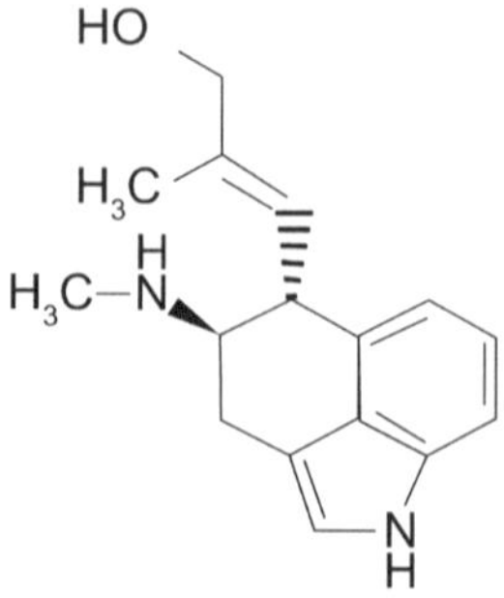

Chanoclavine

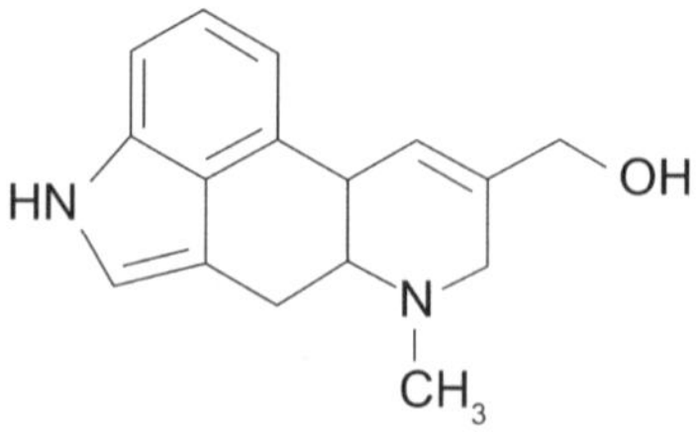

Elymoclavine

Drowsiness, apathy, and mental detachment seem to be the major effects of *ololiuqui.* The derivatives of lysergic acid present in *ololiuqui* are widely distributed throughout the genus *Ipomoea* and other Convolvulaceae species. About 50 plant species from this family are used for medicinal purpose in Asia and the Pacific.

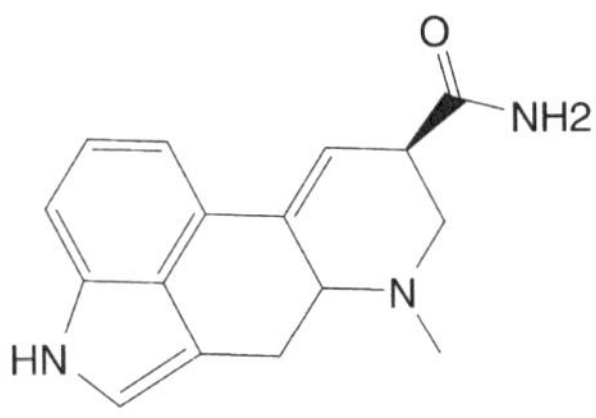

Ergine

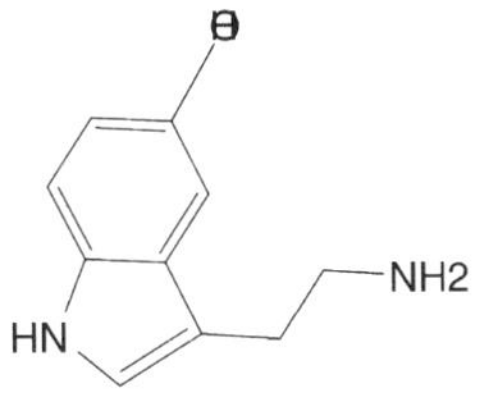

Serotonin

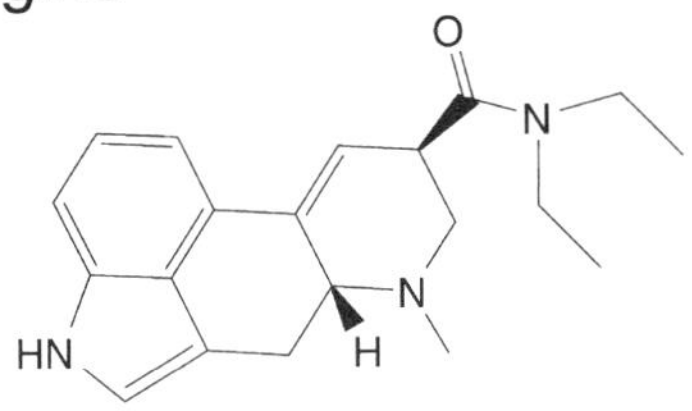

Lysergic acid diethylamide

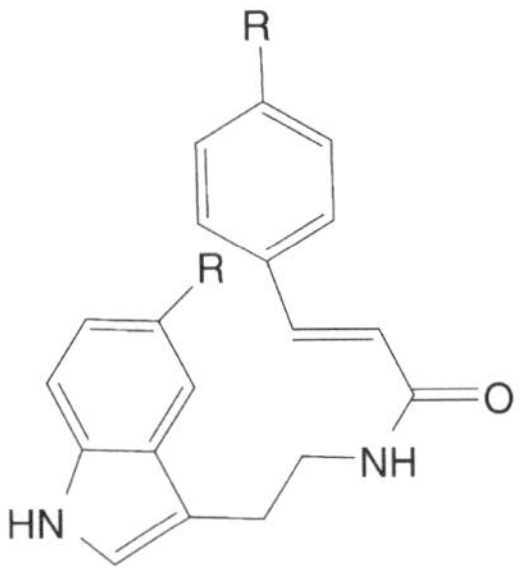

Macrolactam indole alkaloid

Ipomoea obscura (L.) Ker-Gawl., or obscure morning glory, is a slender climber common on fences. It is native to tropical East Africa, the Mascarene Islands, tropical Asia, throughout the Malay Archipelago, to northern Australia and Fiji. The leaves are cordate to 5 cm long and the flowers are infundibuliform and creamy white (Fig. 35).

In Indonesia, a paste of leaves is applied on sores, ulcers, hemorrhoids, and swellings. The seeds of *Ipomoea obscura* (L.) Ker-Gawl are known to contain unusual indole alkaloids including ipobscurines B-D, being unique structural types characterized as serotonin hydroxycinnamic acid amide-type conjugates with a second phenylpropanoid moiety forming an ether with the 5-OH position of the indole nucleus *(10)*. It would be interesting to know whether or not these alkaloids hold some potential as promoters of serotoninergic neurotransmission.

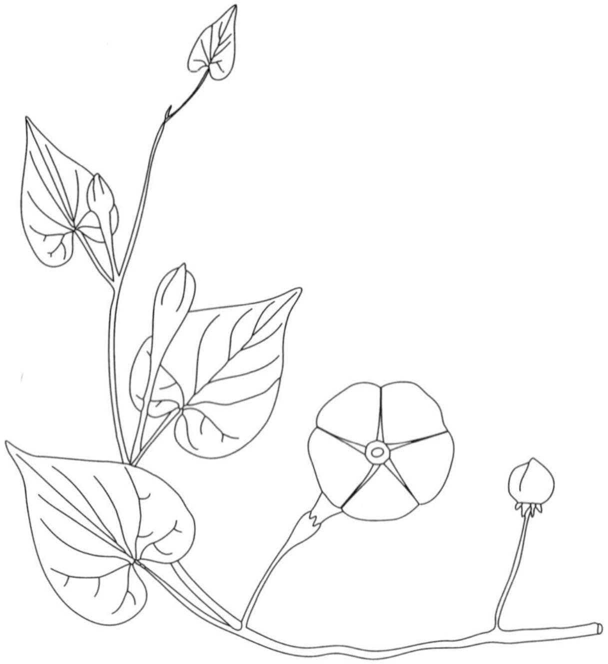

Fig. 35. *Ipomoea obscura* (L.) Ker–Gawl. Flora of Malaya. FRI No 27419. Geographical localization: Kuala Selangor, Malaysia November 10, 1983. Collector: F.S.B Ng. Botanical identification: F.S.B Ng, 4.2.1986.

Ipomoea digitata L. (*Ipomoea paniculata* var. *digitata* Kuntze, *Quamoclit digitata* [L.] G. Don, *Convolvulus paniculatus* [Burm. f.] Kuntze, *Ipomoea paniculata* [L.] R. Br, *Ipomoea mauritiana* Jacq.), or alligator yam, *vidari, bhumy kushmanda* (Sanskrit), or *jari buaya* (Malay), is found in India and Southeast Asia. The plant is grown for ornamental purposes. The roots are ovoid, large, and tuberous. The leaves are large, palmately five to seven lobed, ovate, lanceolate, acute, or acuminate. The flowers are infundibuliform and purple and campanulate–infundibuliform. The fruits are small and ovoid capsules. There are four seeds in each fruit that are black and woolly (Fig. 36). In Cambodia, Laos, and Vietnam, the tubers are used to invigorate, stimulate venereal desire, prevent obesity, and moderate menses. In India, it is used as a general tonic, to treat diseases of the spleen and liver, for menorrhagia, debility, and fat accumulation. To date, the plant is unstudied for its potential as a source of neuroactive compounds.

Ipomoea indica (*Convolvulus indicus* J. Burman, *Ipomoea congesta* R. Brown), or ocean blue morning, glory, *koaliawa* (Hawaii), is a slender climber native to South America, and is cultivated and naturalized in coastal habitats and moist forests in several tropical countries including Indonesia, Malaysia, Burma, New Guinea, Philippines, Sri Lanka, and Pacific Islands. The leaves are cordate to 10 cm long. The flowers are infundibuliform, grow up to 7 cm long and 5 cm in diameter, and are deep blue in color (Fig. 37).

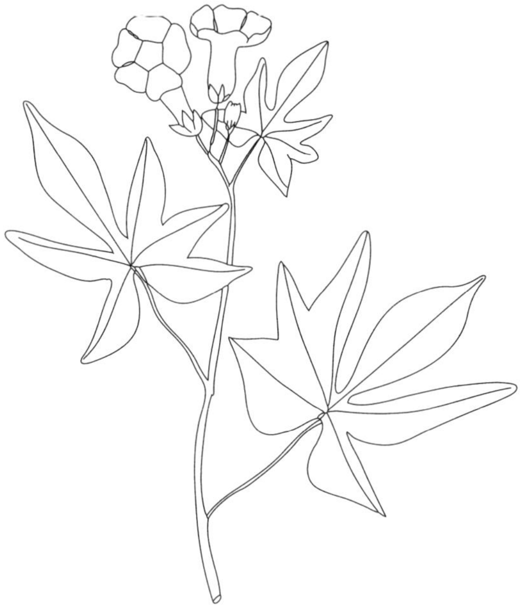

Fig. 36. *Ipomoea digitata* L. Forest Flora, Malay Peninsula. No 37918. Geographical localization: Peteni Hill, Kelantan, 10/16/1934. Collector: C.F. Symington.

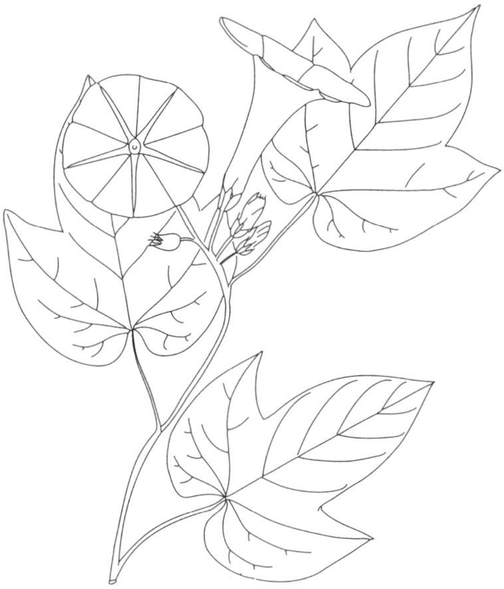

Fig. 37. *Ipomoea indica*. Forest Flora, Malay Peninsula. No 22249. Geographical localization: Gap Sanitarium garden, 1/20/1930. Collector: Symington. Botanical identification: 1958.

In Taiwan, the roots are used to relieve the bowels from costiveness. To date, the pharmacological potential of this plant is unknown.

Medicinal Apocynaceae

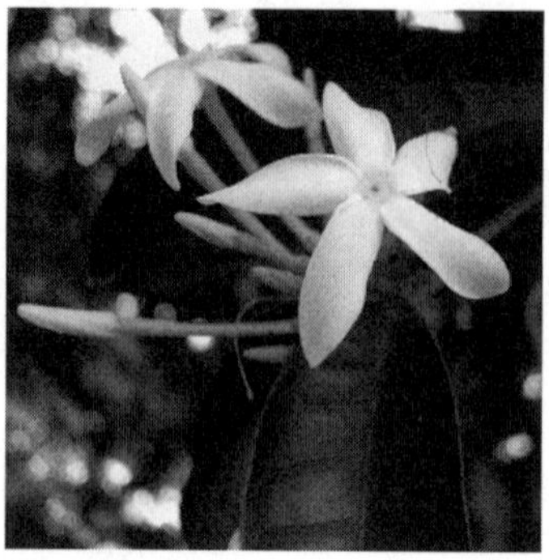

Perhaps no other family of flowering plants has aroused more interest in the field of pharmacological research than the Apocynaceae, the only family that abounds with indole alkaloids of proven clinical value. An interesting aspect in this field of neuropharmacological research is the fact that Apocynaceae elaborate Iboga alkaloids, which are present particularly in the genus *Tabernanthe*, and principally in a Central African shrub *Tabernanthe iboga*. The roots are chewed by the natives to offset hunger and fatigue, and large doses produce excitement, mental confusion, and a drunken madness characterized by prophetic utterances *(11)*.

Tabernanthe iboga contains a series of alkaloids including Ibogaine and tabernanthine. Ibogaine was isolated in 1901, is like serotonin and harmine, and has attracted a great deal of interest on account of its capability to reduce drug craving. The mechanism underlying this effect may result from a regulator of the serotoninergic system that, in turn, regulates dopamine release *(12)*.

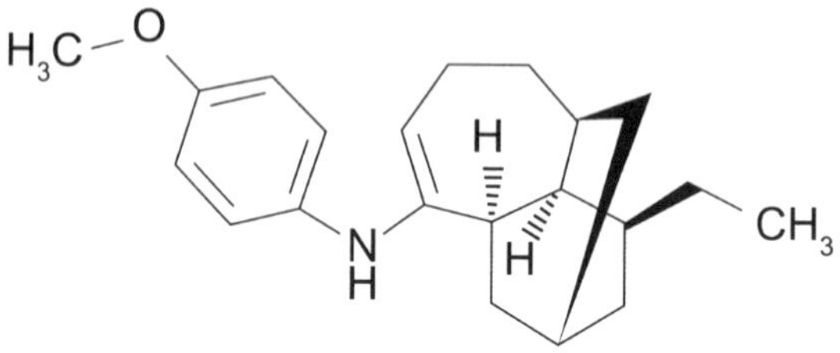

Ibogaine

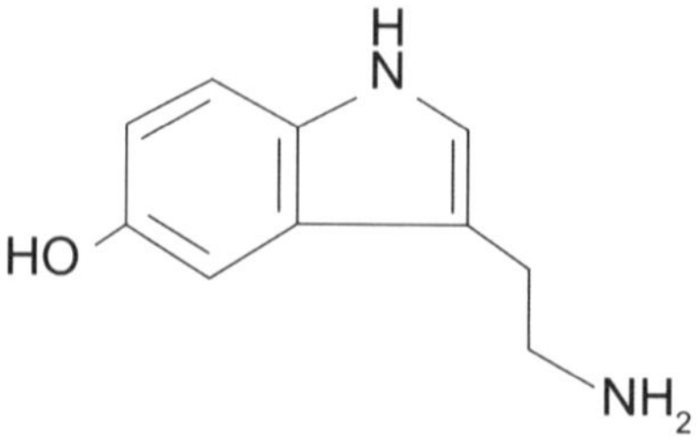

Serotonin

Ibogaine protects the *N*-methyl–D-aspartate neuron receptors against excessive release of excitatory amino acids and represents, therefore, a potential therapeutic agent for the treatment of Alzheimer's disease, Huntington's chorea, and other

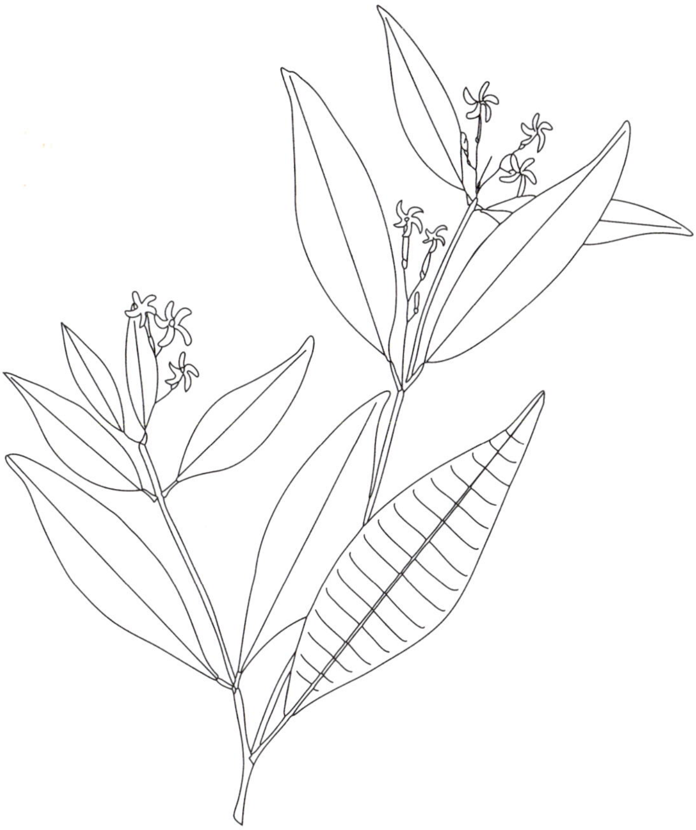

Fig. 38. *Ervatamia pandacaqui* (Poir.) Pichon. Flora of The Philippines. Herbarium Vadense (WAG). Botanical identification: A.J.M. Leuwenberg, 1987. Geographical localization: Pinamalayan, Mindanao. Field collector: Ramos. June, 1922.

brain diseases. The flora of tropical Asia is a rich source of Apocynaceae, including medicinal species, and represents therefore an exciting source of potentially serotoninergic alkaloids for the treatment of depression. In this section, two species belonging to the genus *Ervatamia*, which is closely related to the genus *Tabernanthe*, are described.

Ervatamia pandacaqui (Poir.) Pichon (*Tabernaemontana cuminingiana* A. DC., *Tabernaemontana pandacaqui* Poir., *Tabernaemontana semperflorens* Perr., *Tabernaemontana thailandensis* P. T. Li.), or *ping mai gou ya hua* (Chinese) or *susun kepala* (Philippino), is a shrub that grows to a height of 4 m. The plant grows wild in China, Taiwan, Indonesia, Malaysia, the Philippines, Thailand; Australia, and the Pacific Islands. The leaves are decussate and elliptic. The corolla is white and salver-shaped, with five lobes obliquely oblong and falcate. The fruits are pairs of follicles obliquely ellipsoid (Fig. 38). In the Philippines, the plant is used to soothe bruises and swellings. A decoction of the root and bark is used to treat intestinal disorders and to treat the bites of poisonous animals.

A crude alkaloidal fraction from the stem of *Tabernaemontana pandacaqui* decreased the motor activity, respiratory rate, induced ataxia, antinociception, and loss of screen grip in rats, suggesting a CNS depression. The extract brought about the prolongation of pentobarbital sleeping time and the oxotremorine-induced salivation, hence possible cholinergic effects *(13)*.

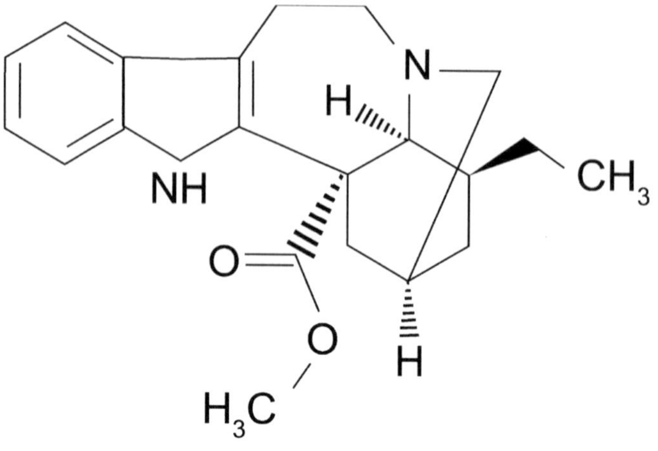

Coronaridine

The active constituent involved here is currently unknown, but the plant is known to produce indole alkaloids including voacangine and coronaridine, which exhibited significant analgesic and hypothermic effects in mice at a dose of 25 mg/kg, orally *(14,15)*. Because *Ervatamia pandacaqui* (Poir.) Pichon elaborates iboga alkaloids, such as ibogamine and tabernanthine, and congeners, such as coronaridine, could it be a source of serotonin re-uptake inhibitors *(16)*?

***Ervatamia corymbosa* (Roxb.) King & Gamble** (*Tabernaemontana corymbosa* Roxb. ex Wall, *Pagiantha peninsularis* Kerr, *Pagiantha peninsularis* var. *brevituba* Kerr, *Ervatamia chinensis* [Merrill] Tsiang, *Tabernaemontana chinensis* Merrill, *Tabernaemontana yunnanensis* [Tsiang] P. T. Li), or *san fang gou ya hua* (Chinese) or *pelir kambing* (Malay), is a shrub that grows to a height of 3 m tall in China, Indonesia, Laos, Malaysia, Burma, Thailand, and Vietnam. The leaves are decussate, papery, and acuminate at apex. The flowers are white, with five obliquely elliptic, mostly falcate lobes. The fruits are pairs of follicles obliquely ellipsoid (Fig. 39).

In China, the bark and leaves are used for the treatment of fractures. The roots are used in Malaysia to recover from childbirth and exhaustion, and a paste of the plant is used to treat orchitis. The plant contains indole alkaloids such as conodurinine, 19′(*S*) hydroxyconoduramin, 19′(*S*)-hydroxyervahanine A, and related iboga alkaloid congeners, and like the species mentioned earlier, and in fact the genera *Ervatamia*, in general, would be worth investigating for serotoninergic activities *(17)*.

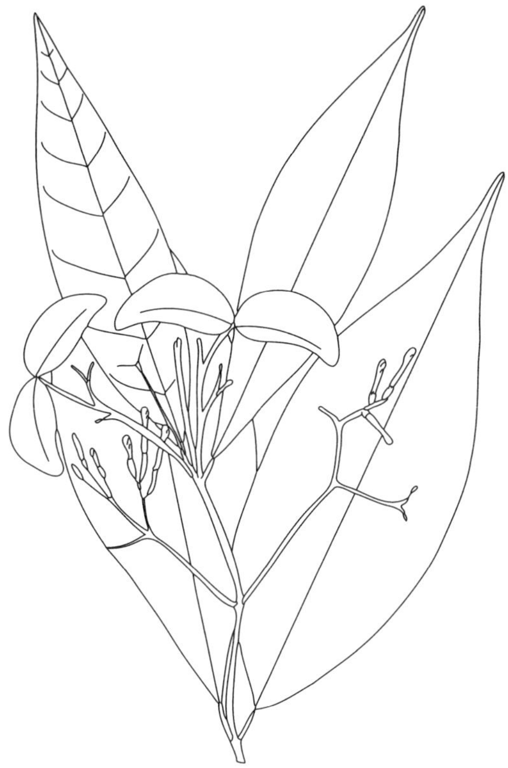

Fig. 39. *Ervatamia corymbosa* (Roxb.) King & Gamble. Flora of Malaya. Field No 104429. Geographical localization: Krau Game Reserve, G. Benom, Central Pahang in primary forest hillside, altitude: 1000 feet. Field collector: S. Chelliah, 7/14/1967. Botanical identification: A.J.M Leeuwenberg, 1986. Herbarium Vadense.

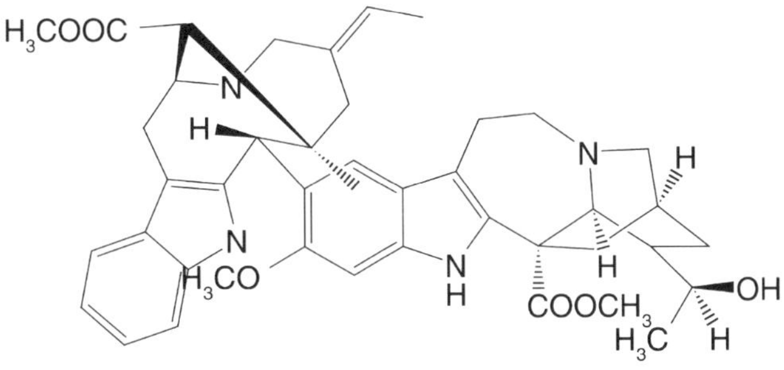

19′ (S) hydroxyconoduramine

Medicinal Zygophyllaceae

The family Zygophyllaceae is made up of 30 genera and 250 species of shrubs known to have the tendency to elaborate a series of serotonin-like psychedelic indole alkaloids such as harmine, harmol, and harmaline, notably found in the seeds of a medicinal plant that grows in the arid regions northern Africa to northern India and Manchuria, *Peganum harmala* L., or Turkey red or Syrian rue (peganum, *British Pharmaceutical Codex*, 1934). The seeds have been used to induce a psychic excitement comprising of visual distortions that are similar to those induced by LSD.

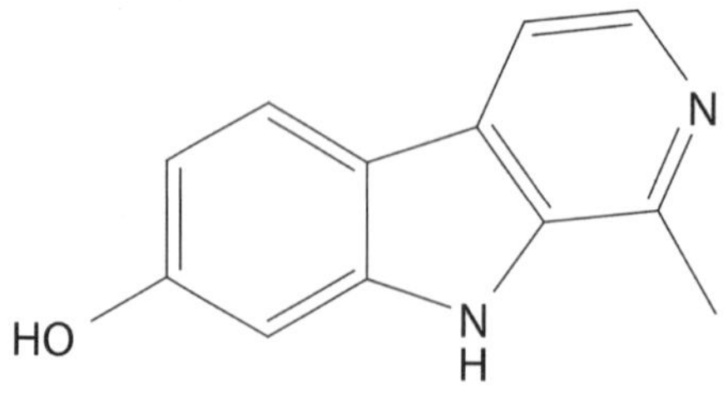

Harmol

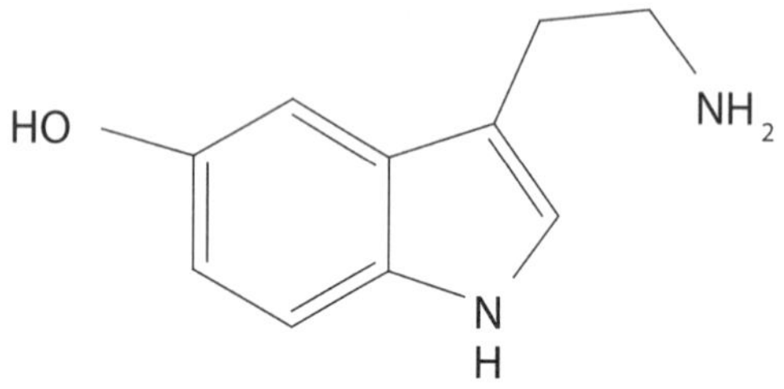

Serotonine

Note that the Malpighiaceae and Zygophyllaceae belong to the orders Polygalales and Sapindales, respectively, with both orders being quite close to the Rosidae, hence the probability of finding such alkaloids near to and in these orders. This type of indole alkaloids, or "harmala alkaloids," are identical to those of *ayahuasca* made from the *Banisteriopsis* species in the Malpighiaceae.

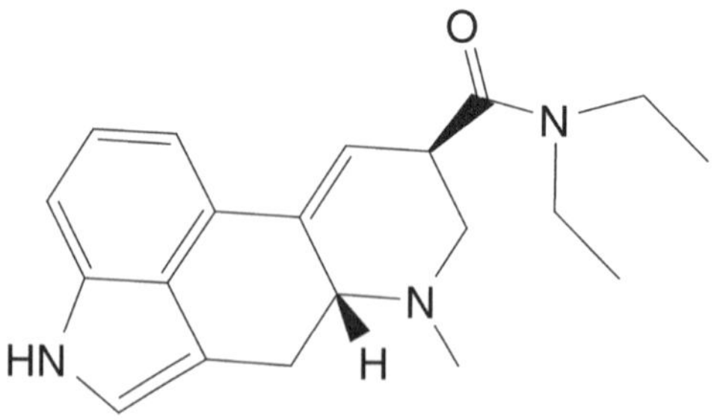

LSD

Tribulus terrestris L. (*Pedalium murex*), or ground burnut, puncture vine, *tzu, chih hsing, tu chi li* (Chinese), is an annual, prostrate dwarf shrubbish herb that grows to a height of 60 cm. The plant grows in disturbed areas, roadsides, railways, cultivated

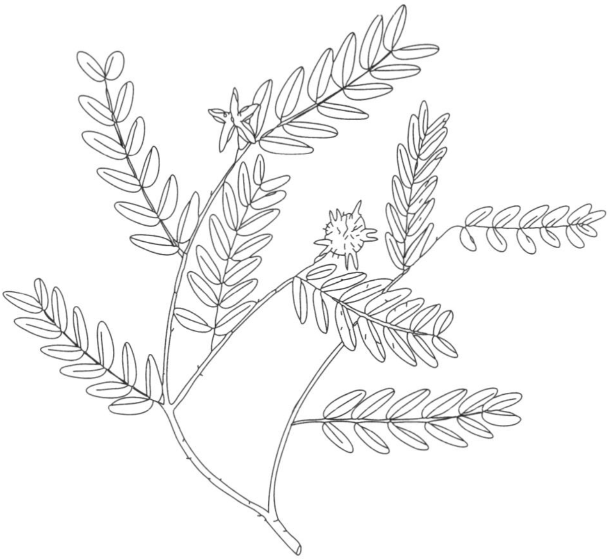

Fig. 40. *Tribulus terrestris* L.

fields, and abandoned gardens in Europe, the United States, and the Asia–Pacific region. The stems are terete, pilose, minute, and green to reddish-brown, and produce numerous stout burrs that can injure people and animals and puncture bicycle tires. The leaves are opposite and pinnate (Fig. 40). In China, the seeds are used as diuretic, tonic, abortifacient, galactagogue, and an alternative anthelmintic. The flowers are used to treat leprosy and a decoction is used to treat skin diseases. The activity of the plant as male aphrodisiac as been demonstrated experimentally in rodents *(18)*.

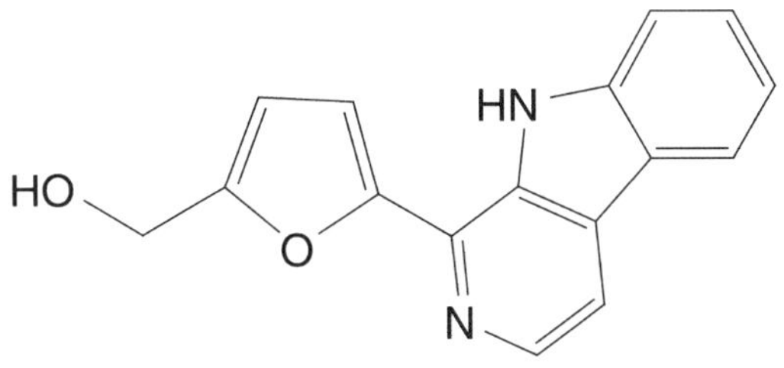

Perlolyrine

The plant is known to elaborate a β-carboline alkaloid, such as tribulusterine, shown by synthesis and spectroscopic analysis to be the (5-hydroxymethyl)-2-furyl analog perlolyrine *(19,20)*. An interesting development from this observation would be to assess the serotoninergic activity of perlolyrine. One might suppose that the diuretic property mentioned previously might involve some levels of serotoninergic activity because serotonin re-uptake has been associated with the development of severe hyponatremia *(21)*. Note that perlolyrine is present in several members of the Polygalaceae family.

Medicinal Polygalaceae

The family Polygalaceae consists of 10 families and 750 species of herbs, shrubs, or woody climbers that have attracted a great deal of interest on account of their ability to produce a series of neuroactive oleanane saponins known as polygalasaponins. In addition, Polygalaceae, like the Malpighiaceae, are member of the Polygalales and elaborate also a series of indole alkaloids that are of neuropharmacological interest. In Asia and the Pacific, about 10 species of plants classified within the family Polygalaceae are of medicinal value. Note that these plants are often used to counteract putrefaction, to treat cough, asthma, and bronchitis, to promote fertility, and to treat cerebral dysfunctions.

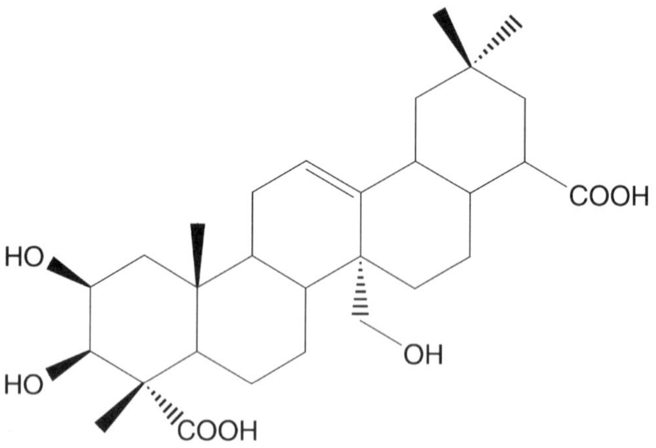

Polygalasaponin aglycone

Polygala tenuifolia (*Polygala sibirica*), or slender lobe milkwort, *yuan chih, yao jao, hsiao ts'ao* (Chinese), is a very slender perennial herb that grows to a height of 20 cm on sun-exposed hillsides, roadsides, and stony slopes of Korea, China, and Mongolia. The leaves are linear and the flowers are whitish (Fig. 41).

In China, the plant is known to promote mental powers. It is used to treat cough, jaundice, hysteria, convulsions, mammary abscess, and gonorrhea. The leaves are used for sperm leaking. The roots and leaves are used to promote urination. In Cambodia, Laos, and Vietnam the roots are used to calm and to treat cough. In Korea, the plant is used to treat psychotic illnesses. In vitro binding studies suggested a potential mechanism for its antipsychotic action, as saponins known as polygalasaponins bind to both dopamine and serotonin receptors. Polygalasaponins (25–500 mg/kg) showed receptor antagonist properties, and their possible utility as antipsychotic agents has been subjected *(22)*. It would be interesting to know whether further study on the precise molecular activity of polygalasaponin discloses any original molecular pathways in the

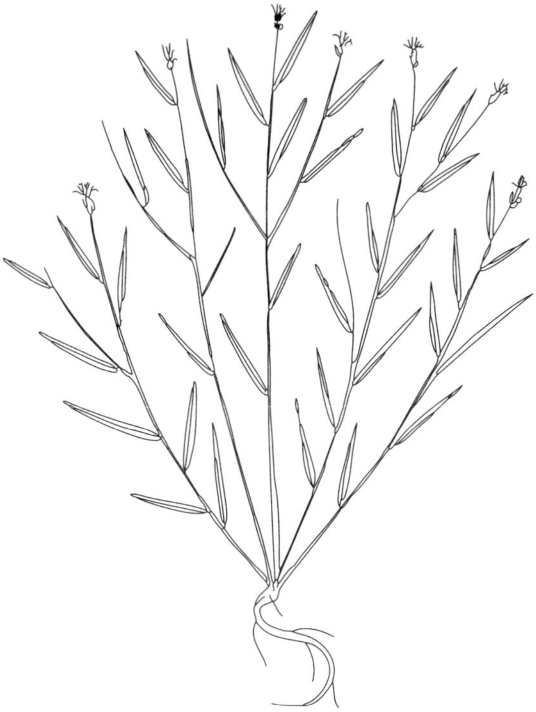

Fig. 41. *Polygala tenuifolia.*

search for serotonin re-uptake inhibitors. Because saponins are very polar, how could it cross the hemato-encephalic barrier and reach the brain unless injected intracranially? Is the genin instead neuroactive?

Note that the plant elaborates a series of carboline alkaloids including 1-carbobutoxy-β-carboline, N9-formylharman, 1-carboethoxy-β-carboline, 1-carbomethoxy- β-carboline, perlolyrine, harman, and norharman *(23)*. An interesting development would be to assess these alkaloids for central nervous activity.

***Polygala japonica* Houtt.** (*Polygala sibirica* non L.), or dwarf milkwort, *himehagi* (Japanese), is a little perennial herb of Australasia. The leaves are tiny and broadly elliptic, and the flowers are purplish-blue (Fig. 42).

It is medicinally used from Korea to Cambodia, Laos, and Vietnam. In Korea, the plant is used as an aphrodisiac for males and the elderly. In Japan, a decoction of the root is drunk to treat cough, invigorate, and treat tuberculosis. In Taiwan, the plant is an external remedy for snake bites. In Cambodia, Laos, and Vietnam, the roots are used to treat bronchitis, amnesia, and to stimulate memory and urination. The antitussive property is very probably owed to polygalasaponins, which are known to abound in the plant *(24–26)*. It would be interesting to know whether the tonic properties mentioned here are owed to serotoninergic mechanisms. What is the alkaloidal content of this herb?

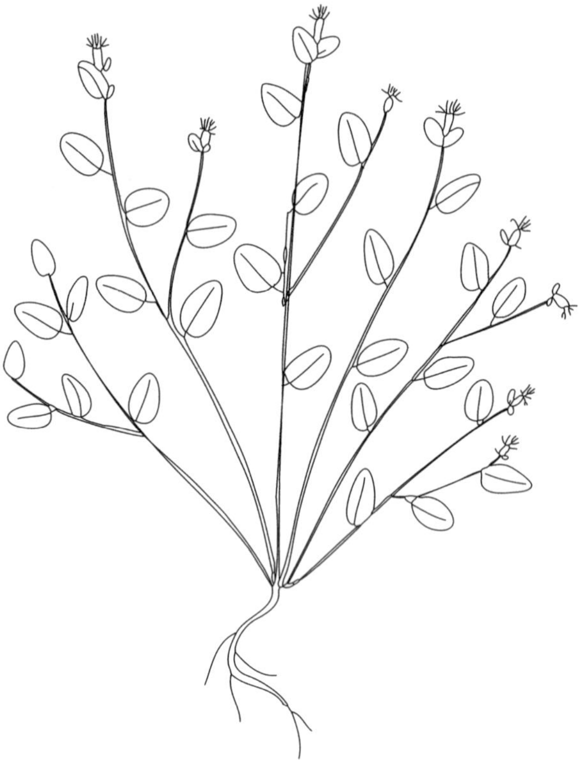

Fig. 42. *Polygala japonica.*

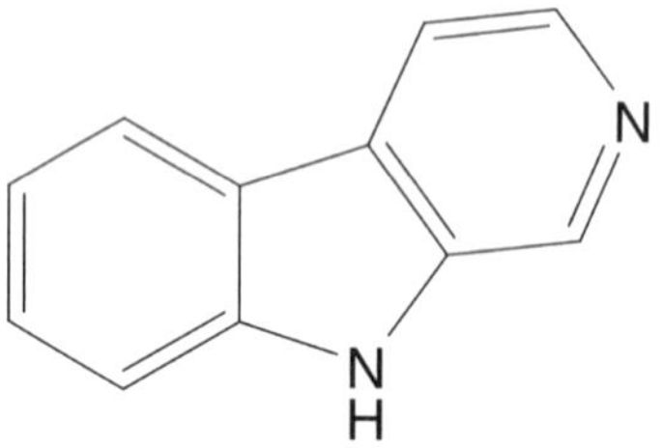

Norharman

Polygala glomerata Lour. (*Polygala chinensis* L., *Polygala densiflora* Blume, *Polygala glomerata* Lour. var. *pygmaea* C.Y. Wu & S.K. Chen, *Polygala glomerata* Lour. var. *villosa* C.Y. Wu & S.K. Chen, *Polygala subopposita* S.K. Chen), or *hua nan yuan zhi* (Chinese), is an annual herb that grows to a height of 25 cm in grasslands, shrub forests, and on slopes of hills in China, Taiwan, India, Bhutan, Cambodia, Indonesia, Laos, Malaya, New Guinea, Philippines, Thailand, and Vietnam. The leaves are obovate, elliptic, or lanceolate. The flowers are 4.5 mm long, yellowish, or white with pink. The fruits are globose, 2 mm in diameter, narrowly winged capsules.

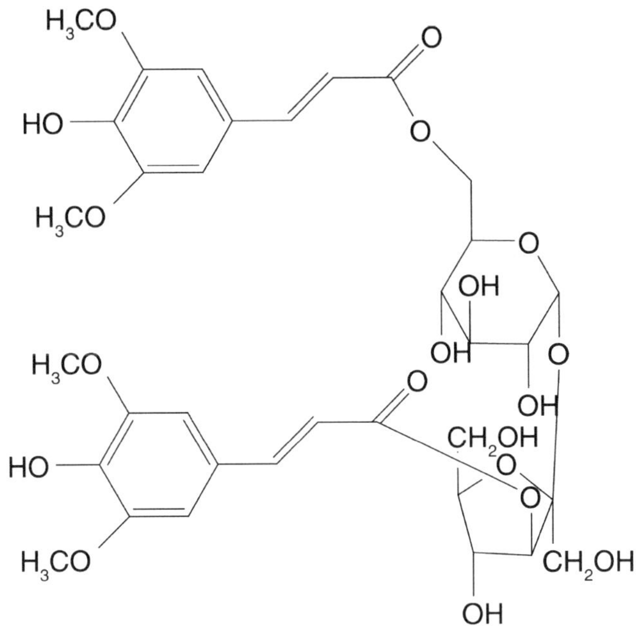

Oligosaccharides of Polygala glomerata

In Vietnam, Cambodia, and Laos, the roots are used to cure inflamed throat, reduce fever, and remove blood from urine. In Indonesia, a tea of the leaves is drunk to treat asthma and cough. The plant is known to elaborate a series of polygalasaponins including polygalasaponins XLII–XLVI, hence mucolytic properties (*26,27*). The plant elaborates a series of oligosaccharide polyesters, the effects of which would be worth assessment because oligosaccharides, especially from the Caryophyllidae, displayed very encouraging pharmacological potentials as antiviral and immunomodulatory agents.

Medicinal Rubiaceae

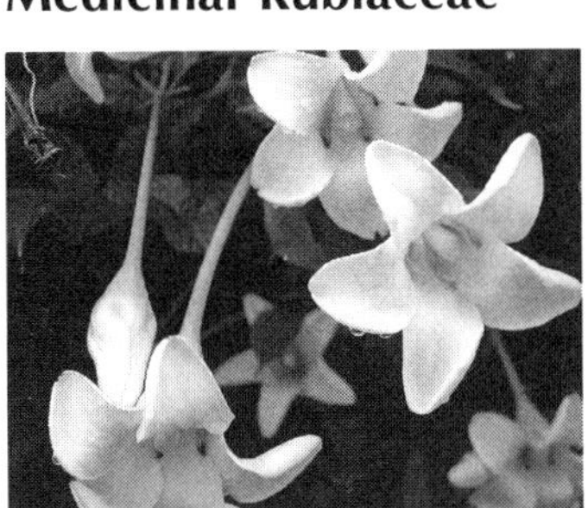

The family Rubiaceae consists of about 450 genera and 6500 species of tropical and sub-tropical trees, shrubs, and climbers that can be quite easily recognized in field collection by their leaves, which are opposite and stipulate, the stipule being interpetiolar. *Cephaelis*, *Nauclea*, *Cinchona*, *Mitragyna*, *Corynanthe*, *Pausinystalia*, *Uncaria*, *Pogonopus*, and *Remijia* species are of particular interest in the family because they produce monoterpenoid indole and quinoline alkaloids, some of which are used as therapeutic alkaloids, such as quinine and emetine. Yohimbine occurs in the genera *Pseudocinchona* and *Yohimbe*. In human subjects, yohimbine at 0.5 mg/kg produces a psychic state stimulating considerable anxiety with tensless, restlessness, irritability, and schizophrenic psychosis.

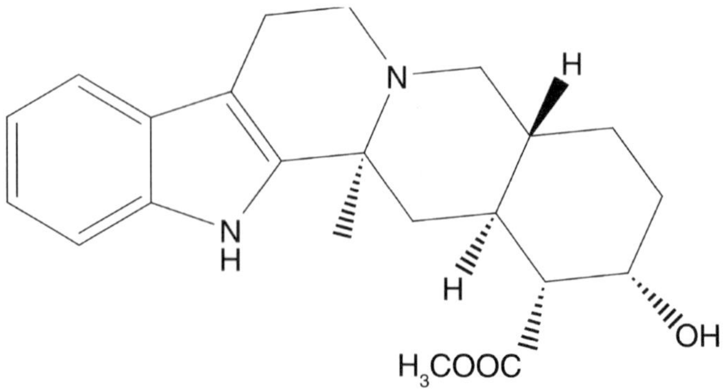

Yohimbine

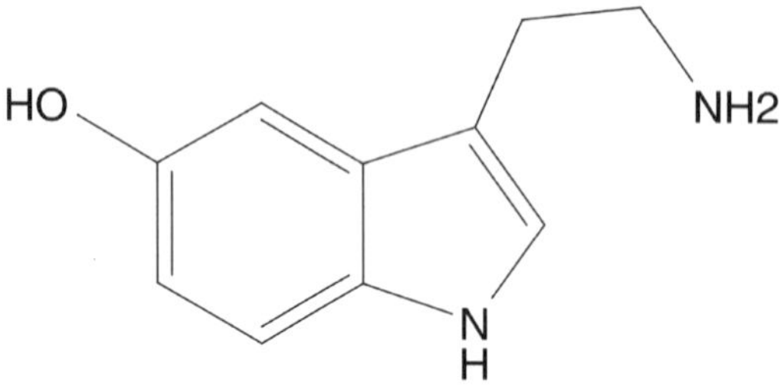

Serotonin

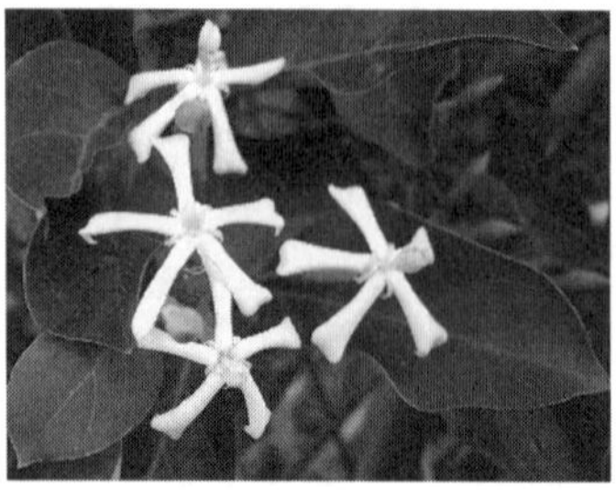

About 120 species of plants classified within the family Rubiaceae are used in traditional medicine of Asia and the Pacific, of which, *Mitragyna speciosa* has been used throughout Southeast Asia, especially in Thailand and Borneo, as an intoxicant. The leaves are chewed alone or mixed with betel, or else prepared for smoking like opium, and its use is legally prescribed in Thailand.

The discovery of natural products of therapeutic value, and especially serotoninergic agents, from this very large family is most probable.

A classical example of medicinal Rubiaceae of Asian origin is *Uncaria gambir* (Hunter) Roxb., from which is extracted an astringent extract (catechu, *British Pharmaceutical Codex*, 1963), employed for the treatment of diarrhea.

***Psychotria adenophylla* Wall.** (*Psychotria siamensis* Ridl.) is a shrub that grows wild to a height of 1 m in Northeast India, Vietnam, Cambodia, Laos, Malaysia, and Java. The leaves are simple, decussate, and stipulate, and show 15 pairs of secondary nerves. The influorescences are racemose. The flowers are small and tubular. The fruits are globose, glossy, and yellowish. In Vietnam, Cambodia, and Laos, the plant is used to treat maladies of the chest.

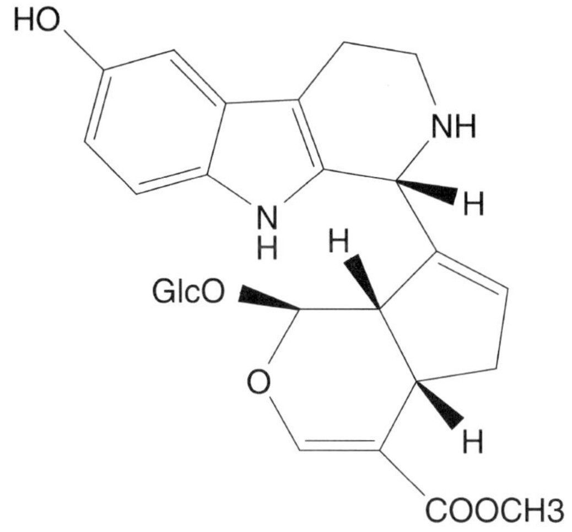

Umbellatine

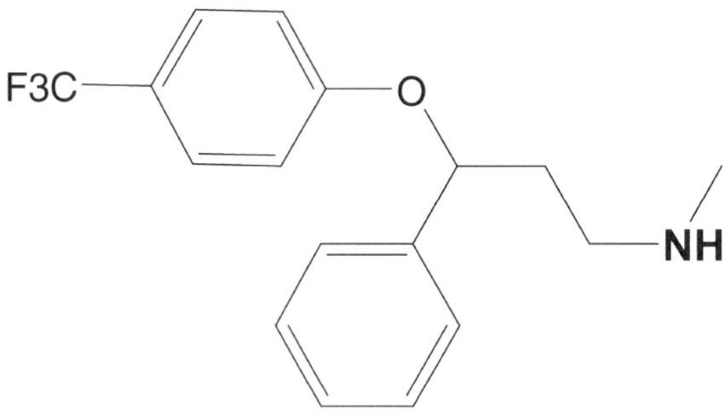

Fluoxetine (Prozac®)

To date, some evidence has already been presented that suggests the genera *Psychotria* to hold potentials as a source of serotoninergic agents. Both et al. drew attention to the fact that psychollatine, an indole alkaloid isolated from Brazilian *Psychotria umbellate*, is centrally active via serotoninergic 5-HT_2 (A/C) receptors *(28)*. In experimental models of anxiety, diazepam (0.75 mg/kg) and psychollatine (7.5 and 15 mg/kg) showed anxiolytic-like effects at doses that do not increase sleeping time nor alter spontaneous locomotor activity. The anxiolytic effect of psychollatine was prevented by ritanserin, indicating the mediation of 5-HT_2 receptors. In the forced swimming model of depression, psychollatine (3 and 7.5 mg/kg) effects were comparable to the antidepressant fluoxetine, or Prozac® (205 mg/kg). Investigating the medicinal flora of the Pacific Rim, and especially the *Psychotria* species, might possibly result in the characterization of antidepressants of clinical value.

Rubia cordifolia (*Rubia cordifolia* var. *mungista* [Roxb.] Miq, *Rubia cordifolia* var. *stenophylla* Franch, *Rubia akane* Nak.), or Indian madder, Bengal Madder, *ch'ien ts'ao, ti hsueh, jan fei ts'ao, hsueh chien-ch'ou*. (Chinese), *munjette, mandjuchaka* (Sanskrit), *guo*

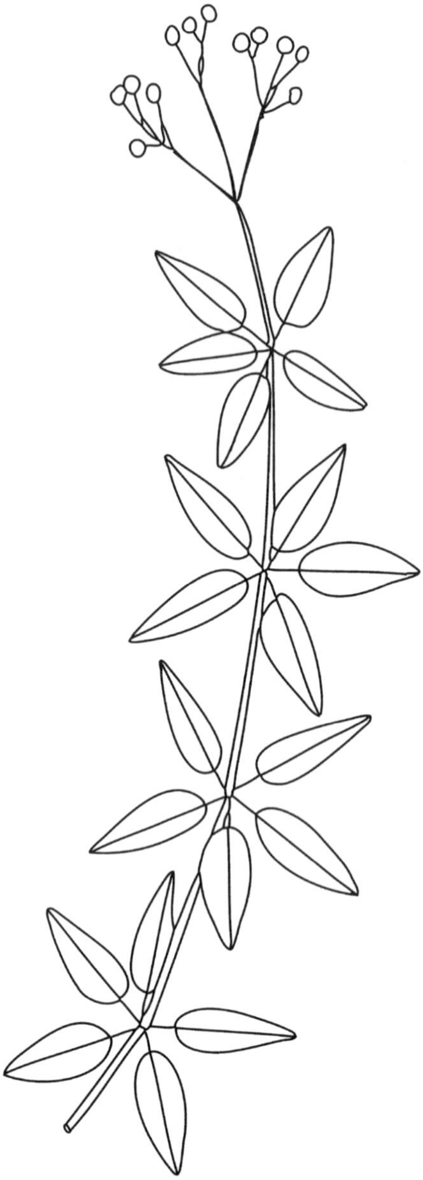

Fig. 43. *Rubia cordifolia* L.

shan long (Taiwan), or *nihon akane*. (Japanese), is a perennial creeping or climbing herb that grows to a length of 3 m in the Himalayas (up to 2000 m), Japan, and China. The stem is quadrangular and minutely prickly. The leaves are cordate and in whorls of four to five (Fig. 43). The plant abounds with purpurin, an anthraquinone, and is used for dyeing a deep red color in China, Tibet, and Japan *(29)*.

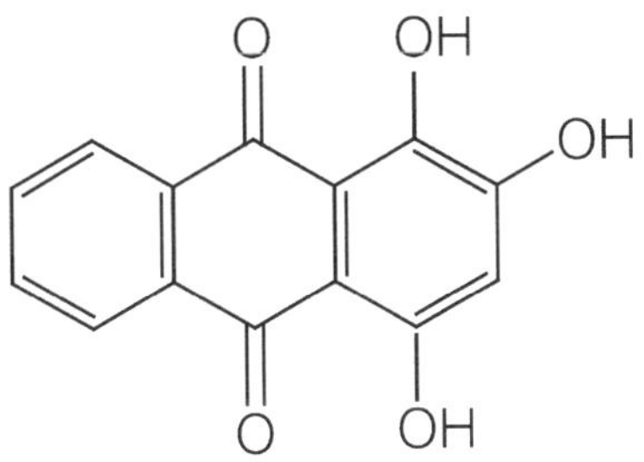

Purpurin

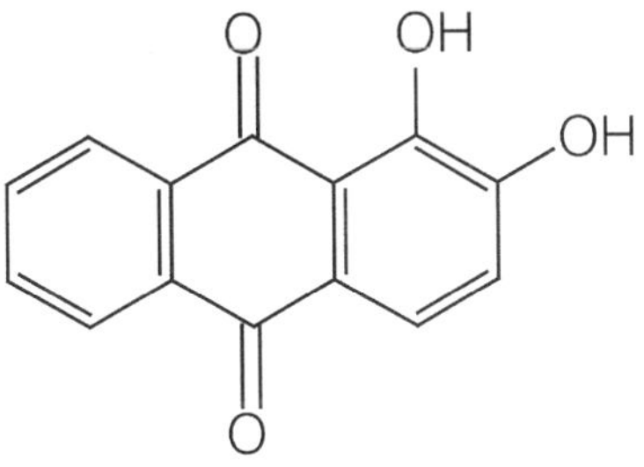

Alizarin

In China and Tibet, the plant is held in great esteem. It was believed that the color of the plant was caused by transformed human blood. The root is used to treat rheumatism, jaundice, hemorrhages, and all sorts of exhausting discharges. In Korea, the root is used to treat rheumatism, jaundice and menstrual disorders. In the Philippines, a decoction of roots is drunk as a remedy for urinary disorders. One might have observed the obvious relationship between the red color of the sap and the blood-related medicinal uses of the plant; it illustrates the "doctrine of signatures" of Paracelsus.

In regard to the experimental evidence available, a substantial number of reports on the chemical constituents of the plant are available, but much less work has been done with the pharmacological properties. Kasture et al., however, made the important observation that a triterpene isolated from *R. cordifolia* induces anxiety in rodents, an effect accompanied with an increase in serotonin contents in the brain *(30)*. An interesting development from that observation would be to explore further the molecular–pharmacological pathway and the effect of this agent on the serotoninergic system because terpenes, compared with indole alkaloids, are seldom reported for serotoninergic activities.

***Uncaria rhynchophylla* Miq.** (*Ourouparia rynchophylla* Matsum.), or Chinese cat's claw; *kou t'eng*, or *tiao t'eng* (Chinese). The plant is a woody a climber native to China and Japan. The stem is quadrangular, hollowed, and regularly hooked. The leaves are simple, opposite, and stipulate, with the stipules being interpetiolar. The influorescences are globose on long pedicels on leaf axis (Fig. 44). In China, sun-dried pieces of hook-bearing stems are used to reduce fever in children and treat nervous disorders of children. In adults, the plant is used to treat dizziness, motes in vision, and bilious disorders. Hou proposed two phenolic compounds—catechin and epicatechin—to be involved in the neurological properties of *Uncaria rhynchophylla* because these molecules inhibited the enzymatic activity of monoamine oxidase-B with inhibiting concentration $(IC)_{50}$ values of 88.6 and 58.9 μM in vitro *(31)*. Can we reasonably expect phenolic compounds to exert significant CNS activity?

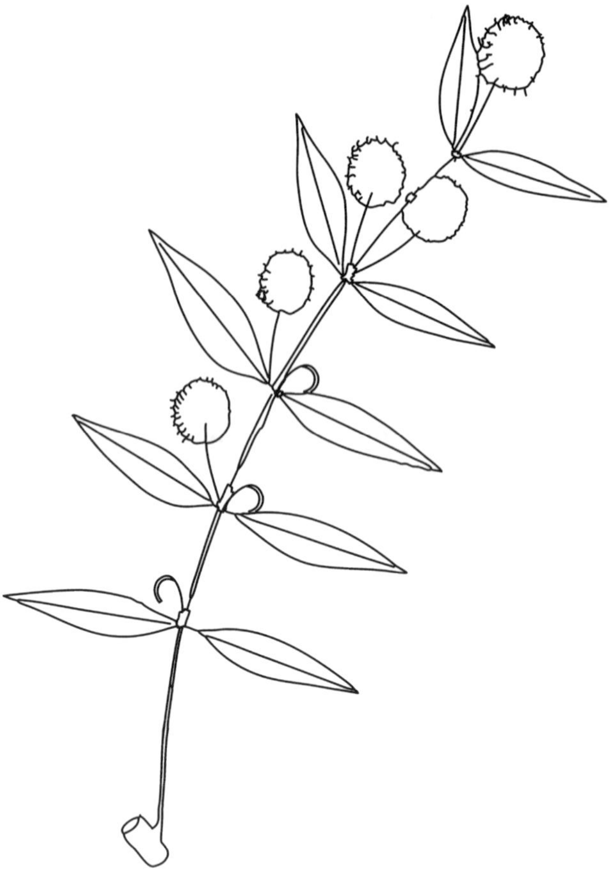

Fig. 44. *Uncaria rynchophylla* Miq.

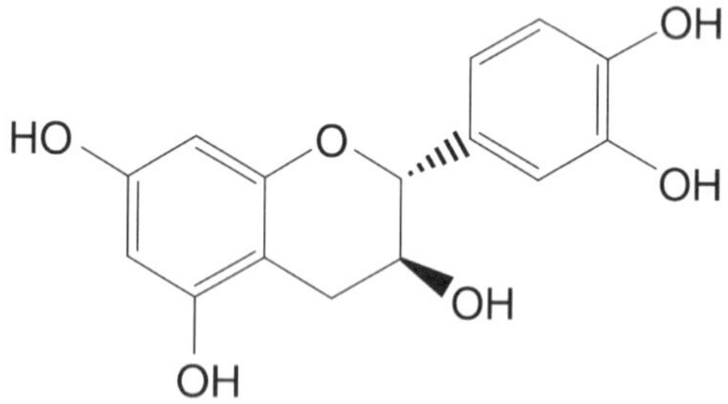

(+) – Catechin

The most likely explanation for these results is that simple phenolics inhibit a very large array of enzymes in vitro. The most likely explanation for the CNS effects of *Uncaria rynchophylla* would be that indole alkaloids, such as dihydrocorynanteine or hirsutine (*32*), interact with the central neurotransmission and possibly the serotoninergic system.

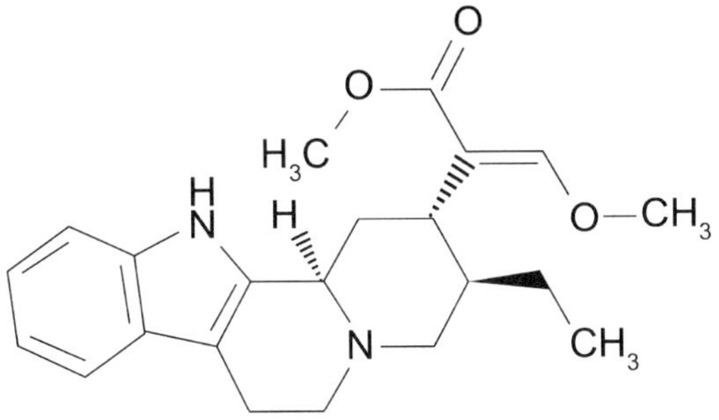

Hirsutine

Evidence in favor of such a hypothesis is given by Jurgensen et al. who have first reported the fact that an alkaloid fraction from *Uncaria tomentosa* (Willd.) DC, a vine used by Peruvian Indians to treat several diseases, given by the intraperitonneal route, dose-dependently suppressed the behavioral response to the chemical stimuli in the models indicated and increased latencies in the thermal stimuli models *(33)*.
The antinociception caused by the fraction in the formalin test was significantly attenuated by intraperitoneal injection of mice with ketanserin (5-HT_2 receptor antagonist), but was not affected by naltrexone (opioid receptor antagonist), atropine (a nonselective muscarinic antagonist), L-arginine (precursor of nitric oxide), prazosin (α_1-adrenoceptor antagonist), yohimbine (α_2-adrenoceptor antagonist), and reserpine (a natural monoamine depletory alkaloid from *Rauvolfia serpentina* [Rubiaceae]). Together, these results indicate that the fraction abrogates, dose-dependently, pain via interaction with 5-HT_2 receptors.

PLANTS AFFECTING THE GABAERGIC NEUROTRANSMISSION

γ-Aminobutyric acid (GABA) is an inhibitory neurotransmitter in the CNS. Neurons using the GABA as neurotransmitter are among the most abundant in the CNS. GABAergic neurones occur mainly as local neurons or interneurons present in all area of the CNS involved in the local modulation of neuron activity and to a lesser extent, as projecting or principal neurones (cerebelar Purkinje cells, striatonigral, striathothalamic, and nigrothalamic pathways). There may be five or more types of GABA receptors, but GABA receptors $GABA_A$ and $GABA_B$ are the most studied. $GABA_A$ receptor blockers, such as bicuculline and picrotoxin, are both $GABA_A$ receptor-blocking agents that impede the GABAergic presynaptic inhibition of excitatory transmission of primary afferent neurones of the spinal cord, hence a general increase in neuronal activity, alertness, anxiety, spasms, seizures, and even death (Fig. 45).

Picrotoxinin is a sesquiterpene, which is found notably in the seeds *Anamirta paniculata* Coleb. (levant berries, Menispermaceae; Fig. 46). This substance is toxic, and as little as 20 mg induces epileptiform convulsions, myosis, and dyspnea with more or less

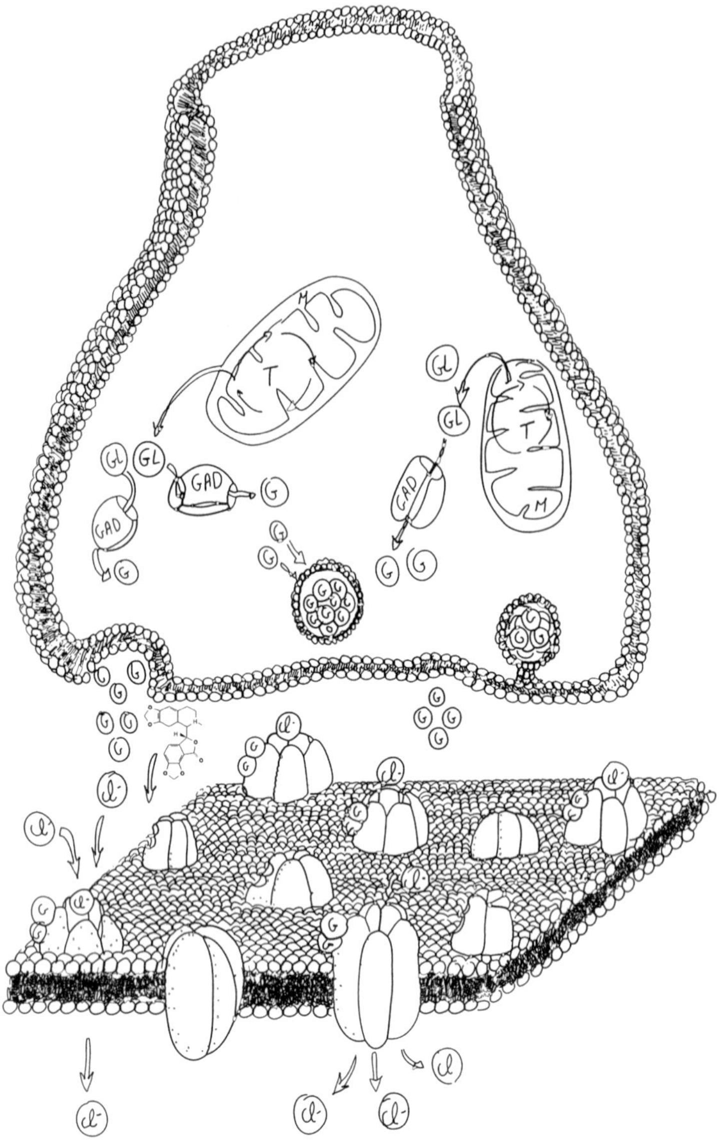

Fig. 45. GABAergic neurone synapse. GAD, glutamic acid decarboxylase; M, mitochondria; G, GABA.

prolonged apnea. Picrotoxin (*British Pharmacopoeia*, 1963) has been used in the treatment of barbiturate poisoning (3–6 mg, intravenously) in Western medicine. Both compounds are elaborated in the Magnolidae (Ranunculales and Papaverales).

Bicuculline is an isoquinoline alkaloid elaborated from members of the family Fumariaceae (Papaverales), especially in *Corydalis*, *Dicentra*, and *Fumaria* species. Bicuculline, like picrotoxin, is a specific GABA receptor-blocking agent that impedes the

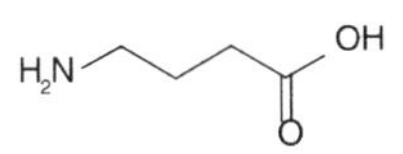

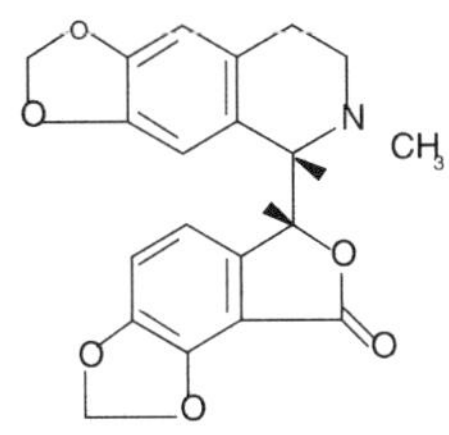

γ – Aminobutyric acid (GABA)

Bicuculline (GABAergic antagonist)

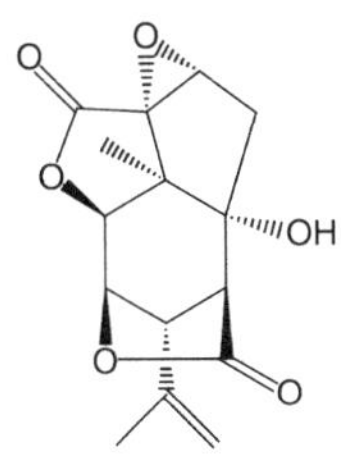

Picrotoxinin (GABAergic antagonist)

Fig. 46. Examples of GABAergic natural products from flowering plants.

GABAergic presynaptic inhibition of excitatory transmission of primary afferent neurones of the spinal cord resulting in epileptiform convulsions, myosis, and dyspnea with more or less prolonged apnea.

One of the most spectacular applications in this field is the development of a $GABA_A$ receptor agonist: the benzodiaxepine. About 15 types of benzodiazepine derivatives are currently available in the United States and marketed as sedatives, anxiolytics, muscle relaxants, intravenous anesthetics, and anticonvulsants. Anxiolytics known as benzodiazepines, which bind to a very specific region of $GABA_A$ receptors. However, benzodiazepines are sedatives that induce serious memory impairment, drowsiness, and dependence, and there is a need for agents with lighter side effects. Experimental observations have led to the suggestion that the etiology of Huntington's chorea, epilepsy, and Alzheimer's disease could be linked to the GABAergic system. The search for $GABA_A$ agonists appears, therefore, as a very exiting quest, and one looking for such agent might look into the medicinal flora of the Asia–Pacific region.

A classic example of a medicinal plant of Asia and the Pacific with GABAergic properties is *Piper methysticum* Forst. (Kava, *British Pharmaceutical Codex*, 1934), or *kava-kava*, the rhizomes of which have been used since a very early period of time by Polynesians to allay anxiety and reduce fatigue. Kava has been marketed in Europe to treat sleep disorders and anxiety. The beverage normally induces a form of euphoria, described as a happy state of complete comfort and peace, with ease of conversation and increased perceptivity, followed by muscular fatigue and restful sleep. Klohs et al. identified the active constituents as series of α-pyrone including kawaine, which mediates anxiolytic effects through $GABA_A$ receptor binding *(34,35)*.

Medicinal Valerianaceae

Valeriana officinalis has been used in traditional medicine for its sedative, hypnotic, and anticonvulsant effects. There are several reports in the literature supporting a GABAergic mechanism of action for valerian. Valerian (*British Pharmaceutical Codex*, 1963) consists of the dried rhizome or roots of *Valeriana officinalis* containing not less than 18% alcohol (60%)-soluble extractive. It has been used in the form of infusion, tinctures (1 in 8 prepared by maceration in alcohol [60%]; dose 4–8 mL, Tinct. Valerian Simp, *British Pharmaceutical Codex*, 1949) to calm. Some evidence has already been presented that indicates that the anxiolytic and sedative effects of valerian involve the GABAergic system. In vitro, the aqueous and hydroalcoholic extracts of *Valeriana officinalis* L. displace [^{3}H]muscimol from $GABA_A$ receptor *(36,37)*. Yuan et al. made the important observation that valerian extract (3 mg/mL) and valerenic acid (100 μM) inhibit the firing rate in most brainstem neurons with IC_{50} values of 240 mg/mL and 23 mM, respectively *(37)*. Bicuculline antagonized the inhibitory effects of both the valerian extract and valerenic acid.

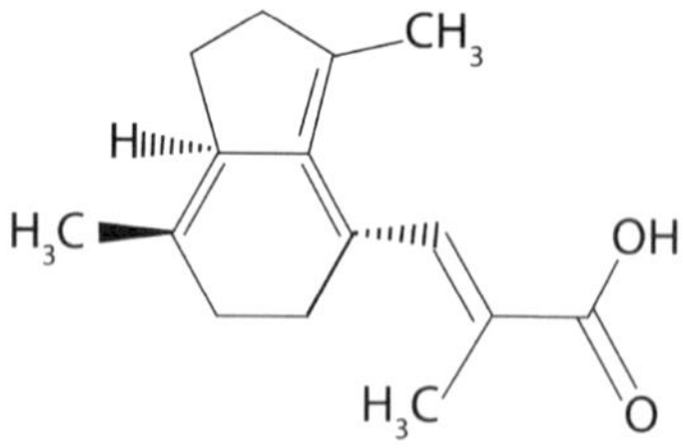

Valerenic acid

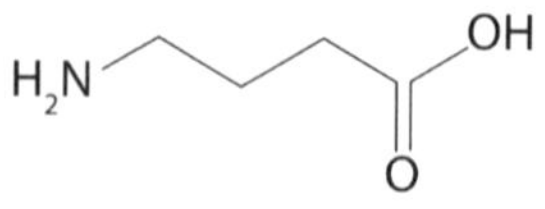

GABA

The rhizomes and roots of *Valeriana wallichii* DC. contain 6-methylapigenin, which is a competitive ligand for $GABA_A$ receptor *(38)*. In the Asia–Pacific region, *Nardostachys chinensis* L., *Nardostachys jatamansis* DC., *Patrinia scabiosaefolia* Link, *Valeriana officinalis* L., *Valeriana dageletiana* Nak. ex Maekawa, and *Valeriana hardwickii* Wall. are used as alternative remedies.

***Nardostachys chinensis* L.** is an herb that grows to a height of 50 cm. The stem is erect and develops from an aromatic rhizome. The leaves are linear and somewhat spathulate. The flowers are small, tubular, and packed in a terminal cyme (Fig. 47). In China, the rhizome is used to treat swollen ankles, assuage toothache, and is given for congested chest and stomach. The plant is interesting because it elaborates a sesquiterpene known as nardosinone, which is an enhancer of the neuritogenic action of dibutyryl cyclic (dbc)AMP and staurosporine, hence the potential as a pharmacological tool for studying the mechanism of action of neuritogenic substances. Nardosinone enhances staurosporine- or dbcAMP-induced neurite growth from PC12D cells in a

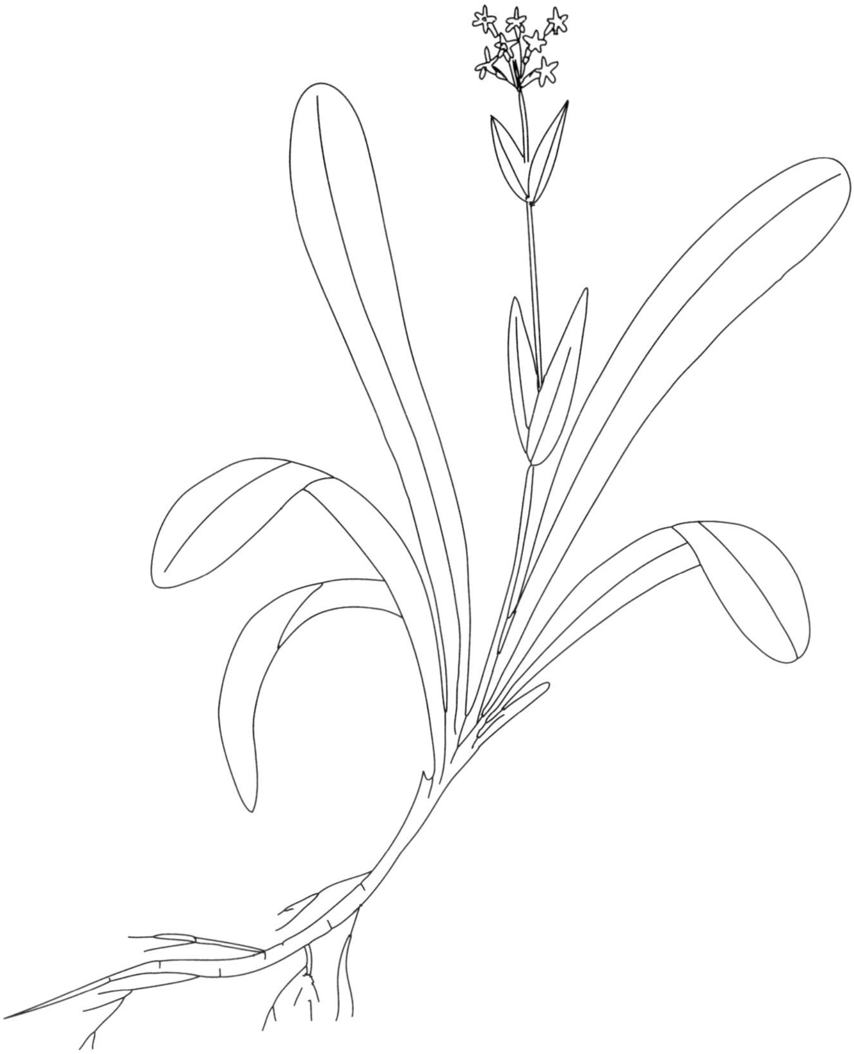

Fig. 47. *Nardostachys chinensis* L.

concentration-dependent manner, possibly by amplifying both the mitogen-activated protein (MAP) kinase-dependent and -independent signaling pathways of dbcAMP and staurosporine. Nardosinone stimulates a downstream step of MAP kinase in the MAP kinase-dependent signaling pathway (39). Note that the pharmacological potentials of this plant for GABAergic properties are unexplored.

Nardostachys jatamansi DC. (*Nardostachys grandiflora* DC.), or spikenard, *jatamansi* (Sanskrit), *jatamansi* (Hindi), *jatamanshi* (Malayalam), *jatamashi* (Tamil); *kan sung shiang* or *ku mi che* (Chinese), is a perennial herb that grows to a height of 60 cm in the Himalayas (from 3000 to 5000 m), Punjab, and Bhutan. The stem is erect, pubescent, and develops from an aromatic rhizome. The flowers are pinkish-blue and arranged in terminal globose cymes (Fig. 48).

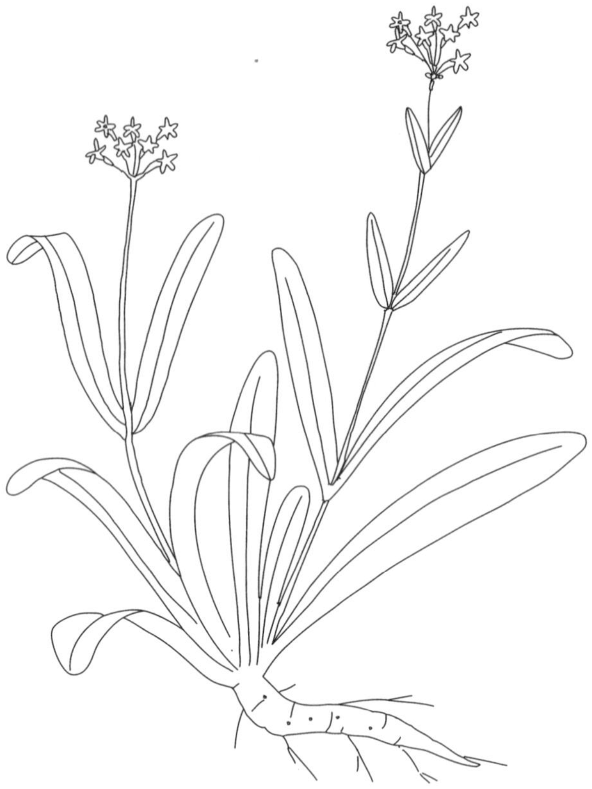

Fig. 48. *Nardostachys jatamansi* DC.

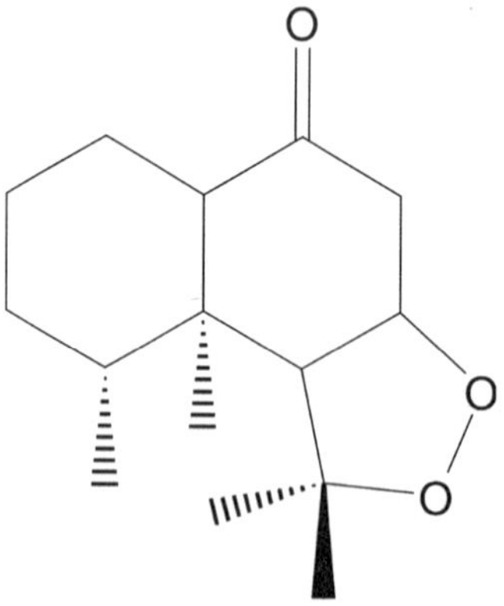

Nardosinone

In China, the rhizome is used as a deodorant, carminative, and stimulant. A decoction is used in various skin affections and in the bath to give fragrance to the body. In India, the rhizome is used to treat depression, hysteria, epilepsy, convulsions, headache, colic, and as a tonic and carminative.

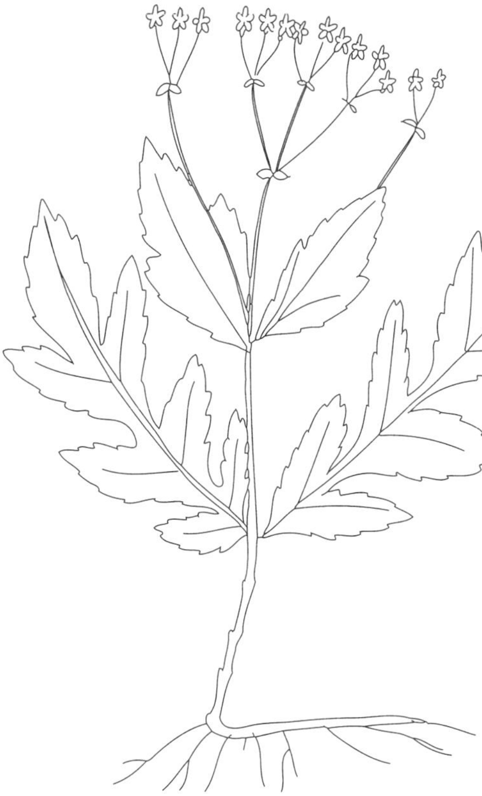

Fig. 49. *Patrinia scabiosaefolia* Link.

The plant has been shown to posses GABAergic properties. Prabhu et al. showed that acute and subchronic administration of an alcoholic extract of the roots *of Nardostachys jatamansi* to male albino Wistar rats resulted in a significant increase in GABA *(40)*. In addition, 2 weeks' oral pretreatment with the plant at a dose of 250 mg/kg abrogated alternations induced by ischemia, including neuronal cell death following middle cerebral artery occlusion *(41)*. Note that the plant exhibits hepatoprotective effects *(42)*. It would be interesting to learn whether further study on this herb discloses any original agent with GABAergic potentials.

Patrinia scabiosaefolia **Link**, or patrinia, *ominameshi* (Japanese), *pai chang, ku chih, ku tu*, or *hai sho* (Chinese), is an erect herb that grows to a height of 1 m in East Asia and in sunny, grassy places in hills and mountains all over Japan. The root of this plant smells like spoiled soy. The leaves are fleshy, soft, whorled, dentate, and serrate. The flowers are small, yellowish-white, and arranged in corymbose cymes (Fig. 49).

The roots are used as an astringent, resolving anodyne and antidotal. It is also used to heal abscesses, assuage postpartum pain, and remove parasites from the skin. The plant was mentioned by Schimmel in the *American Journal of Pharmacy* in 1889. Clinical observation and pharmacological investigation of the sedative and hypnotic effects of the Chinese drug rhizome and root of *Patrinia scabiosaefolia* are discussed by Luo *(43)*.

Note that the plant is known to abound with triterpenoid saponins *(44,45)*. Is the plant holding GABAergic activity? One wonders.

Medicinal Lamiaceae

There is an increasing body of evidence to suggest that flavonoids and diterpenes of Lamiaceae might be of value as source of original antagonists of the GABAergic neurotransmission. Flavonoids in particular possess partial allosteric modulatory action at the $GABA_A$ receptor complex and, therefore, constitute a possibly promising group of naturally occurring agents for the treatment of anxiety disorders. Huen et al. made the interesting discovery that 2′-hydroxyl substitution is a critical moiety on flavonoids with regard to benzodiazepine receptor affinities. Benzodiazepine receptor binding assay-guided fractionation of the methanol extract from sage leaves (*Salvia officinalis* L.), for instance, revealed flavones and abietane diterpenes functioning as benzodiazepine receptor-active components. Apigenin, hispidulin, and cirsimaritin competitively inhibit the binding of 3H-flumazenil to the benzodiazepine receptor with respective IC_{50} values of 30, 1.3, and 350 μM *(46,47)*.

The medicinal Lamiaceae, with about 250 species, represents a vast source of material to explore when looking for anxiolytic agents of clinical value. Among these medicinal species are *Scutellaria baicalensis* Georgi and *Leonotis nepetifolia*, the properties of which are described here.

Scutellaria baicalensis **Georgi** (*Scutellaria micrantha* Fisch, *Scutellaria lanceolaria* Miq.), or Baical scullcap, Chinese scullap, or *huang ch'in* (Chinese), is a perennial herb that grows from a rhizome to a height of 1.20 m. It is common on sunny, grassy slopes, waste and cultivated areas, from 100 to 2000 m in China, Japan, Korea, Mongolia, and the steppes of Siberia. The stems are erect, much branched, quadrangular, and puberulent. The leaves are simple, decussate, and linear-lanceolate. The influorescences are terminal racemes of up to 15 cm long. The flowers are tubular, labiate, dark blue, purple-red to blue, and up to 3 cm long (Fig. 50).

The drug consists of the roots, usually cut into slices is used to promote urination, to quiet pregnant uterus, stimulate respiratory organs, reduce fever, treat jaundice, diarrhea, cancer of the breast, and heal boils. In Korea, the plant is used to treat bacterial infection of respiratory and gastrointestinal tracts and fever. The plant has attracted a great deal of interest as it elaborates a series of flavones: baicalein, wooing, and oroxylina, which bind antagonistly to the benzodiazepine binding site $GABA_A$ receptor *(48–50)*.

5,7-Dihydroxy-6-methoxyflavone (oroxylin A) inhibits the binding of [^{3}H]flunitrazepam to rat cerebral cortical membrane with a IC_{50} value of 1.09 μM. oral administration of oroxylin A (3.75–60 mg/kg) attenuated the anxiolytic, myorelaxant, and motor incoordination elicited by diazepam. Oroxylin A or wogonin given orally to animals (7.5–30 mg/kg) is anxiolytic similarly to diazepam (Valium®) through positive allosteric modulation of the $GABA_A$ receptor complex via interaction at the benzodiazepine site (Fig. 51).

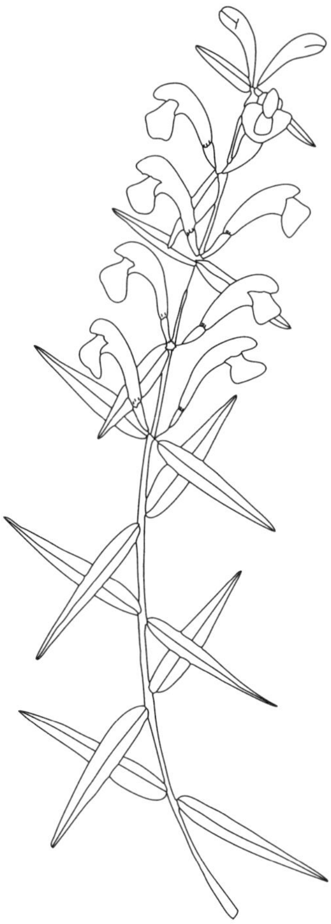

Fig. 50. *Scutellaria baicalensis* Georgi.

It is interesting to note that GABA and glutamine have been characterized from extracts of *Scutellaria lateriflora* L. (American skullcap) at 1.6 and 31 mg/g, respectively *(51)*.
Leonotis nepetifolia **R.Br,** or annual lion's ear, is an annual herb that grows to a height of 2 m. The plant is native to Africa and is commonly grown as an ornamental. The stems are quadrangular. The leaves simple, decussate, and up to 12 cm long. The internodes are 20 cm long. The influorescences are axillary, globular, and spiny (Fig. 52). The flowers are tubular, red, and about 2.5 cm long. In Malaysia, a paste of leaves is applied to wounds. The neuropharmacological potential of this plant is unexplored. Note that an aqueous extract of *Leonotis leonurus* in the doses of 200 and 400 mg/kg, respectively, abbrogated the onset of tonic seizures produced by picrotoxin, hence some GABAergic activities *(52)*. Aqueous extracts of the plant showed some levels of activity on guinea pig smooth muscle and rat cardiac muscle *(53)*. Is 4,6,7-trimethoxy-5-methylchromen-2-one involved here *(54)*? An interesting development from these observations is the fact that flavonoids bind to $GABA_A$ receptors.

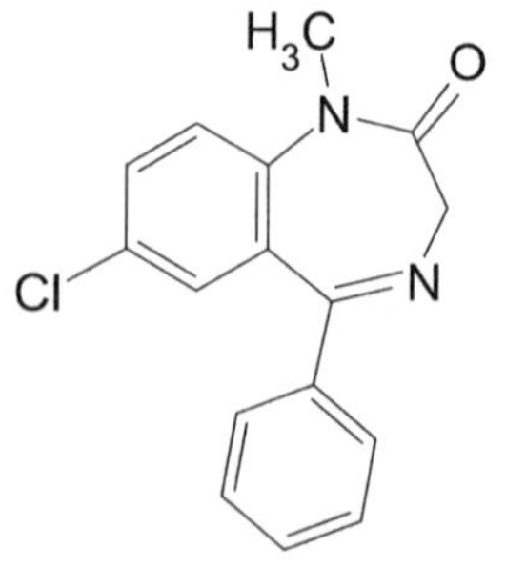

Diazepam (Valiumfi)

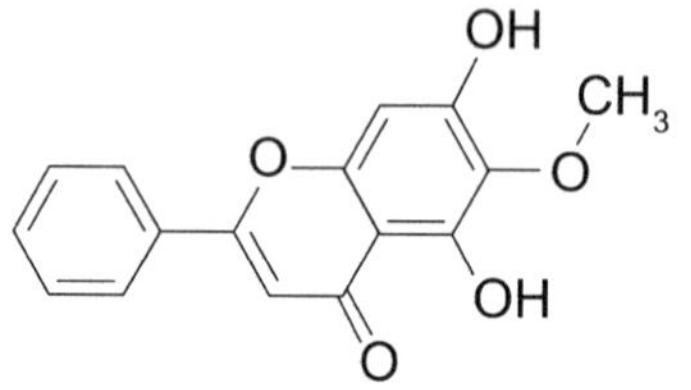

Oroxylin A

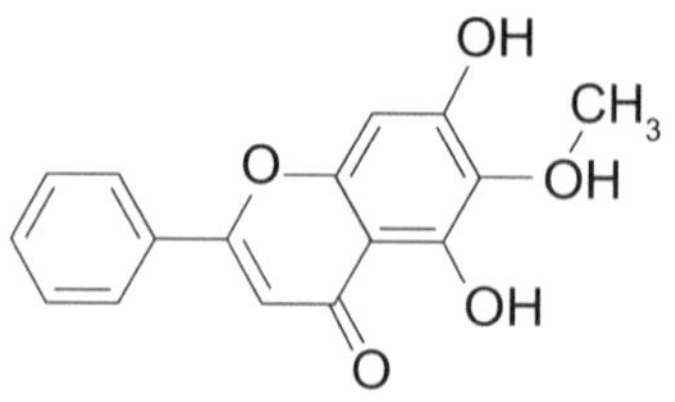

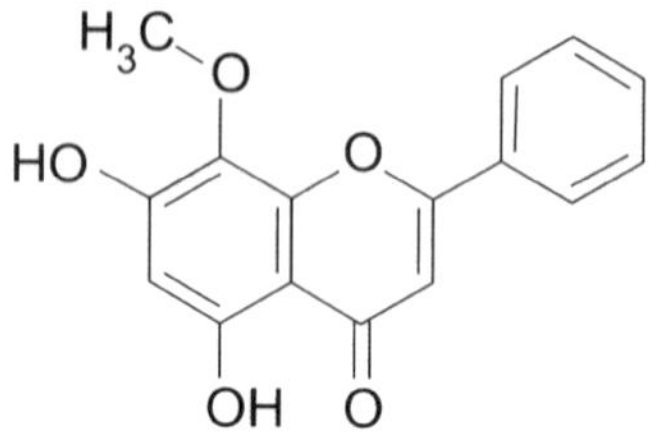

Baicalein Wogonin

Fig. 51. Valium® and GABAergic flavonoids of *Scutellaria baicalensis* Georgi.

Medicinal Asteraceae

A remarkable advance in the neuropharmacological properties of Asteraceae has been provided by Viola et al. and Avallone et al. *(55,56)*. They made the important observation that apigenin blocks the binding of flunitrazepam to $GABA_A$ receptors, displaces flumazenil from the central benzodiazepine binding site, and reduces GABA-activated chloride channels. Apigenin, or 5,7,4′-trihydroxyflavone, is widespread in members of the Asteraceae family and is notably present in *Matricaria chamomilla* L. (*Chamomilla recutita* [L.] Rauschert) or German chamomile (matricaria, *British Pharmaceutical Codex*, 1949).

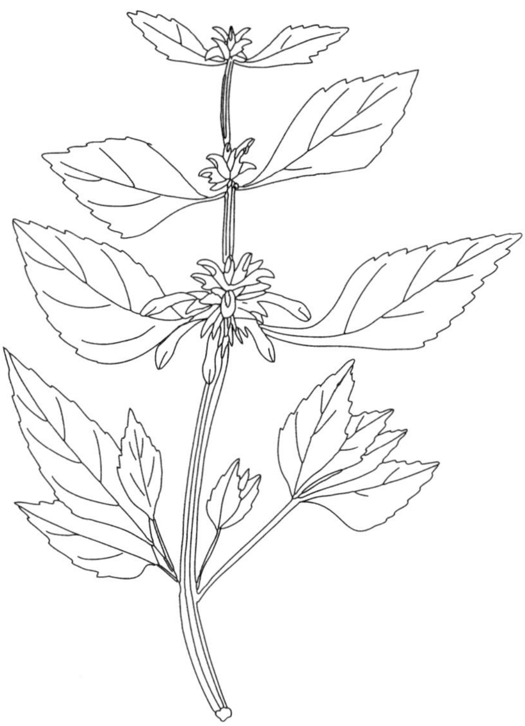

Fig. 52. *Leonotis nepetifolia.*

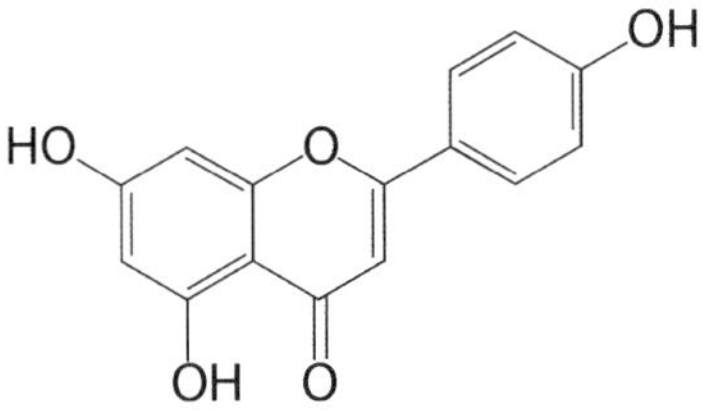

Apigenin

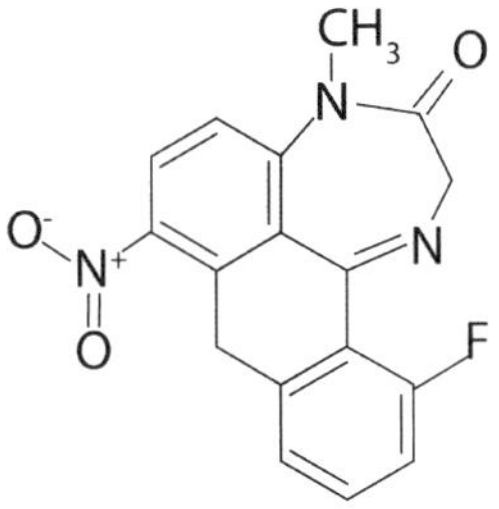

Flunitrazepam

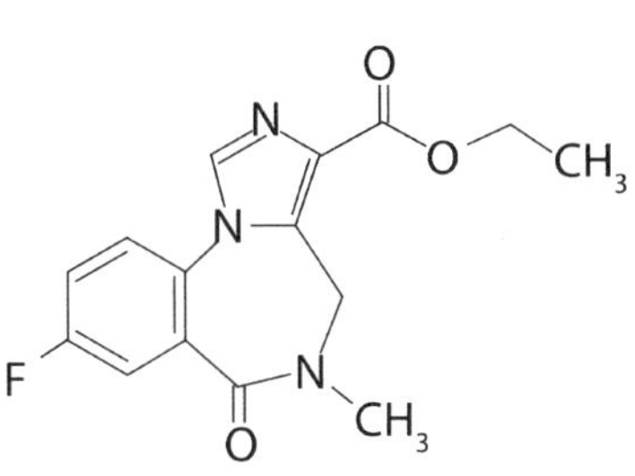

Flumazenil (Ronmazicon®)

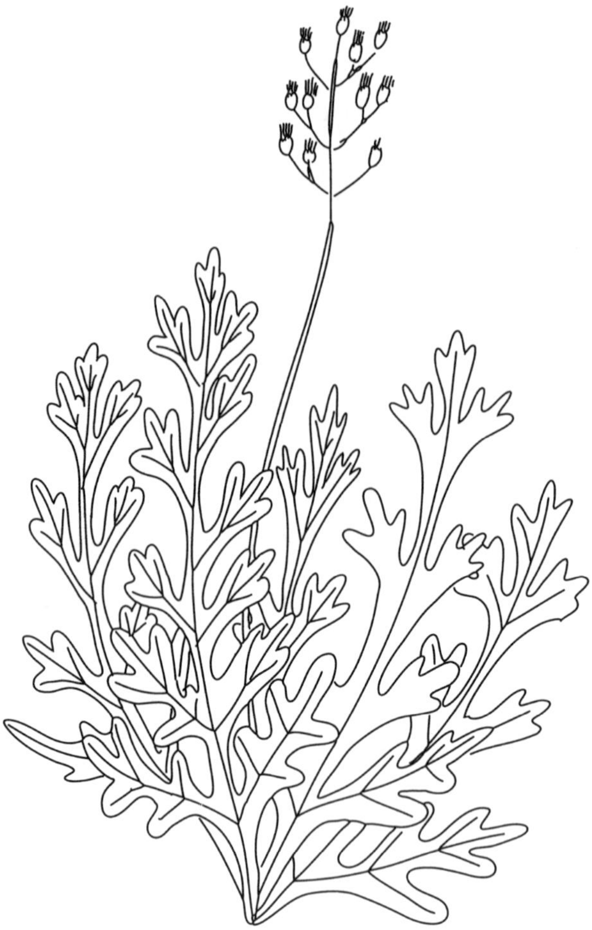

Fig. 53. *Artemisia stelleriana* Bess.

This evidence taken together lends considerable support to the view that sedative Asteraceae owe their activity to the GABAergic property of their flavonoids. One major difficulty seems to be explaining the mechanism by which these polar substances would cross the hemato-encephalic barrier to reach GABA receptors in the brain.

Artemisia stelleriana Bess., or dusty miller sagewort, beach wormwood; old woman, or *pai hao*, *fan*, *lu* (Chinese), is a shrub that grows to 1.20 m in Japan, Korea, China, and Siberia. The whole plant is covered with a glaucous indumentum. The leaves are compound, and the lobes are rounded. The flowers are small, yellowish, and packed in globose capitula (Fig. 53). The medicinal values of *Artemisia stelleriana* Bess. were mentioned by Su Sung (11th century). It has been used internally for food, as carminative, to promote the growth of hair, and to stimulate mental faculties, and externally it provides a remedy for ulcers.

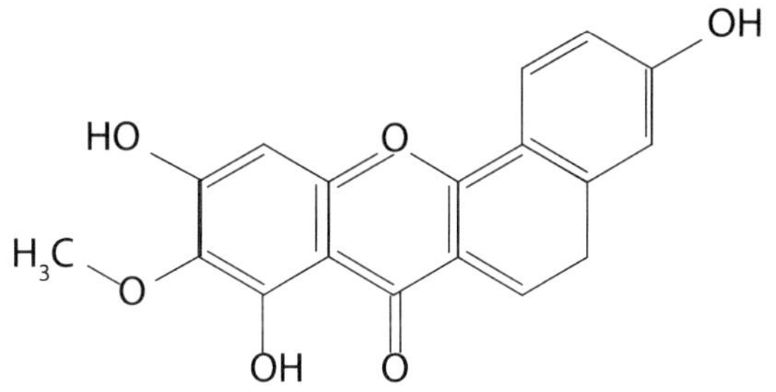

Hispidulin

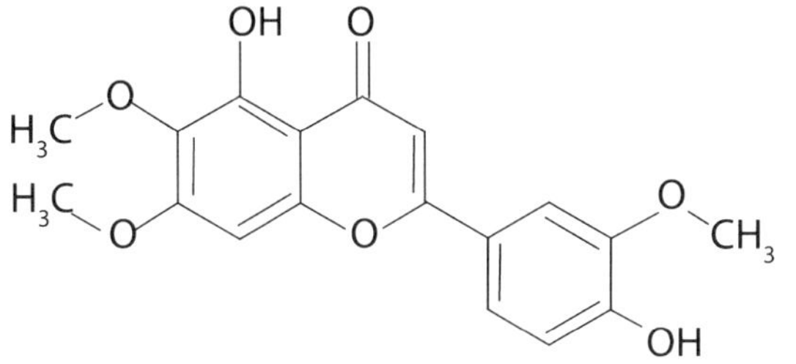

Cirsilineol

The central nervous properties of the plant have not yet been assessed experimentally. One might set the hypothesis that flavonoids could be involved through interference with the GABAergic nervous system as noticed previously. Some evidence has already been presented that suggests that the *Artemisia* species has an affinity to the $GABA_A$ receptor. Such flavonoids could be hispidulin and cirsilineol isolated from an ethyl acetate extract of *Artemisia herba-alba*, which displaces [^{3}H]-flumazenil radioligand assay, have affinity to the $GABA_A$ receptor. Such flavonoids could be hispidulin and cirsilineol isolated from an ethyl acetate extract of *Artemisia herba-alba* which displace [^{3}H]-flumazenil from GABA(A)-benzodiazepine receptor with IC_{50} values of 8 μM and 100 μM, respectively (57,58).

Medicinal Orchidaceae

The family Orchidaceae is a large group that, to date, is known to consist of 1000 genera and about 20,000 species of mycotrophic or epiphytic herbs that are recognized by their flowers, which comprise two whorls of three tepals, including a labellum (Fig. 54). Many orchids are cultivated for their spectacular flowers, and *Vanilla planifolia* is the source of a well-known flavoring material. Members of this family are known to elaborate series of isoquinoline derivatives alkaloids, as well as phenylpropanoids and oligostilbenes. About 120 species of Orchidaceae are used for traditional medicine in Asia and the Pacific region and might hold some potential as starting material for the search for GABA receptor antagonists. One of these plants is *Gastrodia elata* Bl.

***Gastrodia elata* Bl.**, or *ch'ih chien,t'ien ma*, is native to East Asia. The plant develops from a rhizome that is about 7 × 2.5 cm. It consists merely in a stem with few flowers at

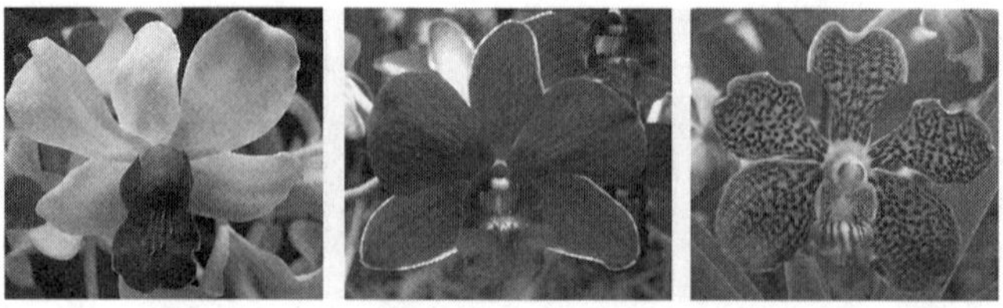

Fig. 54. The botanical hallmark of Orchidaceae: the flowers.

the apex (Fig. 55). In Korea, the plant is used to treat nervous disorders. In China, it had the reputation of being able to "move only in still air," and the tubers are used to treat headaches, vertigo, paralysis, lumbago, neuralgia, and rheumatism. The drug is believed to stimulate physical, mental and sexual vigor. Ha et al. studied the effects of the constituents of *Gastrodia elata* on the GABAergic neurotransmission and made the interesting observation that 4-hydroxybenzaldehyde and 4-hydroxy-3-methoxybenzaldehyde (vanillin) inhibit the activity of GABA transaminase with IC_{50} values of 4.1 and 5.4 μg/mL, respectively, and 4-hydroxy-3-methoxybenzaldehyde dose-dependently increases the binding of [^{3}H]flunitrazepam to GABA receptors *(59,60)*.

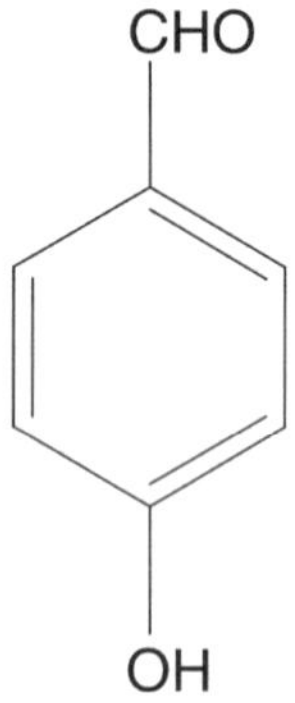

4-hydroxybenzaldehyde.

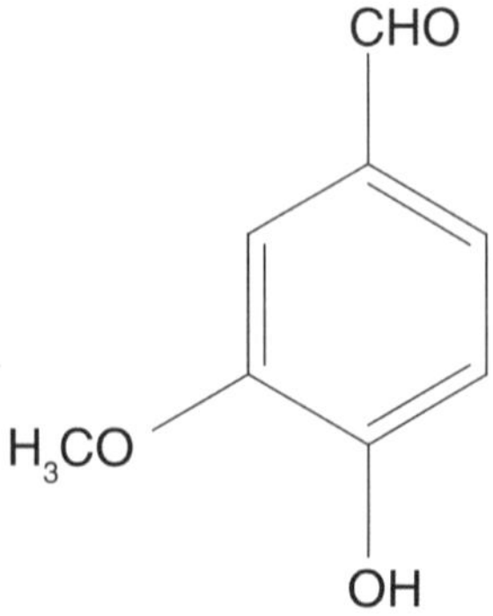

4-hydroxy-3-methoxybenzaldehyde

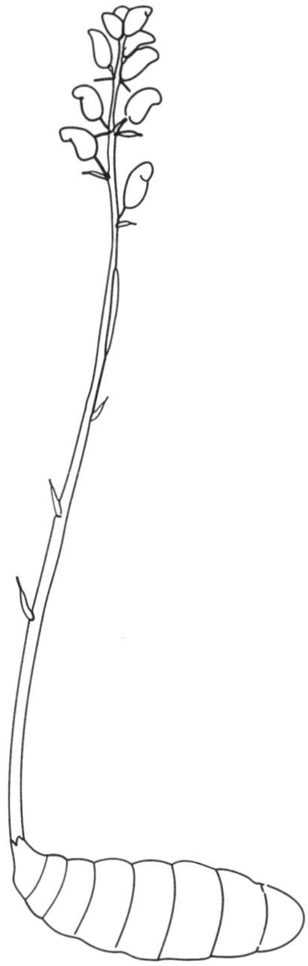

Fig. 55. *Gastrodia elata* Bl.

***Acriopsis javanica* Reinw.** is an epiphyte orchid that grows in Burma, Malaysia, Indonesia, the Philippines, and Papua New Guinea. The pseudobulbs are 5 × 1.5 cm and develop thick roots. Each pseudobulb produces three leaves, which are linear and 25 cm × 9 mm. The influorescences are 60 long and branched panicles. The flowers are 7 mm long and pale purple (Fig. 56).

Malays drink a decoction of the whole plant that is used to reduce fever. In Indonesia, the juice expressed from the pseudobulbs is used to assuage earache, and a paste of the pseudobulb is applied externally to lower blood pressure and reduce fever. The pharmacological potential of this plant is unexplored. Is the antipyretic and analgesic property of *Acriopsis javanica* linked to a dopaminergic effect?

***Bulbophyllum vaginatum* Reich. f.** is an epiphytic orchid that grows in Thailand, Indonesia, and Malaysia. The stems are 3 mm in diameter. The petiole is 2 × 6 mm, swollen, and deeply channeled. The blade is elliptic, thick, spongy, and 8 × 3 cm. The flowers are arranged in clusters of 12–15 pale yellow, 5-cm-long flowers with elongated corollas (Fig. 57).

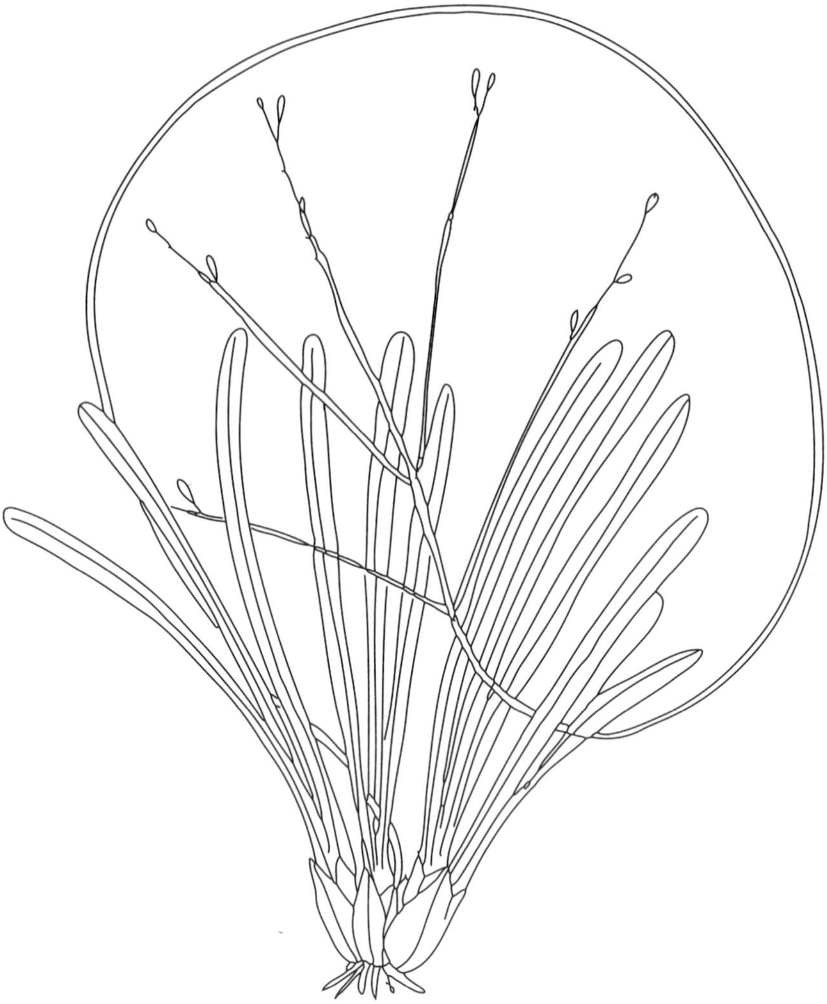

Fig. 56. *Acriopsis javanica*. From Flora of Malaya. Geographical localization: S. Salat on Endau river, Johore. Rocky upper reaches, epiphyte.

In Malaysia, the juice expressed from the plant is warmed and instilled in the ear to mitigate earache. The pharmacological potential of this orchid is unexplored. Note that an interesting development in *Bulbophyllum* species, and Orchidaceae in general, is the search for dopaminergic phenanthrene. Orchidaceae are well known to elaborate bibenzyls, phenanthrenes, and 9,10-dihydrophenanthrenes. Such compounds are found in *Bulbophyllum vaginatum* Reichb., such as 4,6 dimethoxyphenanthrene-2,3,7-triol and 3,4′,5-trihydroxy-3′-methoxybibenzyl *(61)*. An example of a phenanthrenic dopaminergic agent is dihydrexidine, which is a dopamine D_1 receptor agonist *(62)*.

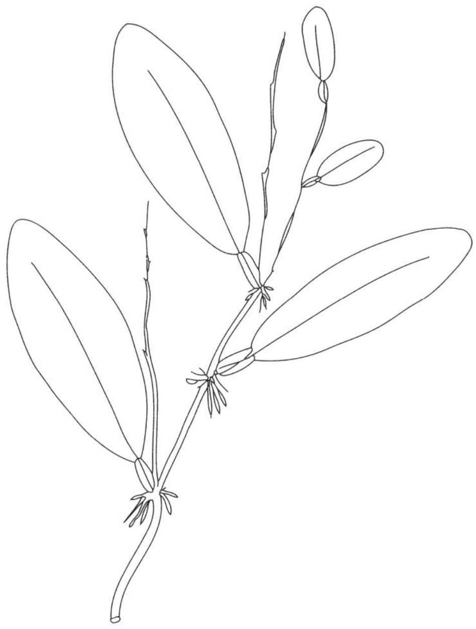

Fig. 57. *Bulbophyllum vaginatum*. From Flora of the Malay Peninsula. Geographical localization: Rantau Panjang, Selangor. 10/30/1930. Field collector: Symington, No: 24330.

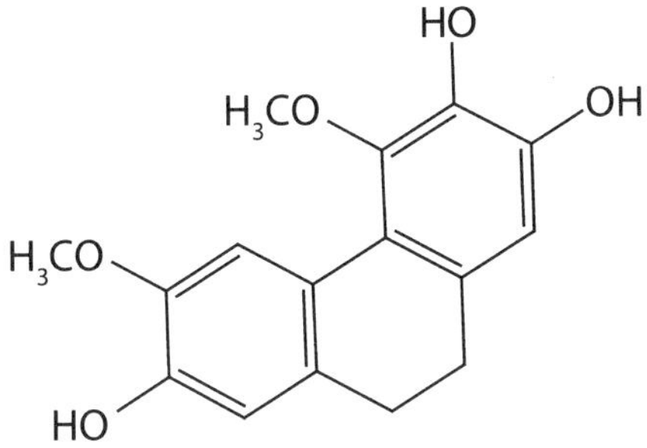

4,6 dimethoxyphenanthrene -2,3,7 -triol

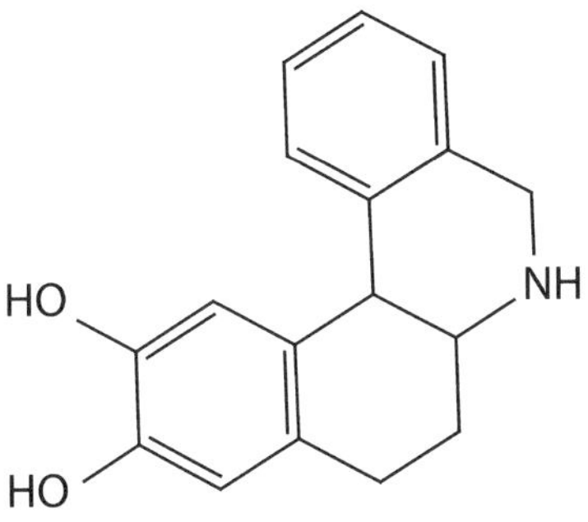

Dihydrexidine

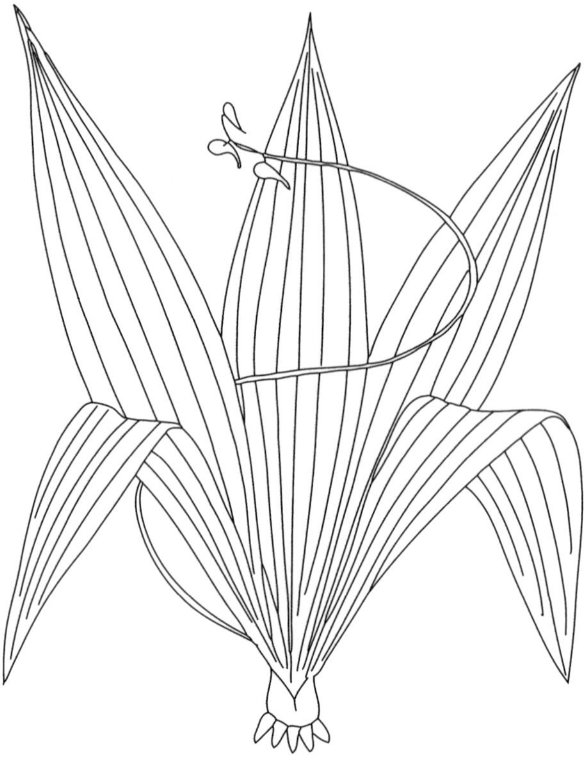

Fig. 58. *Calanthe triplicate.* From Sarawak No 892. Royal Geographical Society, 1977–1978. Mulu Expedition. Field collectors: G. Argent, D Coppins, C. Jermy, 4/5/1978. Geographical localization: Gunong Mulu National Park. 4th Division, Baram District. Hidden Valley (Camp 6). 4° 0.5′ North–114° 53′ East. In lowland alluvial rainforest under towering limestone.

***Calanthe triplicata* (Villem.) Ames** (*Calanthe veratrifolia* R. Br.), or Christmas orchid, is a large terrestrial orchid that grows in Southeast Asia, Papua New Guinea, and Australia. Each pseudobulb develops three or four large pleated leaves, which are 40 × 9 – 50 × 18 cm. The roots are 1.5 cm long and 2 mm in diameter. The influorescence is 50 cm long with numerous 1-cm-long white flowers densely packed in a spike. The flowers show white with green rostrellum and yellow spots at base of labellum, which is forked (Fig. 58). In Indonesia, the roots are used to treat diarrhea and a paste is applied to swollen parts. A paste of flowers is inserted in the hollow of painful caries. A significant advance in the pharmacology of *Calanthes* species has been provided by the work of Yoshikawa et al. Using bioassay-guided fractionation, they isolated calanthoside, glucoindican, calaliukiuenoside, and calaphenanthrenol from *Calanthe discolor* Lindl. and *Calanthe liukiuensis*, which showed an activating effect on skin blood flow and hair restoring activities *(63)*. The dopaminergic and central property of this orchid is unexplored.

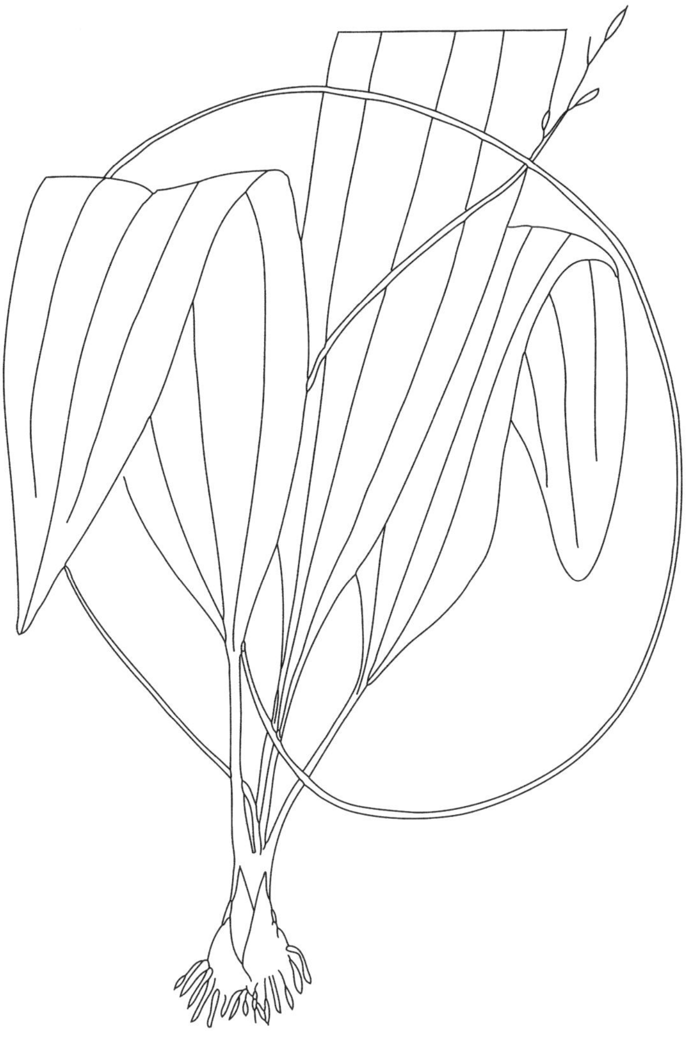

Fig. 59. *Calanthe vestita* Lindl. Flora of Malay Peninsula. Forest Department. Geographical localization: Batu Caves, Selangor. 12/26/1932. Field collector: E.J. Strugnel.

Calanthe vestita Lindl. is a terrestrial orchid that grows in Thailand, Burma, Cambodia, Laos, Vietnam, Malaysia, Sumatra, Java, Borneo, and Celebes. The leaves are 25 × 5 cm. The petiole is 5 cm long. The influorescence is 40 cm long. The flowers are white (Fig. 59). In Cambodia, Laos, and Vietnam, a paste of bulbs is applied to painful bones. The pharmacological properties of this plant are currently unknown.

Dendrobium crumenatum Sw., or pigeon orchid, is an epiphyte orchid that grows in India, China, the Philippines, and Malaysia. The stem is 4 mm in diameter and the bulbs are 2–3 cm around. The leaves are 7 × 1.3 cm, linear, and fleshy. The petiole is 4 × 1 mm. The flowers are white (Fig. 60).

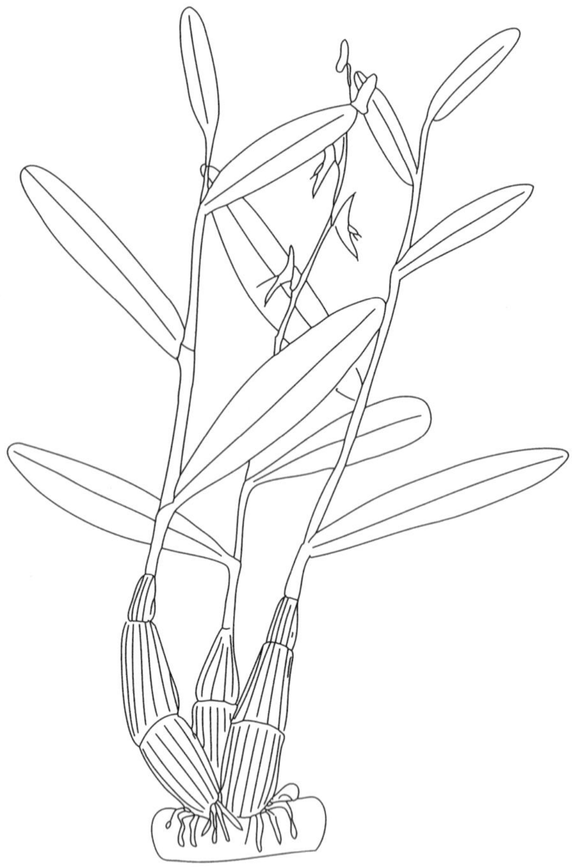

Fig. 60. *Dendrobium crumenatum* l.

The dopaminergic potential of the *Dendrobium* species is, to date, open for exploration. An interesting feature of the *Dendrobium* species is their ability to elaborate sesquiterpene alkaloids, the chemical structure of which resembles the one of strychnine. One such alkaloid is dendrobine, which is widespread in the genus. Kudo et al. noted that dendrobine, isolated from *Dendrobium nobile*, exhibits a strychnine-like presynaptic inhibition in frog spinal cord (*64*).

Dendrobine at a dose of 3×10^{-5} M reduced the dorsal root potential and reflex. It provoked a mild hyperpolarization in both dorsal and ventral roots of frog isolated spinal cord. It affected the β-alanine- and taurine-induced depolarization of primary afferent terminals and reversibly blocked the presynaptic inhibition caused by antidromic conditioning stimulation of the ventral root potential induced by repetitive antidromic stimulation of ventral root and lowered maximum. It would be interesting to learn whether further research of the *Dendrobium* species discloses any alkaloid interfering with the glycinergic system, an aspect discussed under the following heading.

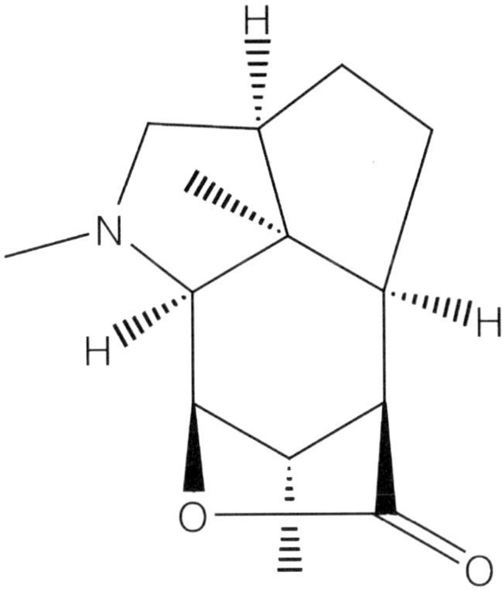

Dendrobine

PLANTS INTERFERING WITH THE GLYCINERGIC SYSTEM

Glycine is an important inhibitory neurotransmitter on moto-neurons that operates via the activation of distinct postsynaptic receptors in the hippocampus the spinal cord and brain stem, the pontine reticular formation, and the substantia gelatinosa. Glycine receptors have also been reported within the nucleus tractus solitarius and the nucleus ambiguus, two medullary areas important for central cardiovascular regulation. An interesting development from the glycinergic neurotransmission is to look into the modulation of glycinergic inputs to neurons that control heart rate. A major determinant of glycinergic activity may be opioids, since Gruol and Smith showed that morphine consistently depressed the postsynaptic currents evoked by glycine in cultured fetal mouse spinal cord neurons (65). Decrease in glycine-mediated neurotransmittion results in pathologies of muscle tone regulation, which cause motor disturbance, increased muscle tone, and hyperactivity of sensory, visual, and acoustic perception, with higher doses resulting in convulsions and death. Select glycine antagonists have emerged from studies on quinolic acid derivatives, and a current tool for glycinergic binding is nipecotic acid (66). Perhaps no other single substance has aroused more interest in the field of glycinergic antagonism that strychnine, an indole alkaloid present in the seeds of *Strychnos* species in the family Loganiaceae, and notably the seeds of an Asian plant: *Strychnos nux-vomica* L. (*nux vomica, British Pharmacopoeia*, 1963). Strychnine causes tremors and slight twitching of the limbs, followed by sudden convulsions of all muscles. The body becomes arched backward in hyperextension, with the legs and arms extended and the feet turned inward in a position called "episthotonos." The facial muscles produce a characteristic grinning expression known as *risus sardonicus*. Death from medullary paralysis usually follows the second or fifth seizure.

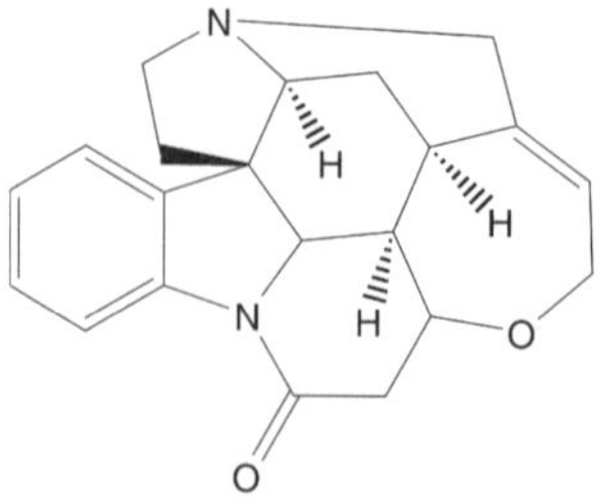

Strychnine

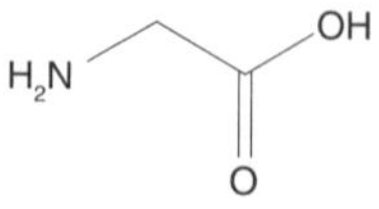

Glycine

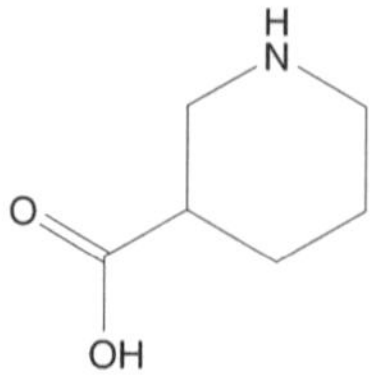

Nipecotic acid

Although there have been many studies on strychnine itself, the evidence available shows that much less work has been done with the search for glycinergic agents from flowering plants, and we can reasonably expect the discovery of major glycinergic agents in the coming decade. An interesting source for such agents is the medicinal flora of Asia and Pacific, which encompasses several *Strychnos* species.

Medicinal Loganiaceae

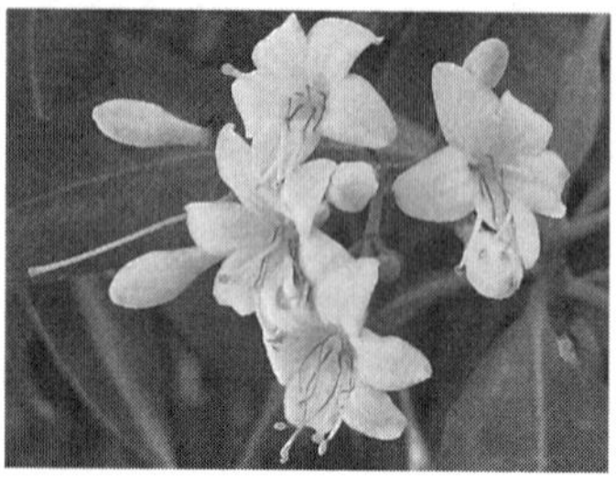

The family Loganiaceae consists of about 20 genera and 500 species of tropical trees, shrubs, or climbers commonly producing iridoids and monoterpenoid indole alkaloids formed by the condensation of tryptamine and secologanin (an iridoid). Examples of pharmaceutical products of loganiaceous origin are the dried ripe seeds of *S. nux-vomica* L. (*nux vomica, British Pharmacopoeia*, 1963) and *Strychnos ignatii* (ignatia, *British Pharmaceutical* Codex, 1934), which have been used as bitter tonic remedies and as ingredients of purgative pills and tablets on account of monoterpenoid indole alkaloids, such as strychnine (*British Pharmaceutical Codex*, 1959), which blocks the glycinergic receptors.

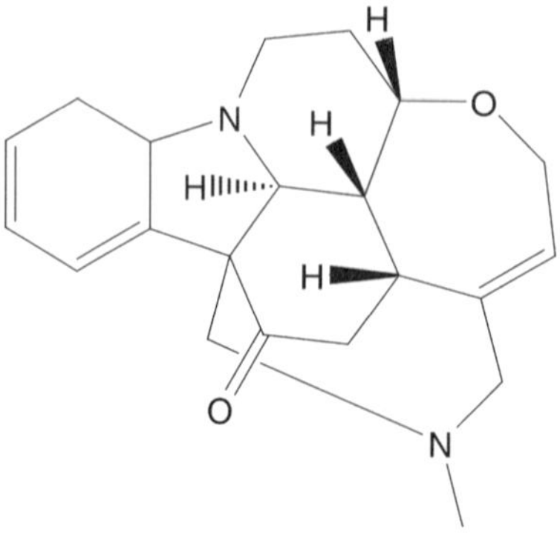

Icajine

Strychnine was elucidated in 1947 owing to the major contribution of H. Leuchs and Sir Robert Robinson. Since then, strychnine has been characterized fro several *Strychnos* species: *Strychnos ignatii* Berg., *Strychnos wallichiana* Steud. Ex DC, and *Strychnos lucida* R. Br. The strong convulsive strychnine is accompanied by series of related alkaloids, such as brucine, colubrine, vomacine, and novacine. Strychnine and related alkaloids could be present in other species, but the complete chemical composition of many *Strychnos* species is as yet unknown (66). In the Pacific Rim, about 20 species of Loganiaceae, including *Strychnos ignatii* Berg., *Strychnos gauthierana* Pierre ex Dop, *Strychnos lucida* R. Br., *Strychnos minor* Dennst., and *Strychnos axillaris* Colebr., are medicinal and often used to invigorate, counteract putrefaction, treat eye diseases, and expel worms from intestines.

Strychnos ignatii Berg. (*Strychnos beccarii* Gilg, *Strychnos cuspidata* A.W. Hills, *Stychnos ovalifolia* Wall, *Strychnos pseudotieute* A.W. Hill, *Strychnos tieute* Lesch. *Ignatia amara* L. f.; *Ignatiana philippinica* Lour., *Strychnos hainanensis* Merr. & Chun, *Strychnos ovalifolia* Wall. ex G. Don.), or *lu sung kuo* (Chinese), *umpas naga*, or *akar ipoh* (Malay), is a climber that grows in open woodlands, on limestone, scrub, or sometimes along river banks up to 800 m in China, Indonesia, Malaysia, the Philippines, Thailand, and Vietnam. The plant grows to a length of 20 m. The stems are grayish-brown, lenticelled, with tendrils. The leaves are simple and opposite; the flowers are yellowish, salver-shaped, 1.7 cm long, and papillose. The fruits are cream-green to orange berries up to 10 cm in diameter, containing several seeds that are ovate and flat (Fig. 61).The dried ripened seeds, or St. Ignatius beans (ignatia, *British Pharmaceutical Codex*, 1934), containing 2.5 to 3% of brucine and strychnine have been used as bitter and tonic in the form of tinctures, cachets, and piles, and the pant is still used in homeotherapy. In China, the seeds were mentioned in the Pentsao for their bitterness and toxicity. The drug is highly valued by the Chinese physicians who call it "precious bean" and who used it as counter-poison in ague, to expel intestinal worms, and treat postpartum difficulties. In Cambodia, Laos, and Vietnam, the seeds are used to invigorate and expel worms from the intestine. In the Philippines, the bark is used to reduce fever and assuage stomach pains. The seeds contain strychnine, brucine, pseudostrychnine, and pseudobrucine (68).

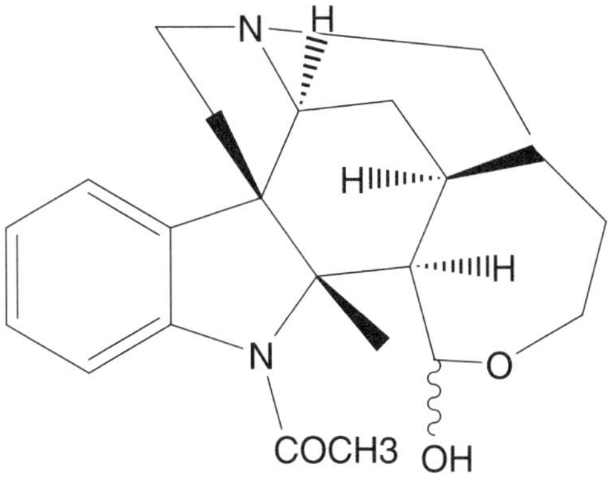

Diaboline

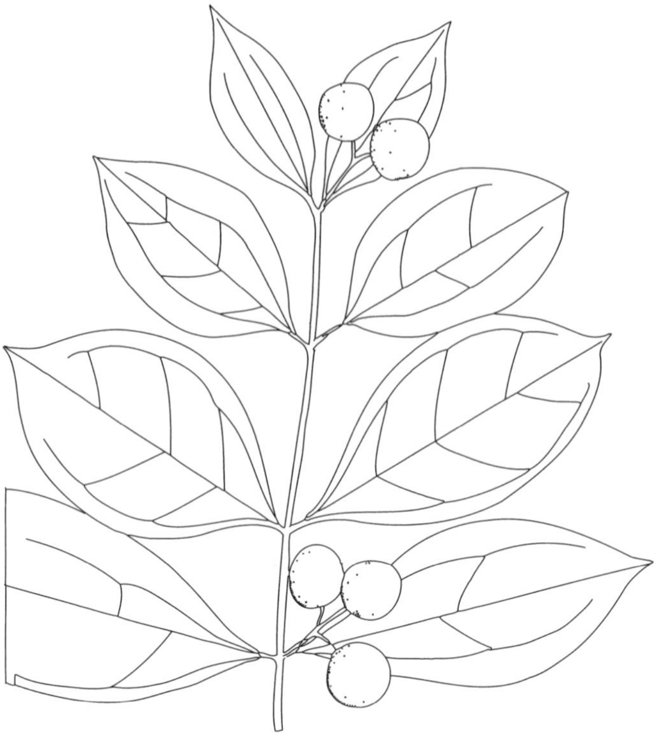

Fig. 61. *Strychnos ignatii Berg.* From Flora of Malaya. Kep: FRI No 15383. 7/21/1970. Field collector: T.C. Whitmore. Geographical localization: National Park, Pahang, Ulu Tembeling. Ridge northwest of Tg Bunhkal in low dense forest.

***Strychnos minor* Dennst.** (*Strychnos multiflora* Benth.) is a climber that grows to a height of 15 m in the rainforests of India, Thailand, Malaysia, Indonesia, and the Philippines. The stems are terete, subglabrous, and develop pairs of hooks at nodes. The leaves are opposite, papery, conspicuously triple-nerved to 10 cm in length. The fruits are berries that are bluish at first and 1.4 cm in diameter (Fig. 62). It is used in the Philippines to treat throat trouble. A decoction of bark is used as an emmenagogue, and the Negritos chew the bark to treat prolapse of the uterus. The seeds are poisonous on probable account of strychnine and congeners.

***Strychnos axillaris* Colebr.** (*Strychnos pubescens* C.B. Clarck), or *ye hua ma qian* (Chinese), *chewong*, or *tenchong gendeng* (Malay), is a climber that grows to 20 m long in mountain forests, forest edges, and to 800 m altitude in a geographical area spanning China, Cambodia, India, Indonesia, Laos, Malaysia, Thailand, Vietnam, and Australia. Stems, petioles, and blades are velvety. The stem shows axillary hooks that are spirally curved. Leaf blades are elliptic, narrowly elliptic, ovate, or suborbicular. The berries are ovoid to globose, and up to 2 cm in diameter and contain one or two seeds (Fig. 63).The seeds have been used to make arrow poison. The chemical composition of the seeds is currently unknown.

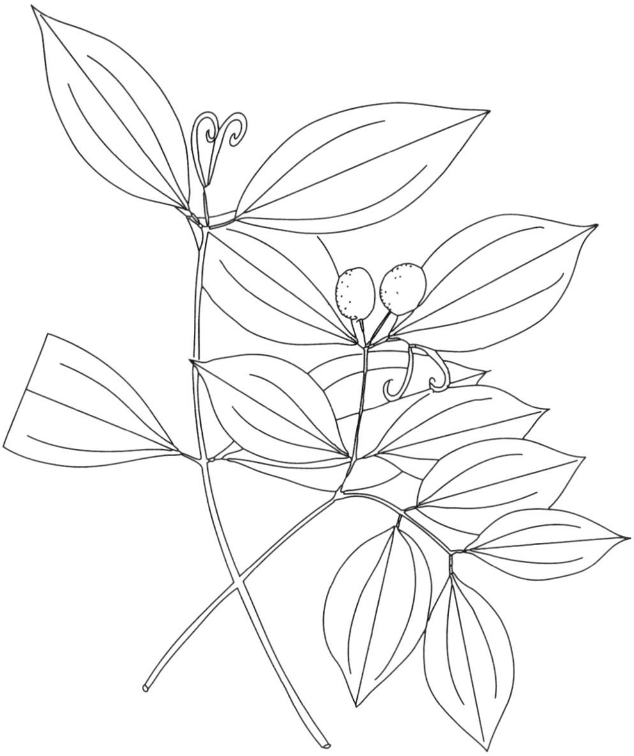

Fig. 62. *Strychnos minor* Dennst. From Plants of South India, C.E. Ridsdale 395. date: 7/12/1976. Geographical localization: Walaiyar Estate, Papanasam, Tamil Nadu. In evergreen forest. Distributed by the Rijskherbarium, Leiden.

Medicinal Apocynaceae

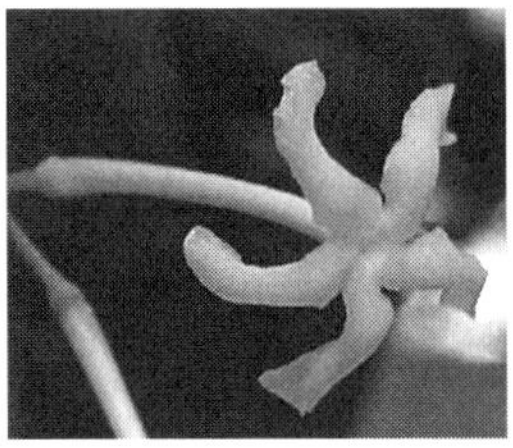

A group of plants of interest when searching for glycine receptor antagonists are the Apocynaceae, the indole alkaloids of which appear to have glycinergic activities. Pathama et al. made the interesting observation that corymine, an indole alkaloid extracted from the leaves of a medicinal plant of Malaysia and Thailand, *Hunteria zeylanica* (Retz.) Gardn. & Thw. (*Hunteria corymbosa* Roxb, *Hunteria roxburghiana* sensu Ridl.), potentiates the convulsions induced by either strychnine or picrotoxin at doses of 2, 8, and 15 mg/kg in mice and inhibits glycine-induced chloride current in *Xenopus* oocytes non-competitively by interacting with a site different from that of 4,4′-diisothiocyanostilbene-2,2′-disulfonic acid, a Cl^- channel blocker (69). All this evidence taken together lends considerable support to the view that monoterpenoid alkaloid-producing families of flowering plants such as Apocynaceae, Loganiaceae, and Rubiaceae represent an exciting reservoir of potential glycinergic agents.

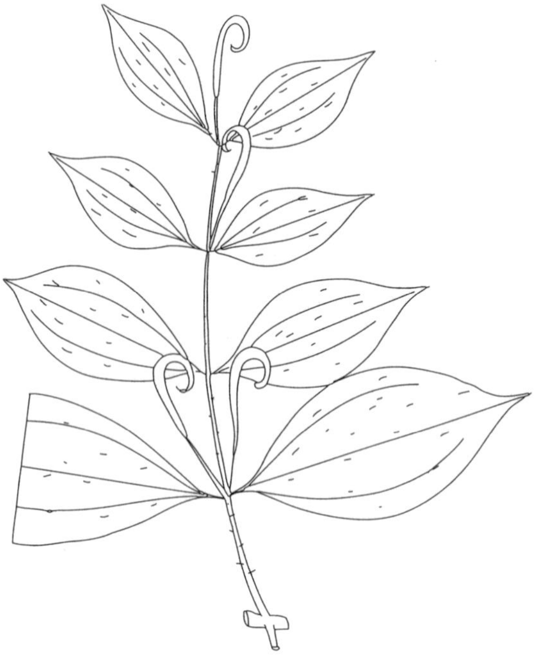

Fig. 63. *Strychnos axillaris* Colebr. Department of Wildlife and National Parks. Plants of Krau. Wildlife Reserve, Malaysia. Field collectors: Hanne Christensen and Rozidan M. Geographical localization: 3° 36′ North–102° 8′ East. In mature forest on level ground.

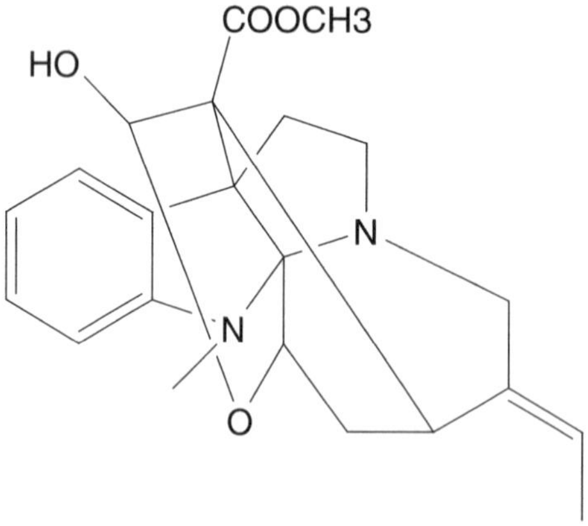

Corymine

PLANTS AFFECTING THE DOPAMINERGIC NEUROTRANSMISSION

Dopamine is a catecholamine neurotransmitter in the CNS and at some ganglia in the autonomic nervous system. To date, three main types of receptors have been found: D_1, D_2, and D_3. The main dopaminergic systems in the brain are the nigro-neostriatal

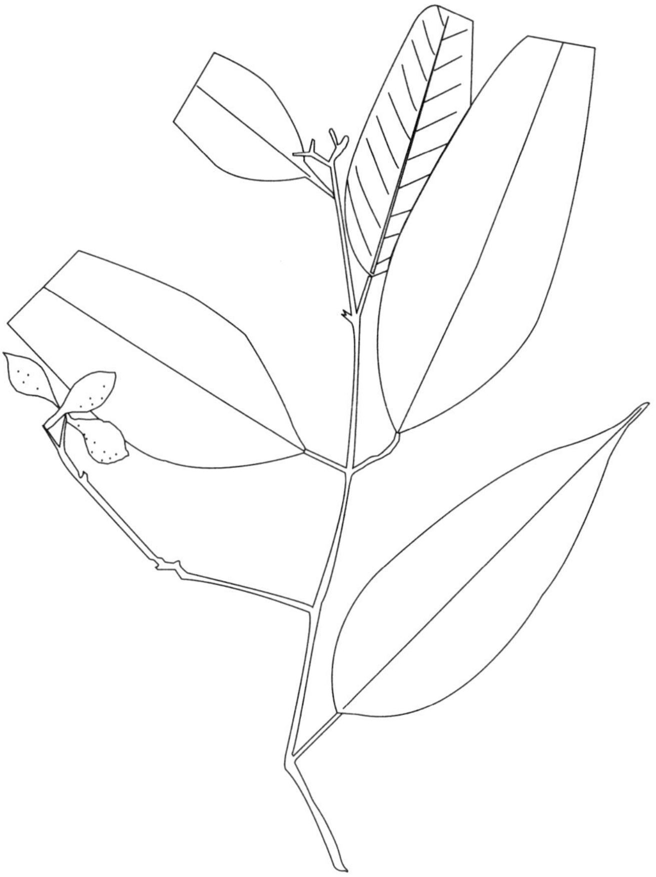

Fig. 64. *Hunteria zeylanica* (Retz.) Gardn. & Thw. From KLU 1658. Field collector: 4/17/1970, E. Soepadmo. Geographical localization: Sempam River, Raub, Pahang, altitude: 2000 feet, Malaysia. Botanical identification: Margraf, 1973.

system, which is concerned with the control of locomotor activity; the midbrain mesolimbic forebrain system, which is involved with behavior; and the tubero-infundibular system of the hypothalamus, which releases dopamine into the portal vessels and thereby inhibits pituitary prolactine disease (Fig. 65).

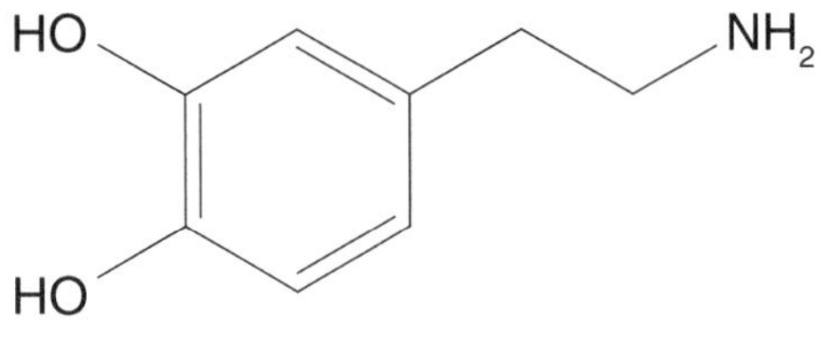

Dopamine

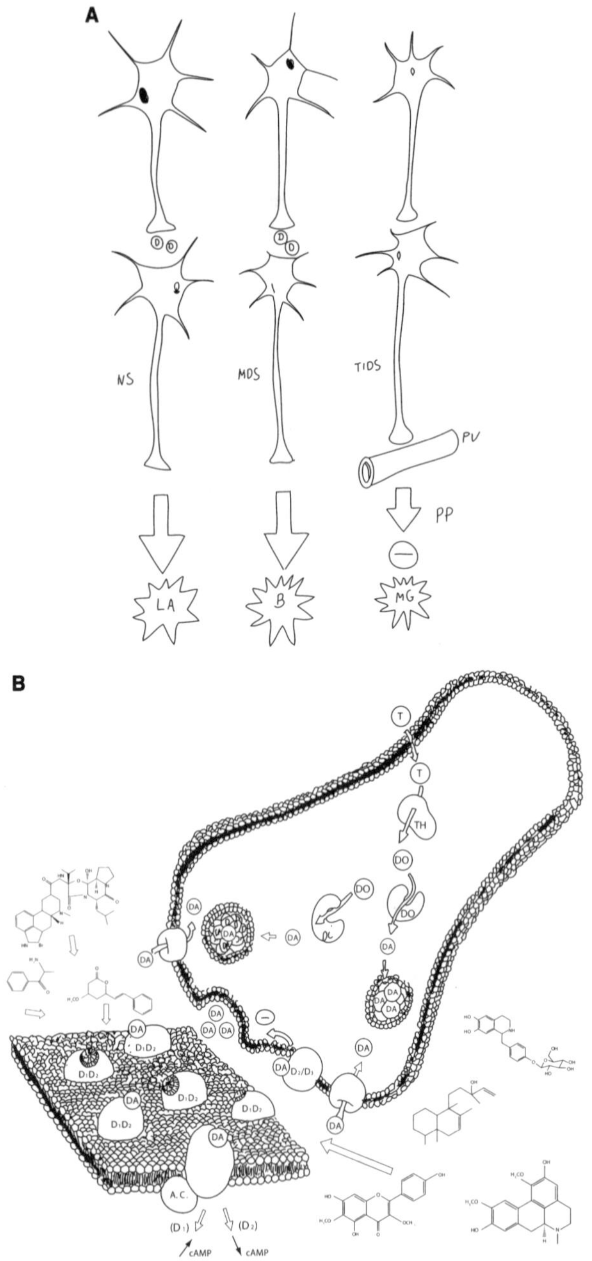

Fig. 65. **(A)** Dopaminergic system: the three important brain dopaminergic systems. **(B)** Dopaminergic system: the dopaminergic neurons. NS, nigrostriatal dopaminergic neurone; PP, prolactin pituitary, PV, portal vein; MG, mammary gland; MDS, mesolimbic dopaminergic system; B, behaviour; LA, locomotor activity; TIDS, tuboinfundibular dopaminergic system; DA, dopamine; DO, DOPA; DC, DOPA decarboxylase; T, tyramine; TH, tyrosine hydroxylase; D1/D2, dopaminergic receptor D_1 or D_2; D2/D3, dopaminergic receptor D_2 or D_3; AC, adenylate cyclase.

In normal physiological conditions, the dopaminergic neurons of the substancia nigra control the cholinergic output but if they do not, as is the case in Parkinsonism, the skeletal muscles experience tremors, rigidity, and akynesia. L-DOPA given by mouth is effective in restoring the ability to initiate movements and is the most effective treatment for this condition; however, high doses are needed that produce nausea, vomiting, and hypotension. Because of the side effects associated with L-DOPA treatment, a number of dopamine receptor agonists have been tried including apomorphine, and ergolines such as bromocriptine. Another alternative to treat Parkinsonism is the use of anticholinergic agents, such as crude extract of *Atropa belladona* L. (Solanaceae) and, more recently, anticholinergic alkaloids and their derivatives, which attenuate the tremor and relieve the muscular rigidity but are better to be used sparingly in elderly, as these these induce heavy nervous side effects. In summary, the drugs developed for the last 30 years have led to a significant reduction in the mortality of patients with Parkinsonism, but fail to prevent the progression of the disease.

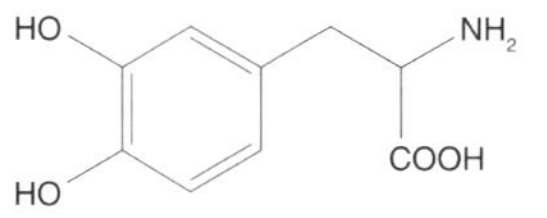

Dopa

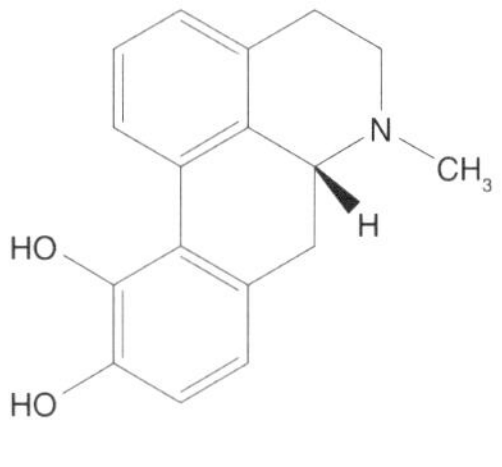

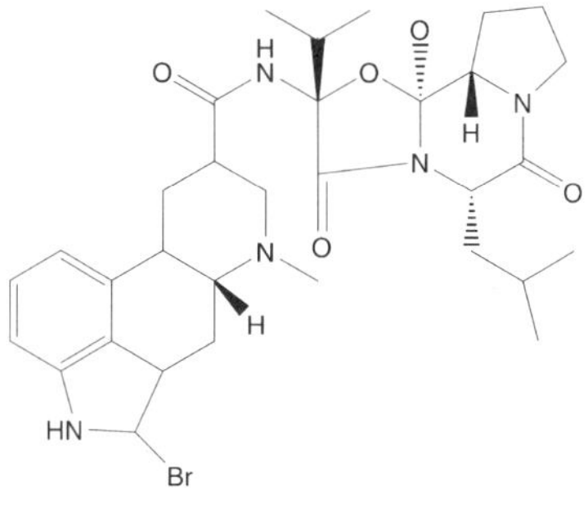

Apomorphine Bromocriptine

An interesting development from dopaminergic agents is the search for drugs for the treatment of premenstrual syndrome because pituitary prolactine release is under tonic hypothalamic inhibition by dopamine. Besides, the dopaminergic system plays an important role in physiopathology of migraine, and a dopamine antagonist such as prochlorperazine has exhibited antimigraine properties in animals by possible central amplification of cholinergic transmission. There is therefore a need for original dopaminergic agents, and one of the possible more exciting sources for such agents is the medicinal flora of Asia and the Pacific. The evidence available so far suggests that such agents would be present in the following medicinal plants.

Medicinal Araliaceae

The traditional systems of medicine of Asia and the Pacific use about 50 species of plant species classified within the family Araliaceae that are of medicinal value and notably used as tonic. Examples od such plants are of *Panax ginseng* C. A. Meyer (ginseng), *Panax notoginseng* Burk. (*san chi* ginseng), *Panax japonicus* C. A. Meyer (Japanese ginseng), and *Acanthopanax senticosus* (Siberian ginseng). The evidence for the existence of immunostimulating and anabolic saponins in *Panax* and *Acanthopanax* species is strong and well documented, but much less work has been done with the dopaminergic potentials of these saponins.

Acanthopanax gracilistylus **W. W. Sm.** (*Acanthopanax spinosus* Miq, *Eleutherococcus gracilistylus*), or *wu chia* (Chinese), *gokahi* (Japanese), or *ogap'i* (Korean), is a deciduous shrub growing to 3 m wild in East Asia and China. The leaves are palmatilobed and show five folioles that are elliptic lanceolate, fleshy, and serrate. The influorescence consists of small umbels up to 6 cm long. The drug consists of the root bark found in Chinese pharmacies in the form of yellowish-brown pieces; it is used for rheumatism, general debility, impotency, and muscular pains. In Malaysia, the plant is used as carminative.

Fujikawa et al. made the interesting observation that an extract from the stem bark given orally at a dose of 250 mg/kg once a day for 2 weeks protects rats against MPTP-induced Parkinsonian bradykinesia and catalepsy and inhibited neuronal loss of dopamine *(70)*. The active constituents involved here are unknown. Note that the plant abounds with pentacyclic oleanene saponins *(71–73)*. Note that *Acanthopanax* species are known to elaborate a series of diterpenes, a group that has the potency to bind to dopamine receptors, as reported in *Vitex agnus-castus*. Are diterpenes involved in the dopaminergic properties of *Acanthopanax gracilistylus* W. W. Sm.?

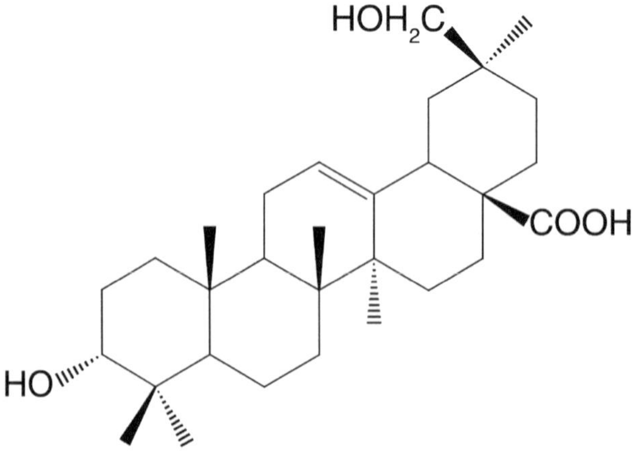

Oleanene aglycone

There is an expanding body of evidence to suggest that ginsenosides have a protective effect on the dopaminergic system. Radad et al. made a careful study on the effects of ginsenosides Rb1 and Rg1 on dopaminergic neurones from embryonic mouse mesencephalon and showed that these saponins protect neurons against the degenerative effects of 1-methyl-4-phenylpyridinium-iodide *(74)*. In addition, pretreatment with ginseng total saponin prevents the methamphetamine-induced striatal dopaminergic depletions *(75)*.

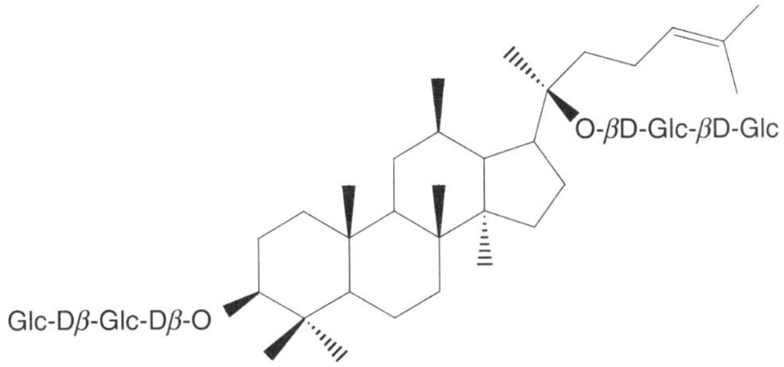

Ginsenoside Rb - (1)

Acanthopanax trifoliatus (L.) Merr. (*Acanthopanax aculeatus* Seem, *Eleutherococcus trifoliatus*) is a deciduous shrub that grows up to 6 m in a geographical area ranging from the eastern Himalayas to Japan and south into Cambodia, Laos, Vietnam, and the Philippines. The stems are light brown and smooth. The leaves are spiral and trifoliolate; the folioles are broadly elliptic, grayish-green, and glossy. The folioles are 5 × 3 cm and show four pairs of secondary nerves. The apex is acuminate, the base is rounded, and the margin is crenate at the apex. The inflorescences are globose umbels, which are 3 cm in diameter and bear about eight flowers (Fig. 66).

The plant is used to treat leprosy; the roots are used to heal ulcers and to cure ringworm infection. A decoction of the leaves is drunk to treat tuberculosis and to improve general weakness. In Cambodia, Laos, and Vietnam, an infusion of the bark is used to correct nervous affections. The plant is known to elaborate lupane triterpene saponins and kaurane diterpenes including 16-αH, 17-isovalerate-ent-kauran-19-oic acid, which strongly inhibited the enzymatic activity of cyclooxygenase in vitro *(76,77)*.

Acanthopanax ricinifolius Seem. (*Kalopanax ricinifolius* [Sieb. & Zucc.] Miq, *Kalopanax pictus* [Thunb.] Nakai, *Acer pictum* [Thunb], *Acanthopanax ricinifolium* [Sieb. & Zucc.] Seem, *Kalopanax septemlobus* Koidz. *var septemlobus*, *Panax ricinifolium* Siebold & Zucc, *Kalopanax ricinifolium* Miq, *Kalopanax pictum* Nakai), or prickly ginseng, castor Aralia, prickly castor oil tree, or *tzu ch'iu-shu* (Chinese), is a deciduous tree that grows to 25 m in Siberia, Korea, Japan, and China. The bark is gray mottled with yellowish-white; the stems are thorny and the leaves simple and palmate (Fig. 67).

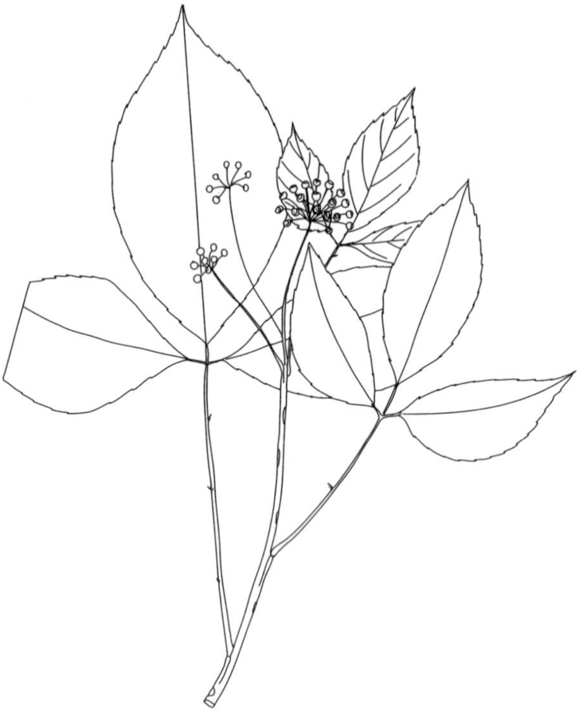

Fig. 66. Acanthopanax trifoliatus (L.) Merr.

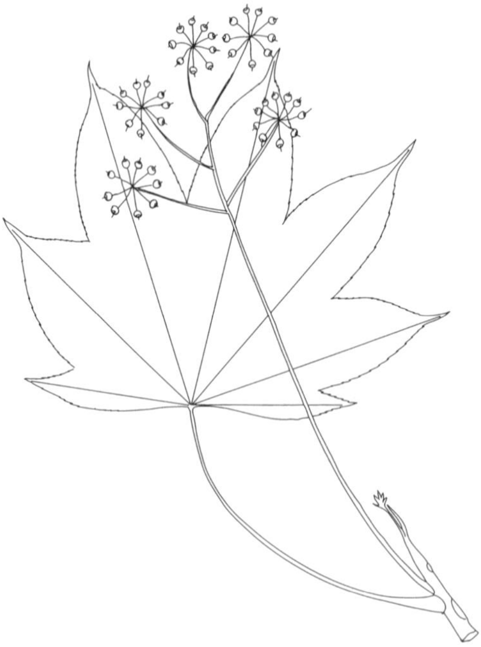

Fig. 67. Acanthopanax ricinifolius Seem.

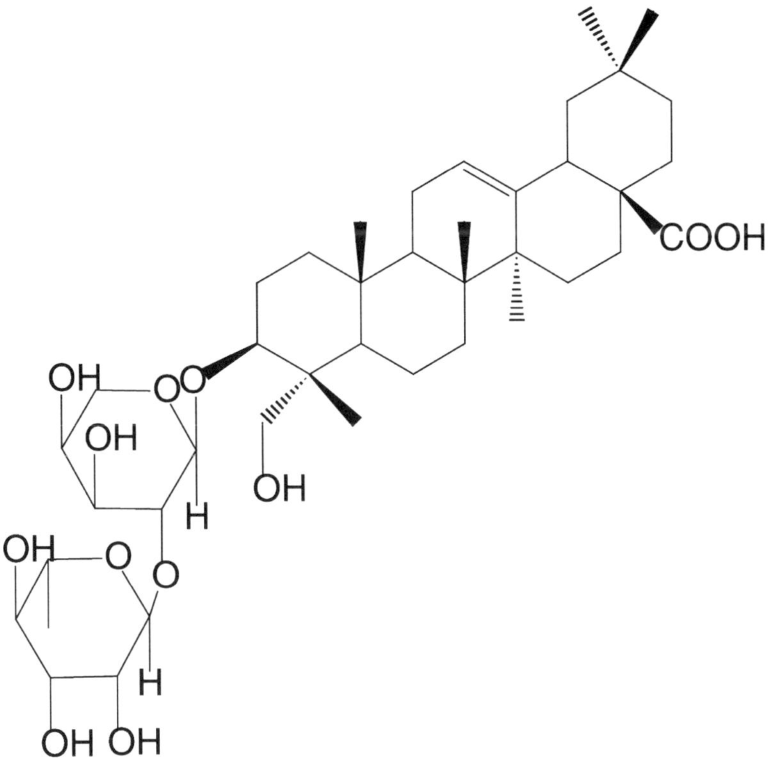

Kalopanaxsaponin A

The wood is valuable as timber. In China, the bark and leaves are used for insecticide, for the treatment of skin diseases, and to heal sores and ulcers. In Korea, the bark is used for the treatment of rheumatisms, cold, and cough. In Cambodia, Laos, and Vietnam, an infusion of leaves is drunk to promote digestion. The anti-inflammatory property of the plan is confirmed in vitro and thought to be imparted by saponins, including kalopanaxsaponin A and pictoside A, which elicited significant anti-inflammatory and anti-oxidant activity in rodents *(78–82)*. What is the dopaminergic activity of kalopanaxsaponin A and pictoside A?

Medicinal Verbenaceae

An interesting feature of the genus *Vitex* is used in several traditional systems of medicine as birth control and to treat gynecological disorders. Most of these plants contain ecdysteroids, the hormonal and especially gynecological effect of which remains to be clarified. Clinical trials showed that the fruits of *Vitex agnus-castus* (chaste tree) are effective in the treatment of the premenstrual syndrome *(83)*. The question that might arise is to know whether the *Vitex* species owes these premenstrual and gynecological properties to a mechanism involving the dopaminergic system. At present, it is not possible to answer this question but some clinical evidence has already

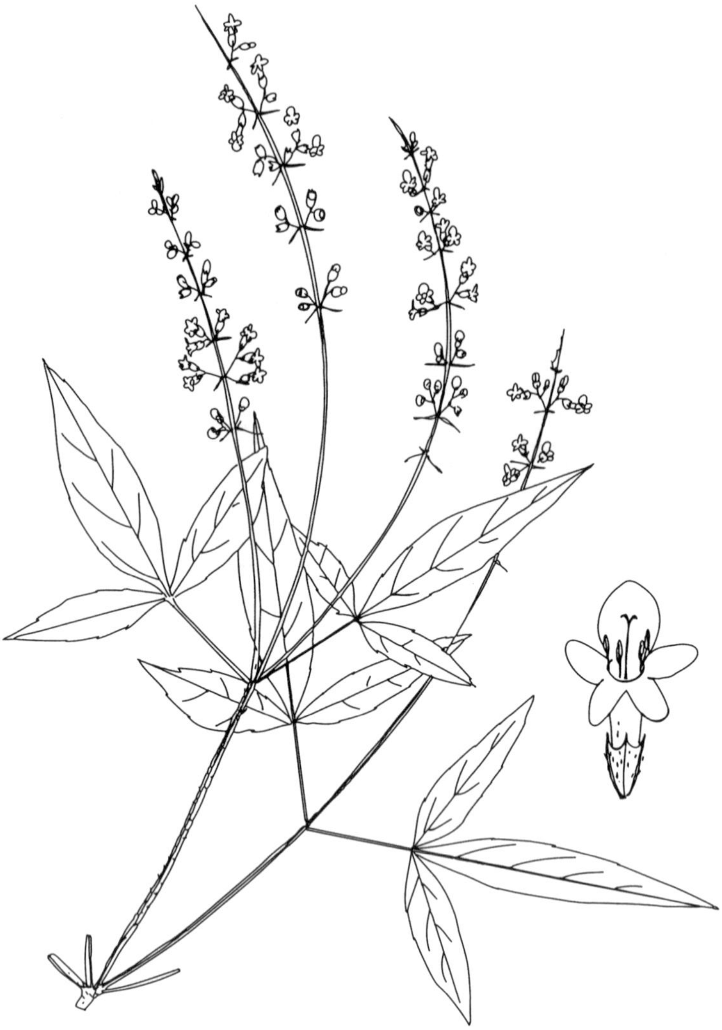

Fig. 68. *Vitex negundo* L.

been presented indicating that premenstrual mastodynia (mastalgia) is improved by intake of *V. agnus-castus* via inhibition of prolactine secretion. Further research in this topic is obviously needed.

Vitex negundo L. (*Vitex spicata* Lour., *Vitex paniculata* Lamk., *Vitex incisa* Lam.), or Indian privet, five-leaved chaste tree *kiyubantin* (Burmese), *mu ching* (Chinese), *agno-casto* (Philippino), *nochi* (Tamil), or *suvaha* (Sanskrit), is a treelet of the Asia–Pacific region. The stems are quadrangular and velvety. The leaves are decussate, exstipulate, three- to five-foliolate, and glaucous below, and show 9–13 pairs of secondary nerves. The influorescences are terminal, with panicles of about 20 cm long of several bluish-purple flowers. The fruits are black berries (Fig. 68). In China, the flowers are used to treat rheumatic difficulties, colds, cough, angina, and gonorrhea. The leaves are used to calm itchiness of eczematous eruptions. The roots are used to treat colds and rheumatisms, and the stems are used to sooth burns and scalds. An infusion of the stems is drunk to treat headache, dizziness, convulsions of children, cough, mental unrest, and to promote wakefulness. In the Philippines, *Vitex negundo* L. is used to promote milk secretion and menses. In India, the plant is used to soothe inflammation and to calm itching. The anti-inflammatory property of *Vitex negundo* L. is confirmed: a water extract of the leaves protects rats against carrageenan-induced rat paw edema, formaldehyde-induced rat paw edema, and hot-plate test. Although there have been many studies on the anti-inflammatory properties of the plant, much less work has been done on the psychopharmacological and especially dopaminergic properties of this plant (84,85). Note that the fruits of *Vitex agnus-castus* contain dopaminergic diterpenes known as clerodadienols, which exhibit prolactine-suppressive effects (86). What are the diterpenic contents of *Vitex negundo*?

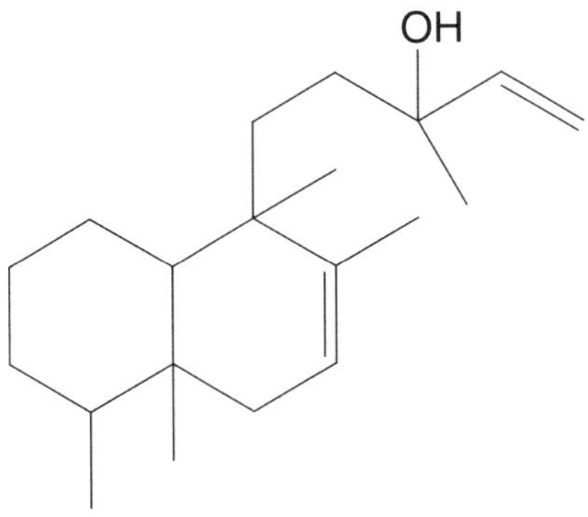

Clerodadienol

Vitex trifolia L. (*Vitex rotundifolia* L.f., *Vitex lagundi* Ridl. *Vitex repens* Blanco), or hand of Mary, *man jing* (Chinese), *dangla* (Philippino), *galumi* (Indonesian), *lenggundi* (Malay), *pitipitikoto* (Papua New Guinea), *khon thiso* (Thai), or *majn kinh* (Vietnamese), is a treelet that grows to a height of 5 m tall in Taiwan, China, Southeast Asia, Australia, and the Pacific Islands. The leaves are three-foliolate, with each foliole lanceolate or obovate, and showing eight pairs of secondary nerves. The flowers are purplish to bluish-purple, and 6 mm to 10 cm long. The fruits are black, subglobose, and with 5-mm-diameter drupes (Fig. 69).

The drug consists of the dried berries that are prescribed for headache, catarrh, watery eyes, and are used to promote beard growth. In Cambodia, Laos, and Vietnam, the berries are used to treat conjunctivis, dropsy, toothache, and as a remedy for swollen breast. In Malaysia, the leaves are used to assuage headache externally, and internally are used to treat tuberculosis and fever.

The plant is attracting a great deal of interest on account of its ability to elaborate labdane diterpenes vitexilactone, 6-acetoxy-9-hydroxy-13(14)-labden-16,15-olide, rotundifuran,

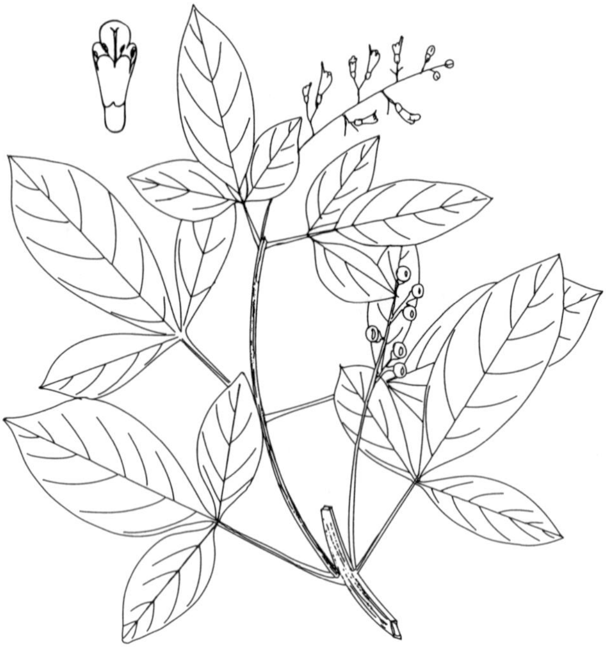

Fig. 69. *Vitex trifolia* L.

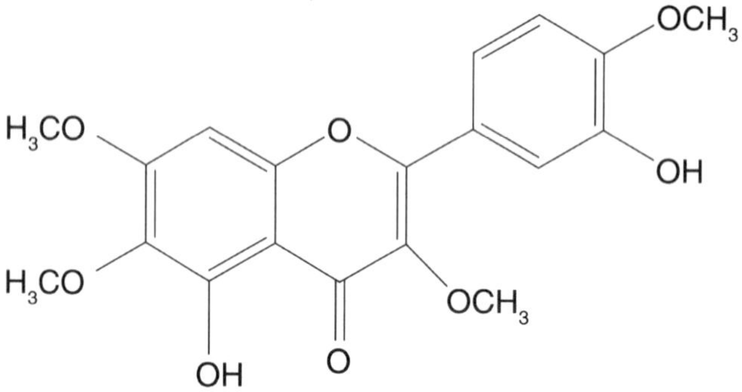

Vitexicarpin

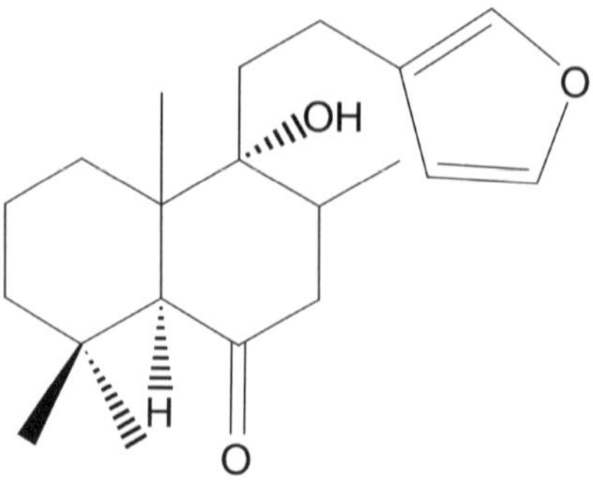

Rotundifuran

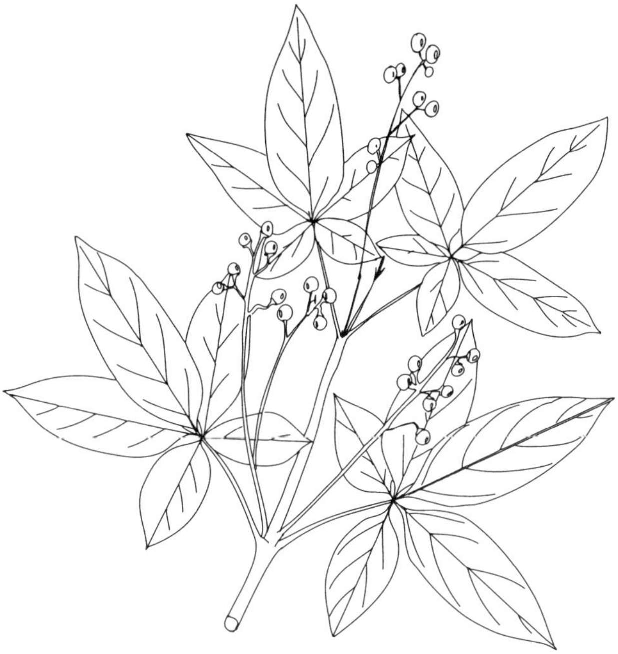

Fig. 70. *Vitex quinata* (Lour.) F.N. Will.

vitetrifolin, and vitetrifolin E, and a flavonoid viteicarpin, which induces apoptosis of both tsFT210 and K562 cell-lines (87,88). Note that the concomitance of use for headache and breast troubles might be indicative of a possible dopaminergic property; however, this remains to be confirmed or infirmed experimentally. Are dopaminergic labdanes involved here or are flavonoids, such as vitexicarpin? Naidu et al. made the exiting suggestion that the analgesic activity of flavonoids, such as quercetin, could be mediated by D_2-dopamine receptors (89). Are flavonoids, especially the liposoluble ones, holding potentials for the treatment of Parkinsonism?

Vitex quinata (Lour.) F.N. Will. (*Vitex heterophylla* Roxb.), or *shan mu jing* (Chinese), is a tree that grows to a height of 12 m in Taiwan, China, India, Indonesia, Japan, Malaysia, the Philippines, and Thailand. The young stems are pubescent and quadrangular. The leaves are decussate and three- to five-foliolate, thinly coriaceous, glossy, and 5–20 cm × 2.5–8.5 cm (Fig. 70). The influorescences are terminal lax, densely yellowish-brown, pubescent panicles of yellowish, bilabiate flowers. The fruits are black drupes. In Taiwan, Cambodia, Laos, and Vietnam, the fruits are used to treat neuralgia and the leaves are used as tea. The bark is used to invigorate and to stimulate appetite. To date, the pharmacological potential of *Vitex quinata* (Lour.) F.N. Will. is unexplored. It would be interesting whether further study results in the characterization of dopaminergic agents from this plant.

Vitex vestita Wallich ex Schauer, or *huang mao mu jing* (Chinese), is a tree that grows to a height of 8 m tall in China and Southeast Asia. The stems are densely yellow-brown and pubescent. Leaves are three-foliolate; the folioles are elliptic-oblong to elliptic, membranous, and 2.5–15 cm × 1.5–8 cm. The influorescence is dichotomous cymes of small yellowish bilabiate flowers. The fruits are black drupes of up to 8 mm long. In Malaysia and Indonesia, the plant is used to cause abortion. The dopaminergic potential of the plant is unknown. Note that some evidence has already been presented indicateing that prolactine disorders might be responsible for habitual abortion. Ando et al. showed that patients with a history of recurrent spontaneous abortion and prolactine disorders without impaired corpus luteum function treated with bromocriptine were able to maintain pregnancy (90). An interesting development from *Vitex vestita* and other plants traditionally used for inducing abortion would be to assess any dopaminergic activities and to characterize the active principles responsible for such activity.

Medicinal Sapindaceae

The family Sapindaceae consists of 140 genera and 1500 species of trees widespread in tropical and subtropical regions. Classic examples of Sapindaceae are the fruit trees *Nephelium lappaceum* L. and *Litchi chinensis* Sonn., which provide *rambutan* and litchi, respectively. Chemically Sapindaceae are well known to abound with saponins and tannins. An example of ornamental Sapindaceae is *Koelreuteria paniculata* L., or golden rain tree, cultivated in temperate regions. The berries of *Sapindus saponaria* L., were used as soap by South American Indians, hence the origin of the word *Sapindus* from *sapo* and *Indus* or the soap of the Indies.

It can be said that the present state of knowledge on the pharmacological potential of this large family is virtually vestigial. A classic example of Sapindaceae of neuropharmacological interest is *Paullinia cupana*, used by the Tapajoz Indians of the Amazon region to make a tonic beverage since very early times. The dried paste prepared from the roasted seeds containing not less that 45% of caffeine has been used for the treatment of headache and astringent in diarrhea (*British Pharmaceutical Codex*, 1934, *Brazilian Pharmacopoeia*, 1959). Today a large number of phytopharmaceutical products containing guarana are on the market. Another example is *Paullinia yopo*, used for the same purpose by Colombian Indians. Caffeine is the most widely consumed psychostimulant substance, being self-administered throughout a wide range of conditions and present in numerous dietary products including coffee, tea, cola drinks, chocolate, candy, and cocoa.

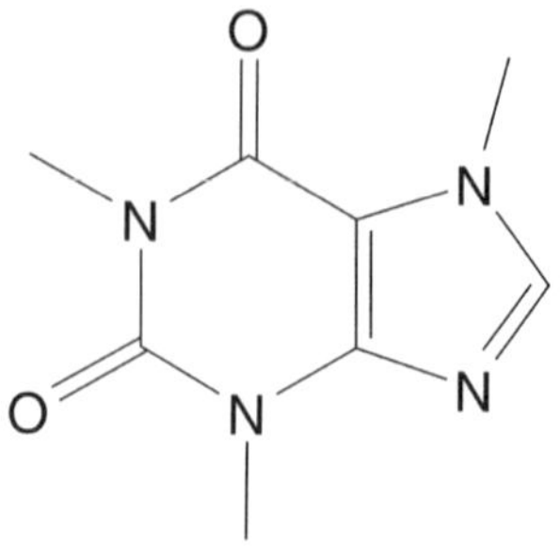

Caffeine

The main mechanism of action of caffeine occurs via the blockade of adenosine receptors in the CNS. Adenosine is an autacoid, which is involved in the modulation of behavior, oxygenation of cells, and dilatation of cerebral and coronary blood vessels and indirectly inhibits the release of dopamine. The blockade of adenosine receptors by caffeine increases the activity of dopamine, which is implicated in the effects of caffeine *(91)*. The question that arises from this observation is to know whether or not adenosine antagonists hold potential for the treatment of Parkinsonism, and further study on the adenosine receptor antagonists from medicinal plants should be encouraged. A possible source for such agents could be the medicinal flora of Asia and the Pacific, among which is the family Sapindaceae.

***Erioglossum rubiginosum* (Roxb.) Bl.** (*Erioglossum edule* Bl, *Sapindus rubiginosus* Roxb, *Lepisanthes rubiginosa* (Roxb.) Leenh. is a treelet that grows up to 10 m tall and is common in coastal forests throughout tropical Asia. The stems are hairy; the leaves are paripinnate without stipules with a woolly rachis. Four to six pairs of folioloes, 10–12.5 cm × 3.5–4.5 cm. The influorescences are terminal panicles of small flowers with four petals and eight stamens. The fruits are blackish, edible, and fleshy. In Malaysia, a decoction of roots is used to mitigate fever and the leaves are used externally to treat skin disease. In Indonesia, the young stems are eaten to induce sleeping. An aqueous extract of pericarp of *the* fruits at intraperitoneal doses of 20 and 100 mg/kg significantly reduced the spontaneous locomotor activity, and at 100 mg/kg, increased the thiopental-induced sleeping time and affinity toward dopaminergic receptors, inhibited the apomorphine-induced climbing behavior in mice, and exhibited affinity toward D_2 receptors, suggesting dopamine D_2 antagonism *(95)*.

***Sapindus mukorossi* Gaertn.**, or soapnut, Indian filbert, china berry, *arishta*, *ritha* (Sanskrit), *wu huan tzu*, *mu huan tzu*, *fei chi tzu*, *p'u ti tzu*, or *kuei chien ch'ou* (Chinese), is a large tree. The leaves are pinnate, grow up to 50 cm long, and show four to six pairs of folioles. The flowers are small, yellowish 3–4 mm long on terminal panicles. The fruits are globose, 2 cm across, and yellowish (Fig. 71). The drug consists of the dried seeds. In China, the seeds are roasted and eaten and the pericarp is used to treat skin diseases, remove tan, and freckles. The seed is also used to treat periodontal abscesses. In Burma, the fruits are used to treat epilepsy. In Taiwan, the flowers are used for heal inflamed eyes. In India, the plant is used to wash hair and delicate silk. In Malaysia, the plant is used as expectorant. The plant abounds with saponins and tannins, hence the antiseptic, anti-inflammatory, cosmetic, and expectorant properties mentioned earlier *(96,97)*. Much less is known about the CNS properties of this plant, especially the anti-epileptic properties. Surprisingly, the physiopathology of epilepsy is poorly understood and so far, there is no clear association between the abnormal function of a specific group of neurons and the genesis of seizures, but Birioukova et al. made the interesting observation that the densities of D_1 and D_2 dopaminergic receptors were different in the striatum of rats with and without genetic predisposition for epilepsy *(98)*. Is *Sapindus mukorossi* Gaertn., and the genus *Sapindus* in general, holding dopaminergic principles of value for the treatment of epilepsy?

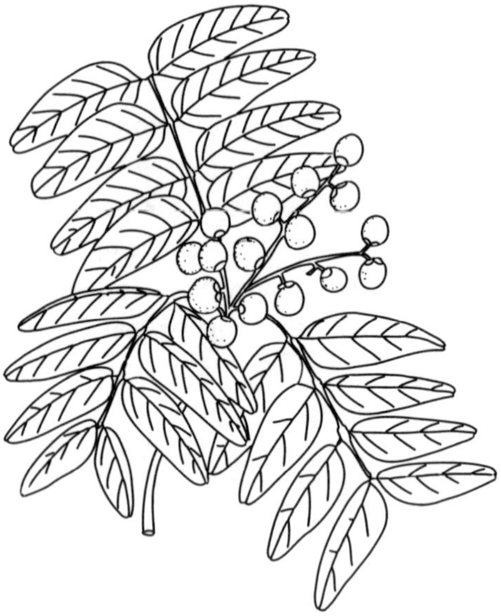

Fig. 71. *Sapindus mukorossi.*

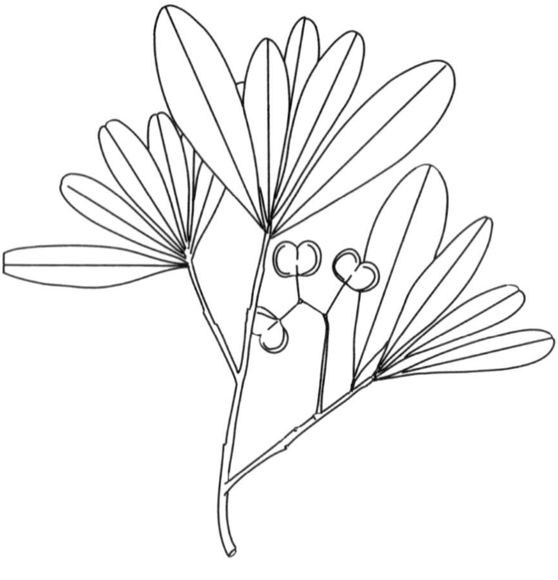

Fig. 72. *Dodonaea viscosa* (L.) Jacq. From Singapore Field No 37952. Distributed by the Botanic Gardens Singapore. Geographical localization: Kedah near Sanitarium Langkawi, in sand near sea. Date: 11/13/ 1941. Field collector: J.C. Naeur. Botanical identification: M.R. Henderson.

***Dodonaea viscosa* (L.) Jacq.**, or Florida hop bush, or *seringan laut* (Malay), is a shrub that grows to a height of 6 m in the sandy shores of the tropical world, including Asia and the Pacific Islands. The leaves are simple, 7.5–12 cm × 2 cm × 3.6 cm. The fruits are 2 cm long, capsular, and dehiscing to expose one to two black seeds in each lobe (Fig. 72).

In Burma, the leaves are used in fomentations. In Taiwan and Palau, the leaves are used to treat eczema, ulcers, and to mitigate fever.
The antipyretic property of the plant is not confirmed yet, but Amabeoku et al. reported that an aqueous extract of *Dodonaea angustifolia* L. reduced fever induced by lipopolysaccharide in rodent *(98)*. The principle involved here is unknown and one might think of 5,7,4,9-trihydroxy-3,6-dimethoxyflavone, which abounds in that plant *(99)*. Flavonoids are able to interact with the dopaminergic system. Is the antipyretic property of *Dodonaeae* species the result of flavonoids via the dopaminergic control of the hypothalamic thermoregulation? What is the antipyretic potential of 9-trihydroxy-3,6-alkylethoxy flavone in general (Fig. 74)?
Pataki et al. showed that apomorphine and bromocriptine enhanced the elevation of body temperature induced by pituitary adenylate cyclase-activating polypeptide in rats and observed that hyperthermia was antagonized by haloperidol, suggesting the involvement of the dopaminergic system *(100)*.

Medicinal Celastraceae

The family Celastraceae consists of about 50 genera and 800 species of trees, shrubs, or climbers known to produce a series of phenethylamine alkaloids that might hold some potentials as sources of dopaminergic agents. About 30 plant species of Celastraceae are medicinal in the Asia–Pacific region.

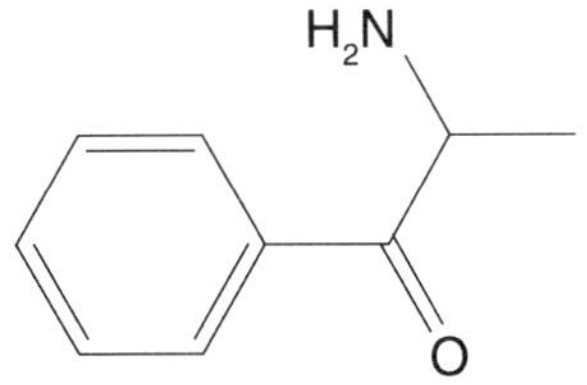

Cathinone

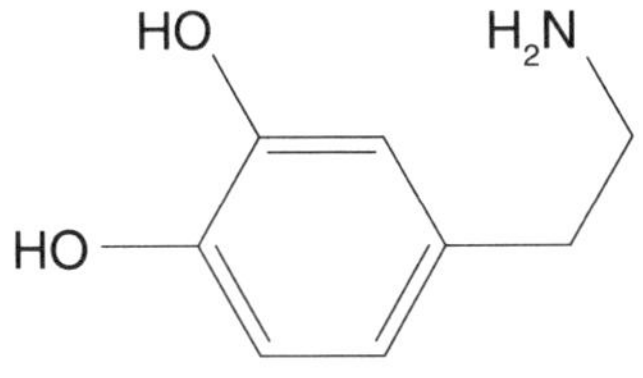

Dopamine

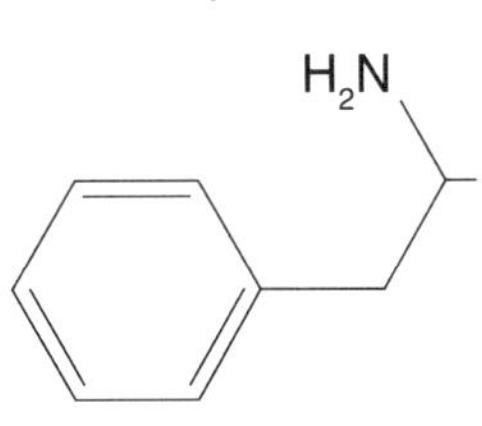

Amphetamine

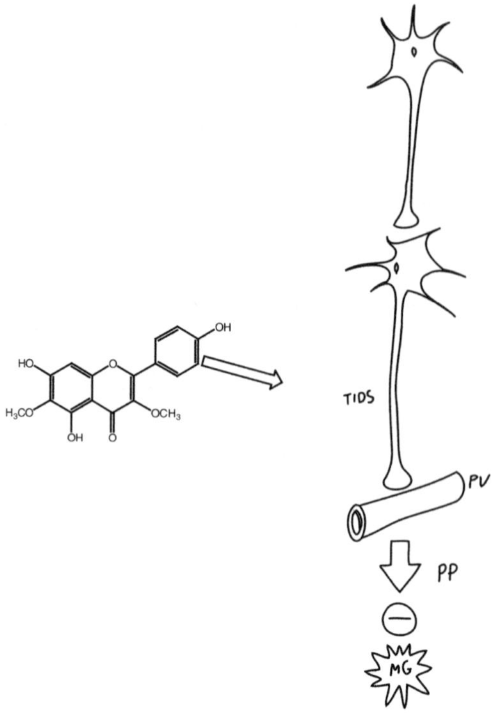

Fig. 73. Hypothetical antipyretic mechanism of 5,7,4,9-trihydroxy-3,6-dimethoxyflavone.

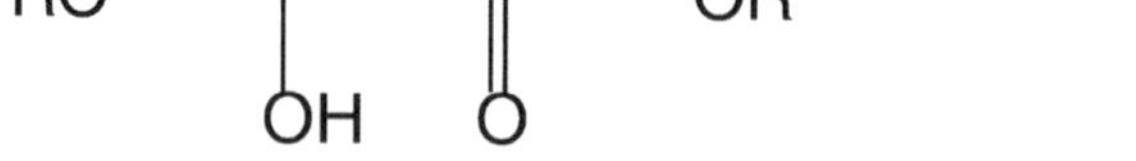

Fig. 74. 9-Trihydroxy-3,6-alkylethoxy flavones: possible antipyretic principle?

A classic example of neuroactive Celastraceae is *Catha edulis* Forsk., or *Khat*, the leaves of which are used daily by millions in a number of African and Arab countries to invigorate the intellect and to assuage hunger. Mounting evidence suggests that that (+)amphetamine and (−)cathinone produce their central stimulant effect via the same dopaminergic mechanism by increasing the levels of dopamine in the brain by acting on the catecholaminergic synapses *(101,102)*.

***Tripterygium wilfordii* Hook f.** (*Tripterygium hypoglaucum*, *Tripterygium forrestii* (Loes.). or thunder God vine or *lei gong teng* (Chinese). is a climber that can reach a length of 10 m from East Asia to South China to Burma. The leaves are simple, crenate-ovate to elliptic, 5–15 cm × 2.5–7 cm. The flowers are whitish with five petals and 9 mm across. The fruits are three-winged and brownish red (Fig. 75).
In China, the plant is used to treat rheumatic inflammation. The anti-inflammatory property is substantiated, and a surprising amount of evidence is available. Note that the main anti-inflammatory principle of *Tripterygium wildfordii* is a diterpene triepoxide known as triptolide, which posseses potent anti-inflammatory and immunosuppressive properties *(103,104)*.

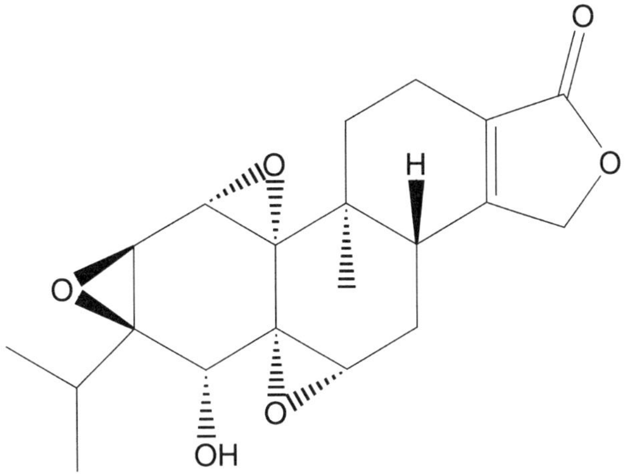

Triptolide

Some evidence suggests glial-mediated inflammation as a possible origin for Parkinson's disease via activation of microglia that release nitric oxide, proteases, and pro-inflammatory cytokines *(105)*. Feng-Qiao et al. made the interesting observation that triptolide concentration dependently attenuated lipopolysaccharide-induced decrease in [^{3}H] dopamine uptake and loss of tyrosine hydroxylase-immunoreactive neurons in primary mesencephalic neuron/glia mixed culture *(106)*. This result suggests that triptolide may protect dopaminergic neurons from lipopolysaccharide-induced degeneration.

Medicinal Lauraceae

The evidence in favor of dopaminergic alkaloids from members of the family Lauraceae is strong and it seems likely that dopaminergic agents of clinical value might be characterized from this family, and to the Magnoliales–Laurales group in general, where isoquinoline abounds. Examples of such alkaloids are boldine and glaucine, which displace specific striatal [^{3}H]-SCH 23390 binding in vitro. In vivo, glaucine at a dose of

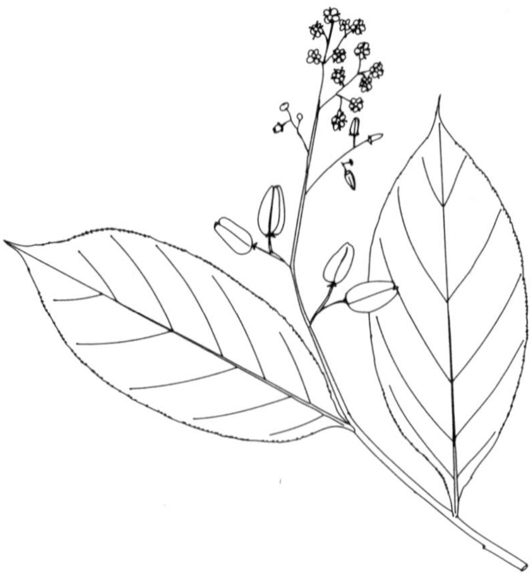

Fig. 75. *Tripterygium wilfordii* Hook f.

40 mg/kg (intraperitoneal) abrogates climbing, sniffing, and grooming elicited by apomorphine in mice *(107)*. In addition, halogenation of boldine in carbon 3 leads to increased affinity for rat brain D_1-ldopaminergic receptors with some selectivity over D_2 receptors, suggesting that a 2-hydroxy group on the aporphine skeleton may determine a binding mode favoring D_1-like over D_2-like receptors *(108)*. An additional example of a dopamine receptor-blocking alkaloid is reticuline, which is found in *Ocotea* species.

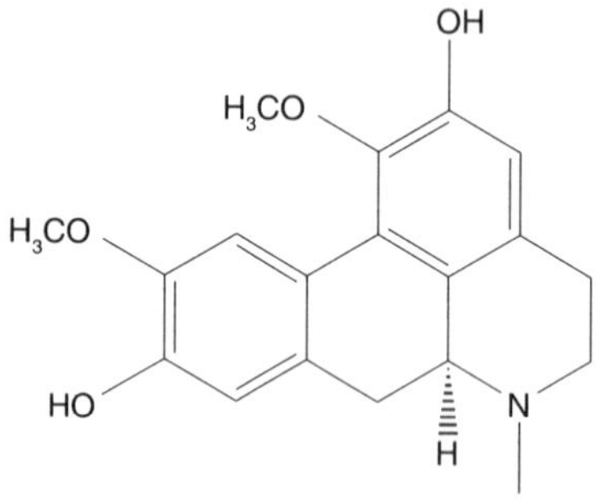

Glaucine

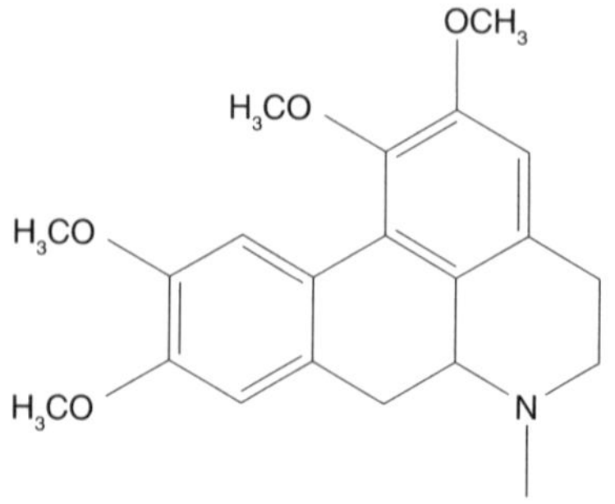

Boldine

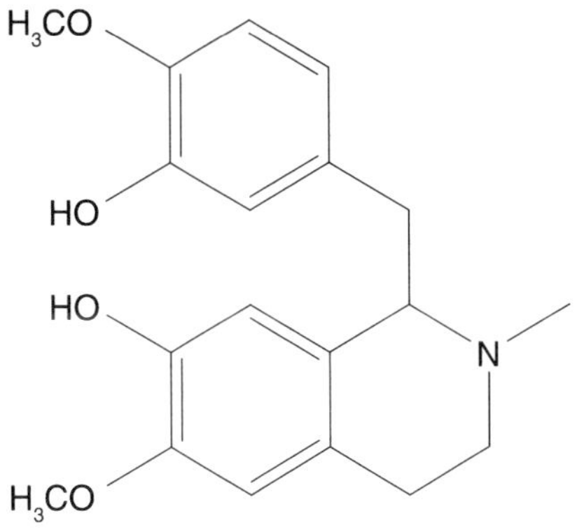

Reticuline

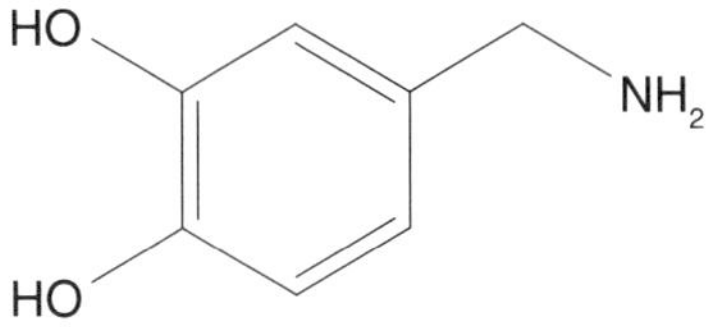

Dopamine

This benzylisoquinoline alkaloid inhibits in vitro the specific bonding of [^{3}H] dopamine to dopamine receptors and abrogates amphetamine-induced circling behavior in rodents with unilateral degeneration of dopaminergic neurons in the corpus striatum *(109)*.

***Cassytha filiformis* L.** (*Cassytha guinensis* Schum.), or dodder-laurel, snotty-gobble, devil's gut, or *chemar batu* (Malay)., is a slender epiphytic climber common on the seashores of Africa and the Asia–Pacific region. At first glance, the plant looks like a bunch of threads, but a closer observation reveals fleshy stems, tiny yellowish flowers, and whitish berries. In Malaysia, the plant is used to promote the growth of hair. Indonesians use the plant internally as vermifuge and laxative. In the Philippines, a decoction of the fresh plant is drunk to precipitate childbirth and to remove blood from saliva. In Taiwan, the stems are used as a diuretic and emmenagogue. In Vietnam, the plant is used to treat syphilis and lung diseases. The plant is known to elaborate series of aporphine alkaloids, including ocoteine, an α_1-adrenoreceptor antagonist.

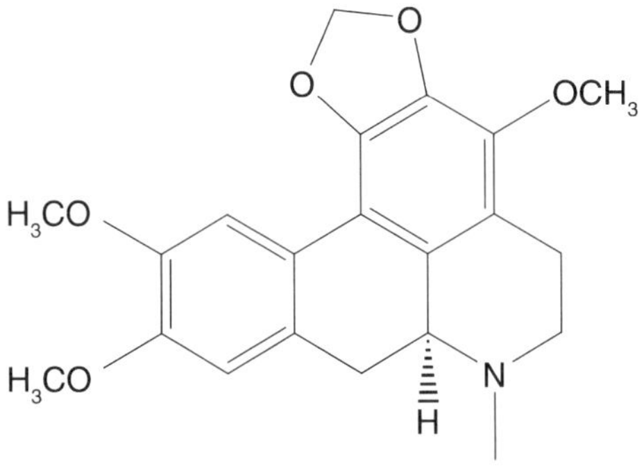

Ocoteine

The plant is known elaborate series of aporphines alkaloids such as glaucine and boldine. Glaucine is cytotoxic against HeLa cells with an IC_{50} value of 8.2 μM thought a cellular mechanism which involves DNA intercalation *(110)*. If the cytotoxic potentials of *Lauraceous aporphines* are well-known, much less evidence is available on their dopaminergic potentials. Hegde et al. made the interesting observation that 5-hydroxy-indoline, a glycosylated tetrahydroisoquinoline analog SCH 71450 from the fruit of *Phoebe chekiangensis*, showed dopaminergic effects, in receptor ligand-binding assay for D_4 receptor *(111)* binding displacement.

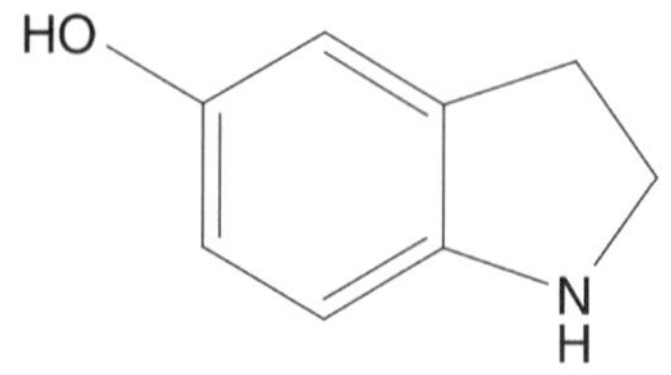

5-Hydroxy -indoline

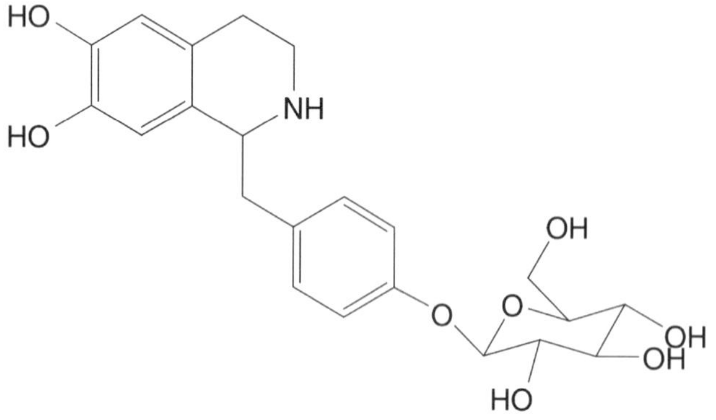

SCH 71450

Is *Cassytha filiformis* L. holding some potential as a source of drugs for the treatment of Parkinson's disease?

***Cryptocarya griffithiana* Wight** is a tree that grows to a height of 20 m in the lowland rainforests of Burma, Thailand, Malaysia, the Philippines, and Indonesia. The stems are stout and covered with a rusty tomentum. The leaves are simple, spiral, exstipulate, leathery, elliptic, and up to 32 cm long. The fruits are globose, glossy, and green (Fig. 76). The bark of this plant has the reputation among Malays and Indonesians of being poisonous.

The pharmacological potential of this tree is unexplored. Note that *Cryptocarya* species are very interesting, as they have the tendency to elaborate a series of stilbenes derivatives known as α-pyrones *(112,113)*. The neuropharmacological potential of such

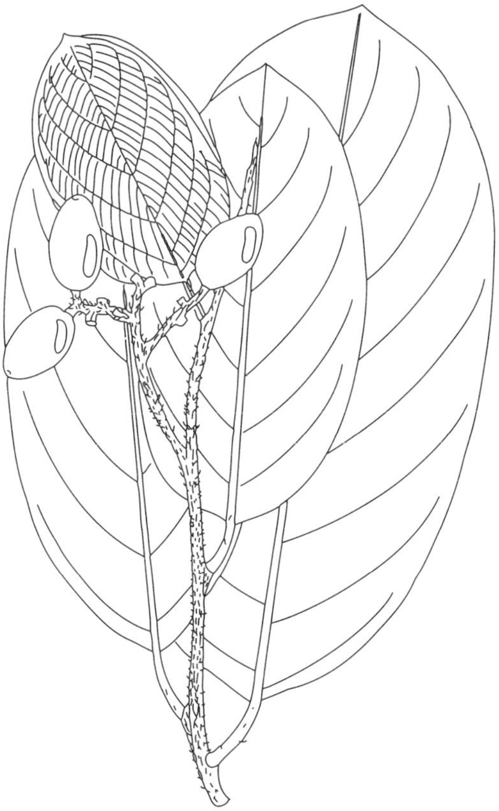

Fig. 76. *Cryptocarya griffithiana.* Distributed by The Botanic Gardens, Singapore, Malay Peninsula. Geographical localization: Kayu River, East Johor, low altitude. 3/9/1937. Det. M.H. Henderson, FSP Ng.

compounds would probably be worth assessment because α-pyrones are known for their anxiolytic properties. Examples of such agents are kavapyrones from a Piperaceae, *Piper methysticum* Forst. (kava, *British Pharmaceutical Codex*, 1934) or *kava-kava*, the rhizomes of which have been used since early times by Polynesians to allay anxiety. Kava is commercially available for relaxation. Baum et al. observed that a small dose of kava extract (120 mg/kg intraperitoneal per killogram of body weight) caused changes in the normal behavior of rats and increased concentrations of dopamine in the nucleus accumbens *(114)*. In addition, Matsumoto et al. recently suggested the possible involvement of cortical GABA neuronal mechanisms in the regional differences of dopamine response to psychological stress, and found that GABAergic neuronal system in the prefrontal cortex plays a key role in the regional differences of the dopaminergic response to psychological stress *(115)*. Are α-pyrones dopaminergic via GABAergic modulation?

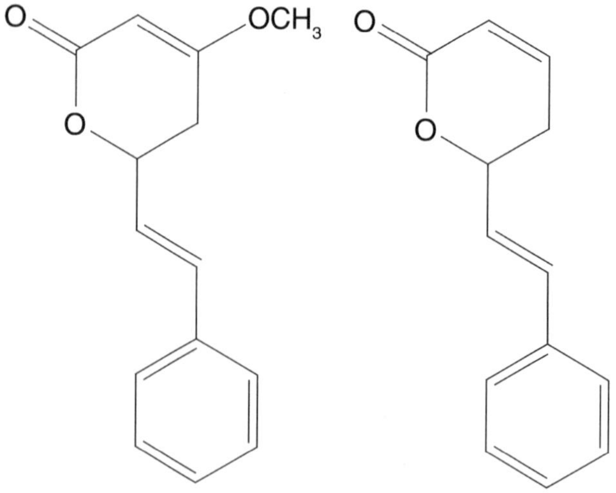

Kavain Goniothalamin

Medicinal Ranunculaceae

Some preliminary evidence has already been presented indicating that alkaloids of Ranunculaceae as a possible source for dopaminergic agents. This large family is classically known to hold a very large amount of ornamental, but drastically poisonous, herbs including for instance *Ranunculus acris* (buttercup), *Helleborus niger* (Christmas rose), *Adonis vernalis* L., *Aquilegia vulgaris*, and *Helleborus orientalis*. Diterpene alkaloids, such as aconitine, elatine, and delphinine, induce tingling of the tongue, mouth, stomach, and skin followed by numbness, anesthesia, nausea, vomiting, diarrhea, excessive salivation, incoordination, muscular weakness, vertigo, and death from paralysis of the heart or the respiratory center. Classic examples of ranunculaceaous alkaloids are berberine and hydrastine.

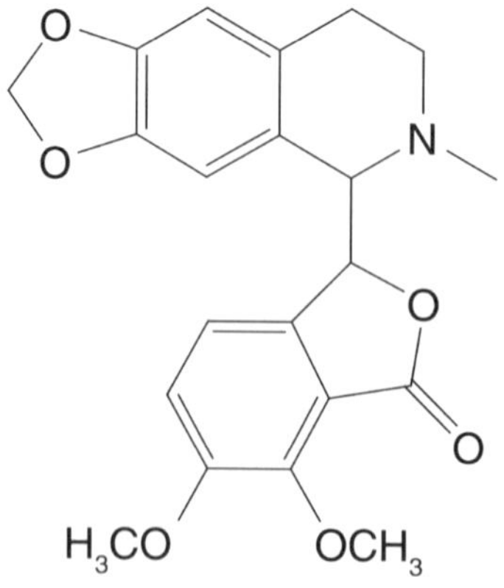

Hydrastine

Aconitum fischeri Reichb., or fischer's monkshood, American aconite, *bao ye wu tou*, or *wu tou* (Chinese), is an herb that grows to a height of 1.6 m tall in China, Korea,

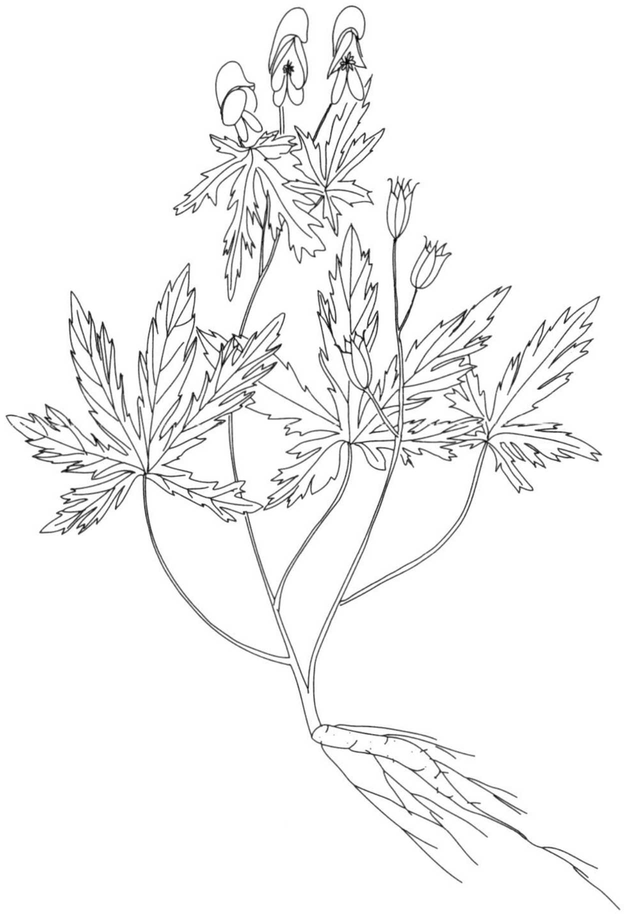

Fig. 77. *Aconitum fischeri* Reichb.

Russia, and the Rocky Mountain region of the United States. The stem is erect and pubescent at apex. The leaves are orbicular 8–12 × 12–15 cm and deeply three- to five-lobed. The flowers are arranged in racemes, deep blue color, 8 mm long, with a spur that is slightly circinate. The fruits are 1.4 cm long follicles (Fig. 77). The drug consists of the dried rhizome. In China, the rhizome is used to treat cold, cause abortion, and as a treatment for lumbago, pox, and ulcers.

The pharmacological potential of this herb is currently unexplored. One might set the hypothesis that the plant contains aconitine and other diterpene alkaloids, such as songorine, which is common in the *Aconitum* species. Interestingly, songorine, is a non competitive antagonist at the $GABA_A$ receptor, which inhibits the specific binding of [^{3}H]muscimol to GABAergic receptors with an IC_{50} value of 7.06 mM *(116)*. Using electrophysiological methods, Ameri showed that songorine (1–100 μM) enhances the excitatory synaptic transmission by agonistic action at D_2 receptors *(117)*. This effect is completely abolished by the selective dopamine D_2 receptor antagonists sulpiride (0.1 μM) and haloperidol (10 μM) and mimicked by amantadine (100 μM).

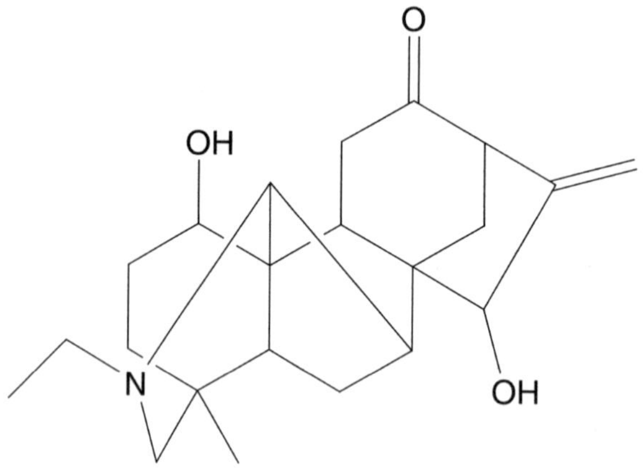

Songorine

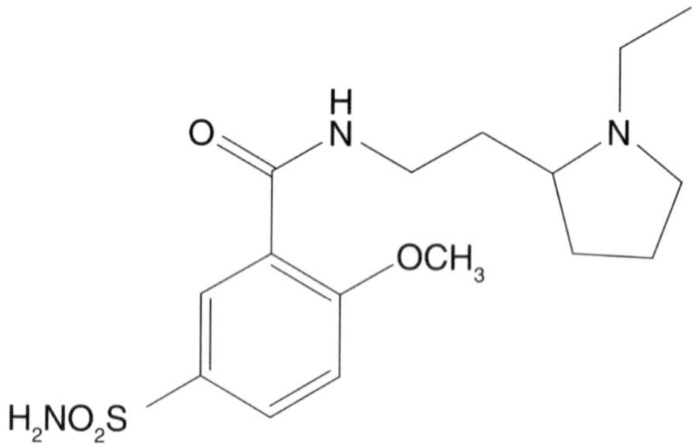

Sulpiride

Coptis teeta Wall. (*Coptis chinensis* Franch, *Coptis teeta* Wall. var. *chinensis* Franch.), or Indian goldthread, *yun nan huang lian, wang lien*, or *chih lien* (Chinese), grows wild in China and is cultivated in Szechuan. It is an herb that grows to a height of 50 cm from a rhizome. The petioles are up to 19 cm glabrous and the blade is ovate-triangular, 6–13 cm × 6–9 cm, and membranaceous. The fruits are papery follicles of about 1 cm long (Fig. 78). The drug consists of the roots, which are said to have a bird's claw appearance. It is bitter, yellow within, and aromatic. In China, the plant is used to soothe inflamed eyes, reduce fever, treat dysentery and diabetes, promote digestion, and counteract poisoning. The root is given to newborns to prevent syphilitic poisoning and mouth sores. In Cambodia, Laos, and Vietnam, the root is used to treat leucorrhea, promote menses, heal mouth sores and ulcers, and treat conjunctivis. The root abounds with berberine and coptisine, which impart to the plant most of its medicinal properties.

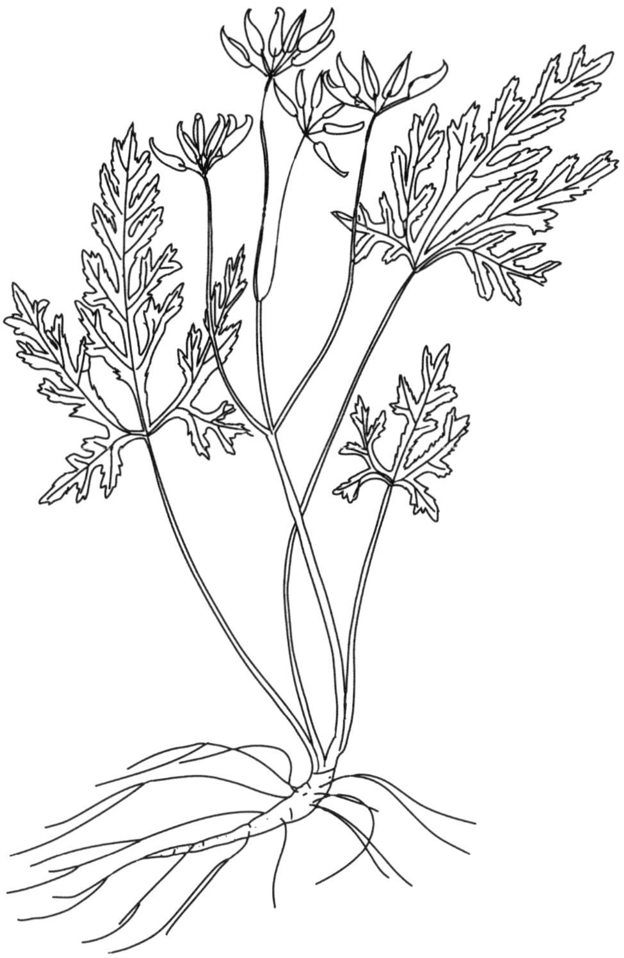

Fig. 78. *Coptis teeta* Wall.

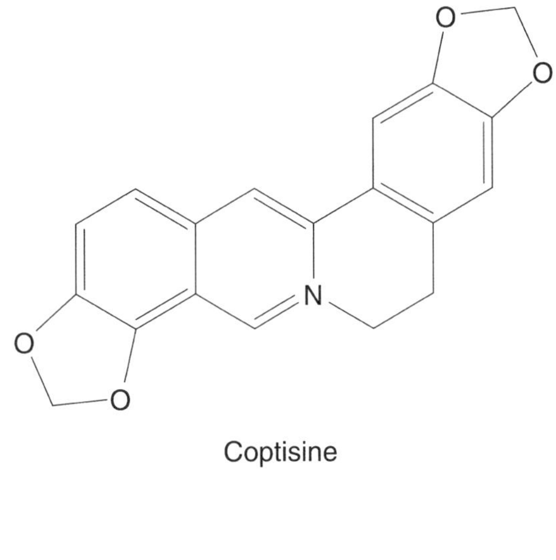

Coptisine

The plant is regarded as a sort of panacea by Chinese doctors, and has attracted a great deal of interest for its cytotoxic and antibacterial properties. The plant was a source of berberine sulphate (*British Pharmacopoeia*, 1949) that was given orally as bitter and in India parenterally for the treatment of oriental sore. Berberine inhibits the enzymatic activity of sortase, with an IC_{50} value of 8.7 μg/mL, and exhibits antibacterial activity against Gram-positive bacteria and could be of value as a source of clinical antiperiodontobacterial agent *(118)*.

Coptis chinensis abrogates the survival of a broad spectrum of cancerous cell-lines—SK-Hep1, HepG2, and Hep3B—and berberine and coptisine inhibit the proliferation of both hepatoma and leukemia cell lines, with IC_{50} values ranging from 1.4 to 15.2 μg/mL and from 0.6 to 14.1 μg/mL, respectively. However, icariin showed no inhibition of either the hepatoma or leukemia cell lines. An extract of *Coptis chinensis* is cytotoxic against a broad spectrum of cancerous cell-lines—SK-Hep1, HepG2, and Hep3B—and berberine and coptisine have potent antineoplastic properties *(119)*. Note that the anti-inflammatory property of the plant is confirmed, as an extract of the plant exhibited free radical scavenging activity *(120)*. Both the cytotoxic and antibacterial properties are known, but much less work has been done however on the dopaminergic potentials of this herb and the genus *Coptis* in general.

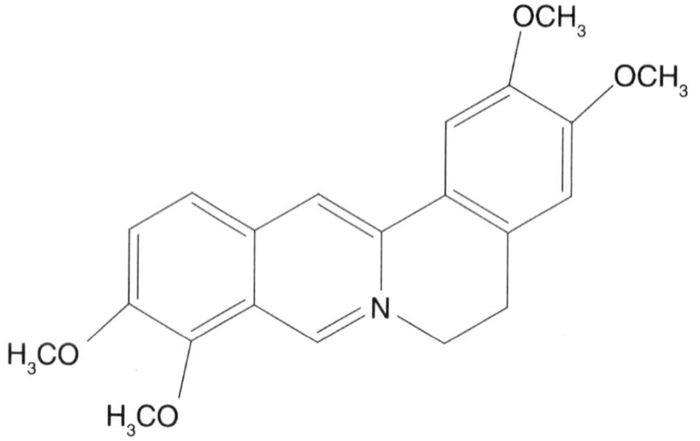

Palmatine

Lee et al. made the first observation that protoberberine alkaloids from *Coptis japonica* Makino, such as berberine and palmatine, induced 77% inhibition on dopamine content in PC12 cells with IC_{50} value of 19.5 μg/mL, and inhibited the biosynthesis catalyzed by tyrosine hydroxylase in PC12 cells with IC_{50} values of berberine and palmatine of 9.5 and 7.7 μg/mL, respectively, indicating that the *Coptis* species—and possibly other protoberberines—and *sensu lato* isoquinoline-containing plants might play some role in the etiology of Parkinsonism *(121)*. It is again interesting to note that both dopaminergic and anti-dopaminergic principles coexist in the same taxonomic group.

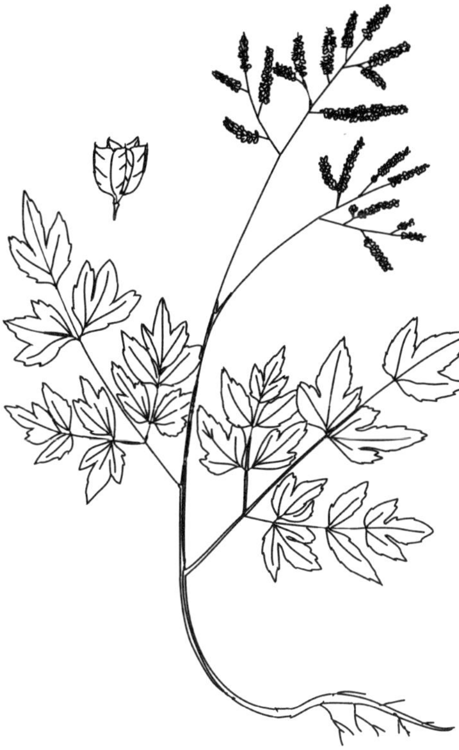

Fig. 79. *Cimicifuga foetida* L.

Surprisingly, C. *chinensis* attenuated the scopolamine-induced amnesia in rats when given orally for 1 week *(122)*.

What is the role of dopamine on memory? The dopamine D_3 receptor has been extensively studied in animal models of drug abuse and psychosis; however, less is known of its possible role in cognitive functions. Laszy et al. investigated the effects of different D_3 antagonists and a partial agonist on spatial learning performance in a water labyrinth test, and clearly demonstrated that D_3 antagonists, such as SB-277011 (24 mg/kg orally) attenuated the memory impairments caused by FG-7142, suggesting that dopamine D_3 receptor antagonists have potentials in improving cognition associated with several psychiatric disorders *(123)*.

***Cimicifuga foetida* L.**, or *sheng ma* (Chinese), is an herb that grows from a rhizome to a height of 2 m in China, Bhutan, India, Kazakhstan, Mongolia, Burma, and Siberia. The leaves are pinnate; the petiole grows up to 15 cm long; and the leaf blade is lobed and serrate. The flowers are 4 mm in diameter and the petals are broadly elliptic. The fruits are 8–14-cm × 2.5–5-mm follicles (Fig. 79). The drug consists of the rhizome, which is used to treat headhaches, sore throat, dysentery, measles, smallpox, ulcers, antidotal, and calming in China. The pharmacological potential of this plant is, to date, unveiled. Note that the plant elaborates a series of triterpenoid saponins and original cycloartane triterpenes, such as neocimicidine of the cycloartane *(124,125)*.

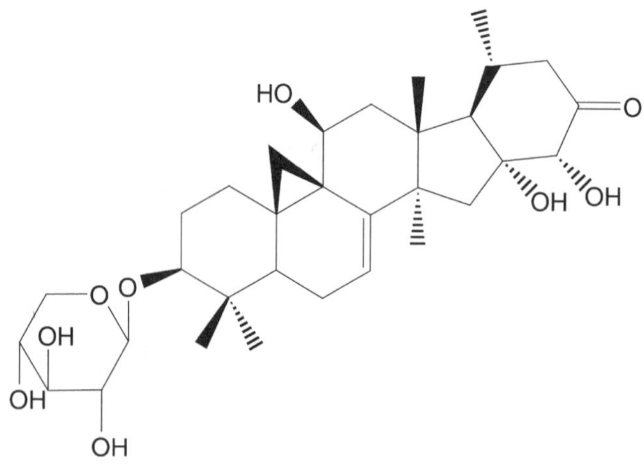

Neocimicidine

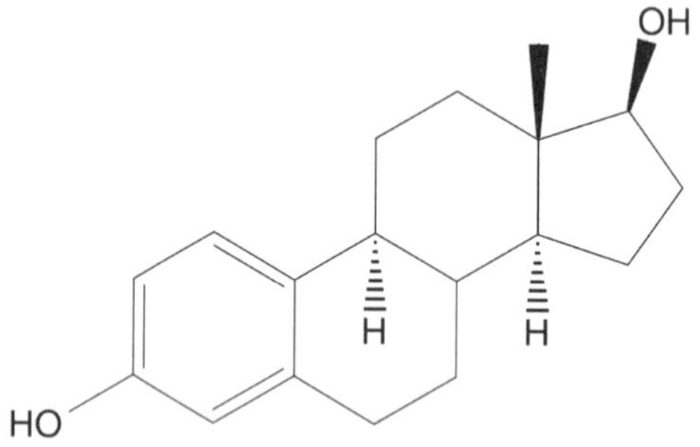

Oestradiol

Note that the dried rhizome of *Cimicifuga racemosa* (*British Pharmaceutical Codex*, 1934; black cohosh) has been used as a bitter and mild expectorant in the form of a liquid alcoholic extract (1 in 1; dose: 0.3–2 mL) and is sold as alternative remedy for the treatment of menopausal syndrome at dose of 40–80 mg/day. The active constituents of black cohosh, and, therefore, the precise molecular mechanism of action involved in the climacteric property of *Cimicifuga racemosa*, are still unknown. The most recent data suggest that the plant is not estrogenic *sensu stricto (126)*.

Jarry et al. showed that the extract of *Cimicifuga racemosa* contains some agents that bind to an unknown estrogen-binding site in the endometrium and dopamine D_2 receptors *(127)*. It will be interesting to learn whether further study on *Cimicifuga foetida* and the *Cimicifuga* species disclose any dopaminergic principles, and whether these are isoquinoline alkaloids. What is the interrelationship between estrogens and dopamine? Can we expect estrogenic compounds as antiparkinson agents?

Medicinal Menispermaceae

The family Menispermaceae consists of 70 genera and about 400 species of tropical climbers that have attracted a great deal of interest on account of their ability to elaborate a series of benzylisoquinoline and aporphine alkaloids. The cardinal features of Menispermaceae are the transversal section of the stem, which shows a yellow wood with broad medullary rays, and muricate and horseshoe-like seeds in glossy little berries. In regard to the pharmaceutical usefulness of Menispermaceae, the dried transverse slices of roots of *Jateorrhiza palmata* Miers (calumba, *British Pharmaceutical Codex*, 1954) and the dried stems of *Tinospora cordifolia* (tinospora, *Indian Pharmaceutical Codex*) have been used to promote appetite and digestion. Examples of drugs obtained from Menispermaceae are picrotoxin and tubocurarine. Tubocurarine, from curare-producing Amazonian Menispermaceae, is anticholinergic at the neuromuscular synapse and abrogates the tone of skeletal muscles, hence its use in general anesthesia (tubocurarine chloride, *British Pharmacopoeia*, 1963).

About 40 plant species in this family are medicinal in the Pacific Rim. Note that many of these are used to reduce fever, promote urination and digestion, and mitigate pains. Although there have been many studies on the phytochemical constituents of Menispermaceae, much less work has been done on the central nervous potential of these isoquinoline-producing plants. An interesting development from Menispermaceae is the search for dopaminergic agents because preliminary evidence suggests that alkaloids such as tetrahydropalmatine bind to dopaminergic D_2 receptors *(128)*.

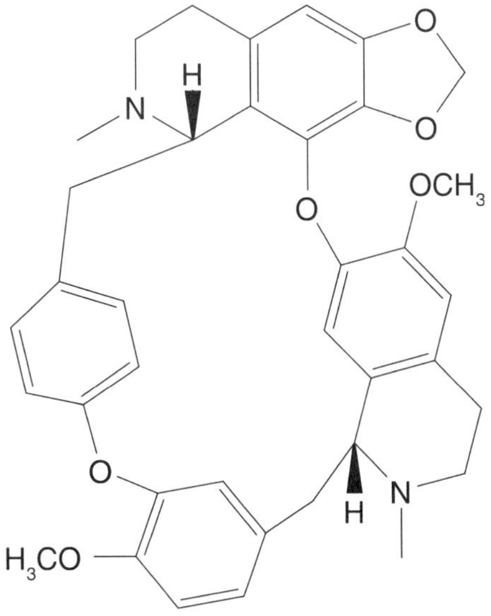

Cepharantine

Stephania cepharantha Hayata (*Stephania tetrandra* S. Moore var. *glabra* Maxim.; *Stephania disciflora* Handel-Mazzetti), or *jin qian diao wu gui* (Chinese), is a climber that grows to 2 m long in open fields and forest edges of China and Taiwan. The roots are tuberous. The stems are purplish-red and prominently lenticelled. The leaves are simple, exstipulate, membranaceous, triangular, and 2–6 cm × 2.5–6.5 cm. The apex of the blade is finely mucronate. The flowers are minute. The fruits consist of drupes that are broadly rotund and 6.5 mm long. In Taiwan, the roots are used to treat epilepsy.

The plant is known to contain cepharantine, which has attracted a great deal of interest on account of its ability to induce apoptosis, fight lung metastasis, and inhibit the replication of HIV *(129–131)*.

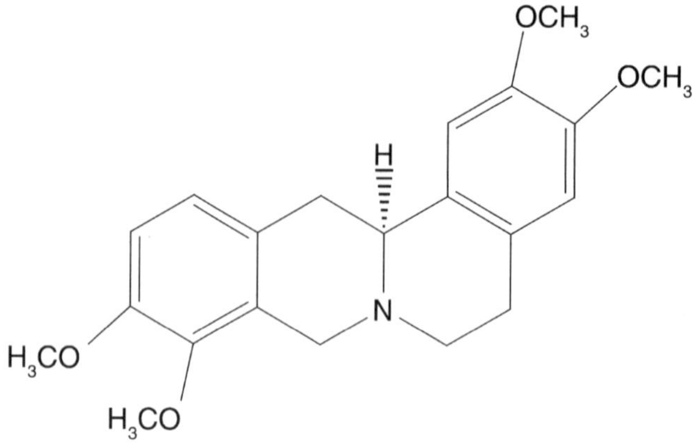

Tetrahydropalmatine

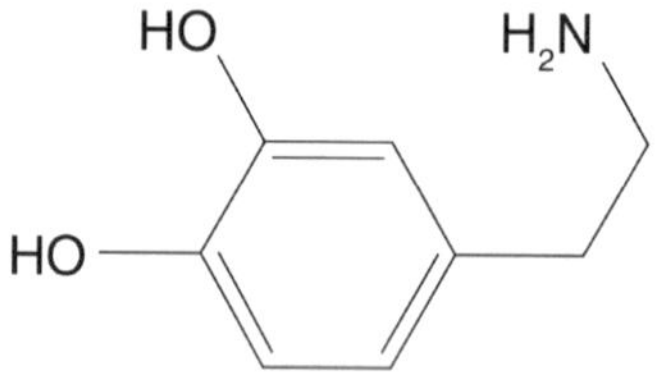

Dopamine

The antiepileptic property of the plant is, however, not substantiated experimentally yet. Vauquelin et al. observed that (±)tetrahydropalmatine binds to dopaminergic D_1 and D_2 dopaminergic receptors in membranes from human putamen *(128)*. Hu et al. noted that intraperitonneal injection of tetrahydropalmatine, as well as D_2 receptor antagonist spiperone, produced dose-dependent antinociceptive effects on the nociception of rats, and suggested that activating the spinal D_2 receptor or blocking the supraspinal D_2 receptor produces antinociception *(132)*. In addition, tetrahydropalmatine abrogates the increase of amygdaloidal release of dopamine in rats treated with 3 mg of picrotoxin per kilogram parentherally *(133)*. The question arises, therefore, whether *Stephania cepharantha* Hayata is antiepileptic through inhibition of amygdaloid dopamine release or not, and if it is, what is the active principle?

CONCLUSION AND FUTURE PROSPECTS

In conclusion, a massive body of evidence has been presented to show that the medicinal plants of the Pacific Rim hold serious potential as source of drugs for the treatment of CNS-related disorders. In summary, the most remarkable feature is the taxonomical and chemical diversity of these drugs. Given the number of medicinal plants in the Pacific Rim, the number of molecules with effects on the CNS is likely to expand in the future, and it is vital to establish a systematic neuropharmacological investigation of these plants in vitro and in vivo. It is likely that in the near future methods will be developed to assess more efficiently the CNS properties of plant secondary metabolites, including in vitro cultures of neurones or neuronal systems and even brains. The availability of original natural products together with the techniques for studying the affinity of plant products to receptors, will contribute significantly to the discovery of centrally active agents. In addition to the knowledge pertinent to the major neuronal systems, one may eventually begin to conceive of strategies for the control of diseases in which serotonin, GABA, glycine, and dopamine, and as of yet unveiled neurotransmittors. In regard to the taxonomic distribution, it appears that alkaloid-producing families are the predominant source of CNS-acting agents, especially in the Magnoliidae and Asteridae *(134)*. One wonders if other sorts of plant metabolites have been skipped.

Note that the families Rubiaceae, Solanaceae, and Convolvulaceae are known to elaborate a series of neuroactive alkaloids, some of clinical value, and represent an interesting pool of potentially centrally active agents. The Rubiaceae in particular has attracted a great deal of interest on account of *Mitragyna speciosa*, from which mitragynine has been characterized , an indole alkaloid of possible value for the treatment of opioid dependence. Górniak et al. studied the effects of *Palicourea marcgravii* (Rubiaceae) leaf on dopamine related behaviors in rats and made the interesting observation that the extract given had a blocking action on a mesostriatal dopamine receptor *(135)*. In the Convolvulaceae–Solanaceae group, some evidence currently available suggests the presence of GABAergic principles. The methanolic extract of stem of *Cuscuta reflexa* (Convolvulaceae) protected rodents against convulsion induced by chemoconvulsive agents in mice, and increased the levels of dopamine and, surprisingly, of GABA in mice brain after a few weeks *(136)*.

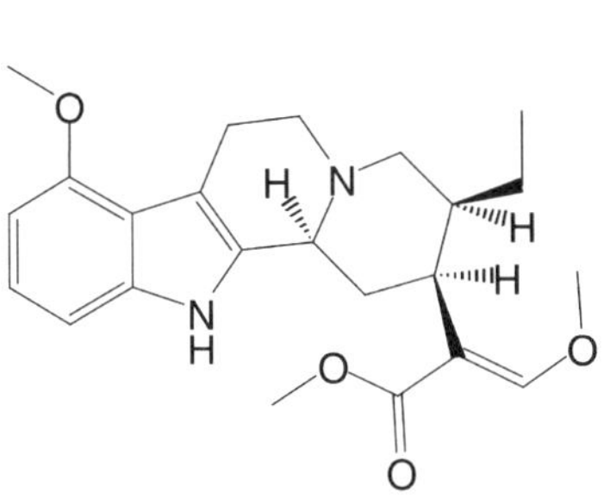

Mitragynine

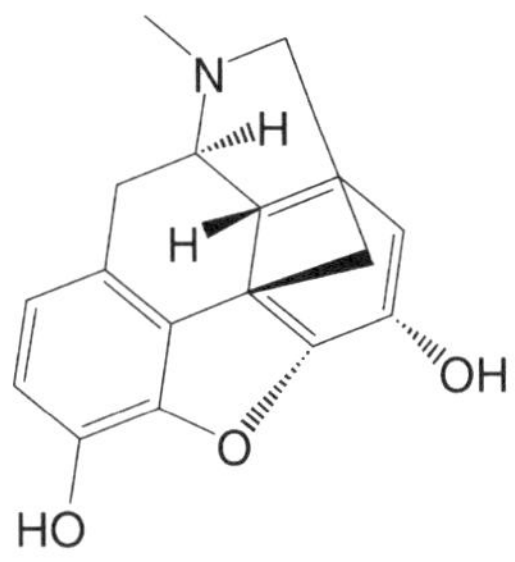

Morphine

Much less work has been done in the Caryophyllidae, Dilleniidae, and Rosidae. In the Rosidae, the family Anacardiaceae would be worth studying for GABAergic activity because Risa et al. observed that extracts of *Rhus tridentate* and *Rhus rehmanniana* are traditionally used to treat epilepsy and convulsions in South Africa, and they have good dose-dependent activity in the $GABA_A$-benzodiazepine receptor binding assay *(137)*. Other Rosidae of interest are Crassulaceae, where *Bryophyllum pinnatum* produced a dose-dependent prolongation of onset and duration of pentobarbitone-induced hypnosis, reduction of exploratory activities in the head-dip and evasion tests in rodents, and delayed onset to convulsion in both strychnine- and picrotoxin-induced seizures *(138)*. Note that Caryophyllidae is still unexplored and the question arises as to whether peptides and oligosaccharides active on the CNS await discovery in this vast taxon.

The evidence for the existence of psychopharmaceutical principles in the Liliopsida is strong, and it seems likely that further research on neuroactive substances from the monocots might pay off sooner or later. An interesting development from Liliopsida is the search of GABAergic and dopaminergic agents from Orchidaceae and Araceae, respectively. A water extract of the dried rhizome of *Acorus gramineus* Soland. dose-dependently inhibits the locomotor activity and the intensity of apomorphine-induced stereotypic behavior, and potentiates pentobarbital-induced sleeping time in rodents at dose 0.5–5.0 g/kg. Receptor binding assays showed that the extract displaced [^{3}H]SCH-23390 and [^{3}H]YM-09151-2 for specific binding to striatal dopamine D_1 and D_2 and competed with [^{3}H]muscimol for specific binding to the GABA binding site of cortex $GABA_A$ receptors *(139)*.

REFERENCES

1. Galien C. De alimentorum facultatibus, Lib. I, cap. 34, De simplicium medicamentorum temperamentis ac facultatibus, Lib VII, cap. 10 edit. Kuhn, Lipsiae, 1826.
2. O'Shaughnessy, W. B. On the preparations of the Indian Hemp, or Gunjah (cannabis indica); their effects on the animal system in health, and their utility in the treatment of tetanus and other convulsive diseases. *Provincial Medical Journal and Retrospect on the Medical Sciences*, London, 1843;5:343–398.
3. Hasrat JA, De Bruyne T, De Backer JP, Vauquelin G, Vlietinck AJ. Isoquinoline derivatives isolated from the fruit of Annona muricata as 5-HTergic $5\text{-}HT_{1A}$ receptor agonists in rats: unexploited antidepressive (lead) products. J Pharm Pharmacol 1997;49:1145–1149.
4. Ko FN, Yu SM, Su MJ, Wu YC, Teng CM. Pharmacological activity of (-)-discretamine, a novel vascular alpha-adrenoceptor and 5-hydroxytryptamine receptor antagonist, isolated from Fissistigma glaucescens. Br J Pharmacol. 1993;110:882–888.
5. Khamis S, Bibby MC, Brown JE, Cooper PA, Scowen I, Wright CW. Phytochemistry and preliminary biological evaluation of Cyathostemma argenteum, a Malaysian plant used traditionally for the treatment of breast cancer. Phytother Res 2004;18:507–510.
6. Lin CH, Chang GJ, Su MJ, Wu YC, Teng CM, Ko FN. Pharmacological characteristics of liriodenine, isolated from Fissistigma glaucescens, a novel muscarinic receptor antagonist in guinea-pigs. Br J Pharmacol 1994;113:275–281.

7. Schultes R.E. Botan. Museum Leaflets, Harvard Univ 1954;16:241.
8. Pinto MMM, Kijjoa A, Tantisewie B, Yoshida M, Gottlieb OR, Arylalkanones from *Horsfieldia glabra*. Phytochemistry 1988;27:3988–3989.
9. Jossang AP, Jossang HA, Hadi H, Bodo B. Horsfiline, an oxindole alkaloid from *Horsfieldia superba*. J. Org. Chem 1991;56:6527.
10. Jenett-Siems K, Weigl R, Kaloga M, Schulz J, Eich E. Ipobscurines C and D: macrolactam-type indole alkaloids from the seeds of *Ipomoea obscura*. Phytochemistry 2003;62:1257–1263.
11. Tyler, V.E. The physiological properties and chemical constituents of some habit-forming plants. Lloydia 1966;29:275.
12. French ED, Dillon K, Ali SF. Effects of Ibogaine, and cocaine and morphine after Ibogaine, on ventral tegmental dopamine neurons. Life Sci 1996;59: 199–205.
13. Taesotikul T, Panthong A, Kanjanapothi D, Verpoorte R, Scheffer JJ. Neuropharmacological activities of the crude alkaloidal fraction from stems of *Tabernaemontana pandacaqui* Poir. J Ethnopharmacol 1998;62:229–234.
14. Abe F, Tatsuo Y, Guevara' BQ. Indole alkaloids from *Tabernaemontana pandacaqui* in the Philippines. Biochem Syst Ecol 1993;21:847–848.
15. Okuyama E, Gao LH, Yamazaki M. Analgesic components from Bornean medicinal plants, *Tabernaemontana pauciflora* Blume and *Tabernaemontana pandacaqui* Poir. Chem Pharm Bull (Tokyo) 1992;40:3358.
16. Van Beek TA, Verpoorte R, Baerheim Svendsen A, Leeuwenberg AJM, Bisset NG. *Tabernaemontana* L. (Apocynaceae): A review of its taxonomy, phytochemistry, ethnobotany and pharmacology. J Ethnopharmacol 1984;10:156.
17. Toh-Seok K, Kooi-Mow S. Conodurine, conoduramine, and ervahanine derivatives from *Tabernaemontana corymbosa*. Phytochemistry 1992;63:625–629.
18. Gauthaman K, Adaikan PG, Prasad RNV. Aphrodisiac properties of *Tribulus terrestris* extract (Protodioscin) in normal and castrated rats. Life Sci 2002;71:1385–1396.
19. Tian-Shung W, Li-Shian S, Shang-Chu K. Alkaloids and other constituents from *Tribulus terrestris*. Phytochemistry 1999;50:1411–1415.
20. Bremner J, Waya S, Southwell I, et al. A revised structure for the alkaloid, tribulusterine, from *Tribulus terrestris* L. Aust J Chem 2004;57:273–276.
21. Rosner MH. Severe hyponatremia associated with the combined use of thiazide diuretics and selective serotonin reuptake inhibitors. Am J Med Sci 2004;327: 109–111.
22. In-Won C, Moore NA, Won-Keun O, et al. Behavioral pharmacology of polygalasaponins indicates potential antipsychotic efficacy. Pharmacol Biochem Behav 2002;71:191–195.
23. Jin B, Park J. Studies on the alkaloidal components of *Polygala tenuifolia* willd. Zhongguo Zhong Yao Za Zhi 1993;18:675–677.
24. Zhang D, Miyase T, Kuroyanagi M, Umehara K, Ueno A. Studies on the constituents of *Polygala japonica* Houtt. I. Structures of polygalasaponins I–X. Chem Pharm Bull (Tokyo) 1995;43:115–120.

25. Zhang D, Miyase T, Kuroyanagi M, Umehara K, Ueno A. Five new triterpene saponins, polygalasaponins XXVIII–XXXII from the root of *Polygala japonica* Houtt. Chem Pharm Bull (Tokyo) 1996;44:810–815.
26. Zhang D, Miyase T, Masanori K, Umehara K, Noguchi H. Polygalasaponins XLII–XLVI from roots of *Polygala glomerata*. Phytochemistry 1998;47:459–466.
27. Zhang D, Miyase T, Kuroyanagi M, Umehara K, Noguchi H. Oligosaccharide polyesters from roots of *Polygala glomerata*. Phytochemistry 1998;47:45–52.
28. Both FL, Meneghini L, Kerber VA, Henriques AT, Elisabetsky E. Psychopharmacological profile of the alkaloid psychollatine as a 5HT2A/C serotonin modulator. J Nat Prod 2005;68:374–80.
29. Beng W, Hesse A, Herramann M, Kraft R. Structure elucidation of a new anthraquinone derivatives from *Rubia tinctorium*. Pharmazie 1975;30:330–334.
30. Kasture VS, Deshmukh VK, Chopde CT. Anticonvulsant and behavioral actions of triterpene isolated from *Rubia cordifolia* Linn. Indian J Exp Biol 2000;38:675–680.
31. Hou WC, Lin RD, Chen CT, Lee MH. Monoamine oxidase B (MAO-B) inhibition by active principles from *Uncaria rhynchophylla*. J Ethnopharmacol 2005;100:216–220.
32. Masumiya H, Saitoh T, Tanaka Y, et al. Effects of hirsutine and dihydrocorynantheine on the action potentials of sino-atrial node, atrium and ventricle. Life Sci 1999;65: 2333–2341.
33. Jürgensen S, Dalbó S, Angers P, Santos AR, Ribeiro-do-Valle RM. Involvement of 5-HT_2 receptors in the antinociceptive effect of *Uncaria tomentosa*. Pharmacol Biochem Behav 2005;81:466–477.
34. Klohs MW, Keller F, Williams RE, Toekes MI, Cronheim GE. A chemical and pharmacological investigation of Piper methysticum Forst. J Med Pharm Chem 1959;1:95–103.
35. Jussofie A, Schmiz A, Hiemke C. Kavapyrone enriched extract from *Piper methysticum* as modulator of the GABA binding site in different regions of rat brain. Psychopharmacology (Berl) 1994;116:469–474.
36. Cavadas C, Araujo I, Cotrim MD, et al. In vitro study on the interaction of *Valeriana officinalis* L. extracts and their amino acids on GABAA receptor in rat brain. Arzneimittelforschung 1995;45:753–755.
37. Yuan CS, Mehendale S, Xiao Y, Aung HH, Xie JT, Ang-Lee MK. The gamma-aminobutyric acidergic effects of valerian and valerenic acid on rat brainstem neuronal activity. Anesth Analg 2004;98:353–358.
38. Wasowski C, Marder M, Viola H, Medina JH, Paladini AC. Isolation and identification of 6-methylapigenin, a competitive ligand for the brain $GABA_A$ receptors, from *Valeriana wallichii*. Planta Med 2002;68:934–936.
39. Ping L, Kimihiro M, Tohru Y, Yasushi O. Nardosinone, the first enhancer of neurite outgrowth-promoting activity of staurosporine and dibutyryl cyclic AMP in PC12D cells. Dev Brain Res 2003;145:177–183.
40. Prabhu V, Karanth KS, Rao A. Effects of *Nardostachys jatamansi* on biogenic amines and inhibitory amino acids in the rat brain. Planta Med 1994;60:114.

41. Sofiyan S, Muzamil A, Khan Shoeb Z, Abdullah S and Fakhrul I. Protective effect of *Nardostachys jatamansi* in rat cerebral ischemia. Pharmacol Biochem Behav 2003;74:481–486.
42. Shakir A, Khursheed A, Ansari MA, Kabeer JH, Diwakar G. *Nardostachys jatamansi* protects against liver damage induced by thioacetamide in rats J Ethnopharmacol 2000;71:359–363.
43. Luo HC, Cui YH, Shen YC, Lou ZQ. Clinical observation and pharmacological investigation of the sedative and hypnotic effects of the Chinese drug rhizome and root of *Patrinia scabiosaefolia* Fisch. J Tradit Chin Med 1986;6:89–94.
44. Won SW, Choi JS, Seligmann O, Wagner H. Sterol and triterpenoid glycosides from the roots of *Patrinia scabiosaefolia*. Phytochemistry 1983;22:1045–1047.
45. Yang B, Tong L, Jin M, Zhao W, Chen Y. Isolation and identification of triterpenoide compound from *Patrinia scabiosaefolia*. Zhong Yao Cai 1998;21:513–514.
46. Huen MSY, Kwok-Min H, Leung JWC, Sigel E, Baur R, Wong JTF. Naturally occurring 2′-hydroxyl-substituted flavonoids as high-affinity benzodiazepine site ligands. Biochem Pharmacol 2003;66:2397–2407.
47. Kavvadias D, Monschein VS, Riederer P, Schreier P. Constituents of sage (*Salvia officinalis*) with in vitro affinity to human brain benzodiazepine receptor. Planta Med 2003;69:113–117.
48. Kwok MH, Huen MSY, Wang HY, et al. Anxiolytic effect of wogonin, a benzodiazepine receptor ligand isolated from *Scutellaria baicalensis* Georgi. Biochem Pharmacol 2002;64:1415–1424.
49. Huen MS, Leung JW, Ng W, et al. Dihydroxy-6-methoxyflavone, a benzodiazepine site ligand isolated from *Scutellaria baicalensis* Georgi, with selective antagonistic properties. Biochem Pharmacol 2003;66:125–127.
50. Huen MSY, Hui KM, Leung JWC, et al. Naturally occurring 2′-hydroxyl-substituted flavonoids as high-affinity benzodiazepine site ligands. Biochem Pharmacol 2003;66:2397–2407.
51. Awad R, Arnason JT, Trudeau V, et al. Phytochemical and biological analysis of skullcap (*Scutellaria lateriflora* L.): a medicinal plant with anxiolytic properties. Phytomedicine 2003;10:640–649.
52. Bienvenu E, Amabeoku GJ, Eagles PK, Scott G, Springfield EP. Anticonvulsant activity of aqueous extract of *Leonotis leonurus*. Phytomedicine 2002; 9:217–223.
53. Calixto JB, Yunes RA, Rae GA. Effect of crude extracts from *Leonotis nepetaefolia* (Labiatae) on rat and guinea-pig smooth muscle and rat cardiac muscle. J Pharm Pharmacol 1991;43:529–534.
54. Purushothaman KK, Vasanth S, Connolly JD, Labbe C. 4,6,7-Trimethoxy-5-methylchromen-2-one, a new coumarin from *Leonotis nepetaefolia*. J Chem Soc 1976;23:2594–2595.
55. Viola H, Wasowski C, Levi de Stein M, et al. Apigenin, a component of *Matricaria recutita* flowers, is a central benzodiazepine receptors-ligand with anxiolytic effects. Planta Med 1995;61:213–216.

56. Avallone R, Zanoli P, Puia G, Kleinschnitz M, Schreier P, Baraldi M. Pharmacological profile of apigenin, a flavonoid isolated from *Matricaria chamomilla*. Biochem Pharmacol 2000;59:1387–1394.
57. Salah SM, Jager AK. Screening of traditionally used Lebanese herbs for neurological activities. J Ethnopharmacol 2005;97:145–159.
58. Salah SM, Jager AK. Two flavonoids from *Artemisia herba-alba* with in vitro $GABA_A$-benzodiazepine receptor activity. J Ethnopharmacol 2005;99:145–146.
59. Jeoung-Hee H, Dong-Ung L, Jae-Tae L, et al. Hydroxybenzaldehyde from *Gastrodia elata* Bl. is active in the antioxidation and GABAergic neuromodulation of the rat brain. J Ethnopharmacol 2000;73:329–333.
60. Ha JH, Shin SM, Lee SK, et al. In vitro effects of hydroxybenzaldehydes from *Gastrodia elata* and their analogues on GABAergic neurotransmission, and a structure –activity correlation. Planta Med 2001;67:877–880.
61. Leong YW, Powell AD. Phenanthrene and other aromatic constituents of *Bulbophyllum vaginatum*. Phytochemistry 1999;50:1237–1241.
62. Salmi P, Isacson R, Kull B. Dihydrexidine—the first full dopamine D1 receptor agonist. CNS Drug Rev 2004;10:230–242.
63. Yoshikawa M, Murakami T, Kishi A, et al. Novel indole S,O-bisdesmoside, calanthoside, the precursor glycoside of tryptanthrin, indirubin, and isatin, with increasing skin blood flow promoting effects, from two Calanthe species (Orchidaceae). Chem Pharm Bull (Tokyo) 1998;46:886–888.
64. Kudo Y, Tanaka A, Yamada K. Dendrobine, an antagonist of beta-alanine, taurine and of presynaptic inhibition in the frog spinal cord. Br J Pharmacol 1983;78:709–715.
65. Gruol DL and Smith TG. Opiate antagonism of glycine-evoked membrane polarizations in cultured mouse spinal cord neurons. Brain Res 1981;223:355–365.
66. Schmieden V, Jezequel S, Betz H. Novel antagonists of the inhibitory glycine receptor derived from quinolinic acid compounds. Mol Pharmacol 1996;50:1200–1206.
67. Philippe G, Angenot L, Tits M, Frédérich M. About the toxicity of some *Strychnos* species and their alkaloids. Toxicon 2004;44:405–416.
68. Bisset NG, Walker MD. Alkaloids from the stem bark of *Strychnos ignatii*. Phytochemistry 1974:13:525–526.
69. Pathama L, Michihisa T, Kinzo M, et al. Inhibitory effects of corymine, an alkaloidal component from the leaves of *Hunteria zeylanica*, on glycine receptors expressed in Xenopus oocytes. Euro J Pharmacol 1997;332:321–326.
70. Fujikawa T, Miguchi S, Kanada N, et al. *Acanthopanax senticosus* Harms as a prophylactic for MPTP-induced Parkinson's disease in rats. J Ethnopharmacol 2005;97: 375–381.
71. Masazumi M, Yoshiteru I, Susumu I, Junzo S. 3α-Hydroxy-oleanane-type triterpene glycosyl esters from leaves of *Acanthopanax spinosus*. Phytochemistry 1993;34: 1599–1602.
72. Masazumi M, Yoshiteru I, Susumu I, Junzo S. Epi-Oleanene type triterpene glycosyl esters from leaves of *Acanthopanax spinosus*. Phytochemistry 1993;33:891–895.

73. Masazumi M, Susumu I, Hirotoshi S, Yasuaki H, Junzo S, Yoshiteru I. 3α-hydroxy-oleanene type triterpene glycosyl esters from leaves of *Acanthopanax spinosus*. Phytochemistry 1997;46:1255–1259.
74. Radad K, Gille G, Moldzio R, Saito H, Ishige K, Rausch WD. Ginsenosides Rb1 and Rg1 effects on survival and neurite growth of MPP+-affected mesencephalic dopaminergic cells. J Neural Transm 2004;111:37–45.
75. Oh KW, Kim HS, Wagner GC. Ginseng total saponin inhibits the dopaminergic depletions induced by methamphetamine. Planta Med 1997;63:80–81.
76. Ty Ph. D, M. Lischewski, H. V. Phiet, A. Preiss, Ph. V. Nguyen, Adam G. 3α, 11 α - Dihydroxy-23-oxo-lup-20(29)-en-28-oic acid from *Acanthopanax trifoliatus*. Phytochemistry 1985;24:867–869 .
77. Kiem PV, Cai XF, Minh CV, Lee JJ, Kim YH. Kaurane-type diterpene glycoside from the stem bark of *Acanthopanax trifoliatus*. Planta Med 2004;70:282–284.
78. Lee EB, Li DW, Hyun JE, Kim IH, Whang WK. Anti-inflammatory activity of methanol extract of *Kalopanax pictus* bark and its fractions. J Ethnopharmacol 2001;77:197–201.
79. Li da W, Lee EB, Kang SS, Hyun JE, Whang WK. Activity-guided isolation of saponins from *Kalopanax pictus* with anti-inflammatory activity. Chem Pharm Bull (Tokyo) 2002;50:900–903.
80. Jongwon C, Keun H, Suk-Hwan K, Kyung-Tae L, Hyeong-Kyu L. Hee-Juhn P. Kalopanaxsaponin A from *Kalopanax pictus*, a potent antioxidant in the rheumatoidal rat treated with Freund's complete adjuvant reagent. J Ethnopharmacol 2002;79:113–118.
81. Kim IT, Park YM, Shin KM, et al. Anti-inflammatory and anti-nociceptive effects of the extract from *Kalopanax pictus*, *Pueraria thunbergiana* and *Rhus verniciflua*. J Ethnopharmacol 2004;94:165–173.
82. Lee MW, Kim SU, Hahn DR. Antifungal activity of modified hederagenin glycosides from the leaves of *Kalopanax pictum* var. chinense. Biol Pharm Bull 2001;24:718–719.
83. Schellenberg R. Treatment for the premenstrual syndrome with *Agnus castus* fruit extract: prospective, randomised, placebo controlled study. BMJ 2001;322:134–137.
84. Dharmasiri MG, Jayakody JR, Galhena G, Liyanage SS, Ratnasooriya WD. Anti-inflammatory and analgesic activities of mature fresh leaves of *Vitex negundo*. J Ethnopharmacol 2003;87:199–206.
85. Alam MI, Gomes A. Snake venom neutralization by Indian medicinal plants (*Vitex negundo* and *Emblica officinalis*) root extracts. J Ethnopharmacol 2003;86:75–80.
86. Wuttke W, Jarry H, Christoffel V, Spengler B, Seidlova-Wuttke D. Chaste tree (*Vitex agnus-castus*)—pharmacology and clinical indications Phytomedicine 2003;10: 348–357.
87. Li WX, Cui CB, Cai B, Yao XS. Labdane-type diterpenes as new cell cycle inhibitors and apoptosis inducers from *Vitex trifolia* L. J Asian Nat Prod Res 2005;7:95–105.
88. Wang HY, Cai B, Cui CB, Zhang DY, Yang BF. Vitexicarpin, a flavonoid from *Vitex trifolia* L, induces apoptosis in K562 cells via mitochondria-controlled apoptotic pathway. Yao Xue Xue Bao 2005;40:27–31.

89. Naidu PS, Singh A, Kulkarni SK. D_2-dopamine receptor and alpha2-adrenoreceptor-mediated analgesic response of quercetin. Indian J Exp Biol 2003;41:1400–1404.
90. Ando N, Gorai I, Hirabuki T, Onose R, Hirahara F, Minaguchi H. Prolactin disorders in patients with habitual abortion. Nippon Sanka Fujinka Gakkai Zasshi 1992;44: 650–656.
91. Cauli O, Morelli M. Caffeine and the dopaminergic system. Behav Pharmacol 2005;16:63–77.
92. Arulmozhi DK, Veeranjaneyulu A, Bodhankar SL, Arora SK. Pharmacological studies of the aqueous extract of *Sapindus trifoliatus* on central nervous system: possible ant migraine mechanisms. J Ethnopharmacol 2005;97:491–496.
93. Arulmozhi DK, Veeranjaneyulu A, Bodhankar SL, Arora SK. Effect of *Sapindus trifoliatus* on hyperalgesic in vivo migraine models. Braz J Med Biol Res 2005;38:469–475.
94. Kuo YH, Huang HC, Yang Kuo LM, et al. New dammarane-type saponins from the galls of *Sapindus mukorossi*. J Agric Food Chem 2005;53:4722–4727.
95. Munavvar AS, Gan EK, Loke SE, Mah KF, Wong WH. Effect of an extract of *Erioglossum edule* on the central nervous system. J Ethnopharmacol 1989;25:217–220.
96. Takagi K, Park EH, Kato H. Anti-inflammatory activities of hederagenin and crude saponin isolated from *Sapindus mukorossi* Gaertn. Chem Pharm Bull (Tokyo) 1980;28:1183–1188.
97. Birioukova LM, Midzyanovskaya IS, Lensu S, Tuomisto L, van Luijtelaar G. Distribution of D_1-like and D_2-like dopamine receptors in the brain of genetic epileptic WAG/Rij rats. Epilepsy Res 2005;63:89–96.
98. Amabeoku GJ, Eagles P, Scott G, Mayeng I, Springfield E. Analgesic and antipyretic effects of *Dodonaea angustifolia* and *Salvia africana-lutea*. J Ethnopharmacol 2001;75:117–124.
99. Heerden FR. van, Viljoen AM, van Wyk BE. The major flavonoid of *Dodonaea angustifolia*. Fitoterapia 2000;71:602–604.
100. Pataki I, Adamik A, Jaszberenyi M, Macsai M, Telegdy G. Involvement of transmitters in pituitary adenylate cyclase-activating polypeptide-induced hyperthermia. Regul Pept 2003;115:187–193.
101. Patel NB. Mechanism of action of cathinone: the active ingredient of khat (*Catha edulis*). East Afr Med J 2000;77:329–332.
102. Connor J. D, Ruston A, Eyasu M. Comparison of effects of khat extract and amphetamine on motor behaviors in mice. J Ethnopharmacol 2002;81:65–71.
103. Zheng J. Screening of active anti-inflammatory, immunosuppressive and anti-fertility components of *Tripterygium wildfordii*: III. A comparison of the anti-inflammatory and immunosuppressive activities of 7 diterpene lactones epoxides compounds in vivo. Zhongguo Yixue Kexueyuan Xuebao 1991;13:391–397.
104. Zhao G, Vaszar LT, Qiu D, Shi I, Kao PN. Anti-inflammatory effects of triptolide in human bronchial epithelial cells. Am J Physiol Lung Cell Mol Physiol 2000; 279:L958–L966.
105. Hirsch EC. Glial cells and Parkinson's disease. J Neurol 2000;247:1158–1162.

106. Feng-Qiao L, Xiu-Zhi L., Xi-Bin L, et al. Triptolide, a Chinese herbal extract, protects dopaminergic neurons from inflammation-mediated damage through inhibition of microglial activation. J Neuroimmunol 2004;148:24–31.
107. Asencio M, Delaquerrière B, Cassels BK, Speisky H, Comoy E, Protais P. Biochemical and behavioral effects of boldine and glaucine on dopamine systems. Pharmacol Biochem Behav 1999;62:7–13.
108. Asencio M, Hurtado-Guzmán C, López JJ, Cassels BK, Protais P, Chagraoui A. Structure–affinity relationships of halogenated predicentrine and glaucine derivatives at D1 and D_2 dopaminergic receptors: halogenation and D_1 receptor selectivity. Bioorg Med Chem 2005;13:3699–3704.
109. Banning, JW, Uretsky NJ, Patil PN, Beal JL. Reticuline: a dopamine receptor blocker. Life Sci 1980;26:2083–2091.
110. Hoet S, Stevigny C, Block S, et al. Alkaloids from *Cassytha filiformis* and related aporphines: anti-trypanosomal activity, cytotoxicity, and interaction with DNA and topoisomerases. Planta Med 2004;70:407–413.
111. Hegde VR, Dai P, Ladislaw C, Patel MG, Puar MS, Pachter JA. D_4 dopamine receptor-selective compounds from the Chinese plant *Phoebe chekiangensis*. Bioorg Med Chem Lett 1997;7:1207–1212.
112. Drewes SE, Horn MM, Scott RS. α-Pyrones and their derivatives from two *Cryptocarya* species. Phytochemistry 1995;40:321–323.
113. Lia DJ, Mariko K, Hiromitsu T, Sjamsul AA, Norio A. A 6-substituted-5,6-dihydro-2-pyrone from *Cryptocarya strictifolia*. Phytochemistry 2000;54:989–993.
114. Baum SS, Hill R, Rommelspacher H. Effect of kava extract and individual kavapyrones on neurotransmitter levels in the nucleus accumbens of rats. Prog Neuropsychopharmacol Biol Psychiatry 1998;22:1105–1120.
115. Matsumoto M, Togashi H, Kaku A, Kanno M, Tahara K, Yoshioka M. Cortical GABAergic regulation of dopaminergic responses to psychological stress in the rat dorsolateral striatum. Synaps 2005;56:117–121.
116. Zhao XY, Wang Y, Li Y, et al. Songorine, a diterpenoid alkaloid of the genus *Aconitum*, is a novel $GABA_A$ receptor antagonist in rat brain. Neurosci Lett 2003;337:33–36.
117. Ameri A. Effects of the Aconitum alkaloid songorine on synaptic transmission and paired-pulse facilitation of CA1 pyramidal cells in rat hippocampal slices. Br J Pharmacol 1998;125:461–468.
118. Kim SH, Shin DS, Oh MN, Chung SC, Lee JS, Oh KB. Inhibition of the bacterial surface protein anchoring transpeptidase sortase by isoquinoline alkaloids. Biosci Biotechnol Biochem 2004;68:421–424.
119. Lin CC, Ng LT, Hsu FF, Shieh DE, Chiang LC. Cytotoxic effects of *Coptis chinensis* and *Epimedium sagittatum* extracts and their major constituents (berberine, coptisine and icariin) on hepatoma and leukaemia cell growth. Clin Exp Pharmacol Physiol 2004;31:65–69.
120. Schinella GR, Tournier HA, Prieto JM, Mordujovich de Buschiazzo P, Rios JL. Antioxidant activity of anti-inflammatory plant extracts. Life Sci 2002;70:1023–1033.

121. Lee MK, Kim HS. Inhibitory effects of protoberberine alkaloids from the roots of *Coptis japonica* on catecholamine biosynthesis in PC12 cells. Planta Med 1996;62: 31–34.
122. Hsieh MT, Peng WH, Wu CR, Wang WH. The ameliorating effects of the cognitive-enhancing Chinese herbs on scopolamine-induced amnesia in rats. Phytother Res 2000;14:375–377.
123. Laszy J, Laszlovszky I, Gyertyan I. Dopamine D_3 receptor antagonists improve the learning performance in memory-impaired rats. Psychopharmacology (Berl) 2005; 179:567–575.
124. Cong-Jun Li, Ying-He Li, Pei-Gen X, Tom JM, Watson WH, Krawiec M. An unusual cycloartane triterpenoid from *Cimicifuga foetida*. Phytochemistry 1996;42:489–494.
125. Pan RL, Chen DH, Si JY, Zhao XH, Shen LG. Studies on the new triterpenoid saponin of the aerial part of *Cimicifuga foetida*. Zhongguo Zhong Yao Za Zhi 2003;8:230–232.
126. Mahady GB. Black cohosh (*Cimicifuga racemosa*): review of the clinical data for safety and efficacy in menopausal symptoms. Treat Endocrinol 2005;4:177–184.
127. Jarry H, Thelen P, Christoffel V, Spengler B, Wuttke W. *Cimicifuga racemosa* extract BNO 1055 inhibits proliferation of the human prostate cancer cell line LNCaP. Phytomedicine 2005;12:178–182.
128. Vauquelin G, De Keyser J, Banyingela K, Vanhaelen M. (±)Tetrahydroanisocycline and (±)tetrahydropalmatine binding to D_1 and D_2 dopaminergic receptors in human putamen. Neurochem Int 1989;15:321–324.
129. Wang Y, Kuroda M, Gao XS, et al. Cepharanthine enhances in vitro and in vivo thermosensitivity of a mouse fibrosarcoma, FSa-II, based on increased apoptosis. Int J Mol Med 2004;13:405–411.
130. Okada K, Sakusabe N, Kobayashi A, Hoshi N, Sato K. Prevention of lung metastasis by intra-tumoural injection of Cepharanthin and staphylococcal enterotoxin B in transplantable rat osteosarcoma. Jpn J Cancer Res 1999;90:928–933.
131. Okamoto M, Ono M, Baba M. Potent inhibition of HIV type 1 replication by an anti-inflammatory alkaloid, cepharanthine, in chronically infected monocytic cells. Res Hum Retroviruses 1998;14:1239–1245.
132. Hu JY, Jin GZ. Supraspinal D_2 receptor involved in antinociception induced by l-tetrahydropalmatine. Zhongguo Yao Li Xue Bao 1999;20:715–719.
133. Chang CK, Lin MT. DL-Tetrahydropalmatine may act through inhibition of amygdaloid release of dopamine to inhibit an epileptic attack in rats. Neurosci Lett 2001;307:163–166.
134. Sousa FCF, Melo CTV, Monteiro AP, et al. Antianxiety and antidepressant effects of riparin III from *Aniba riparia* (Nees) Mez (Lauraceae) in mice. Pharmacol Biochem Behav 2004;78:27–33.
135. Górniak SL, Palermo-Neto J, de Souza-Spinosa H. Effects of a *Palicourea marcgravii* leaf extract on some dopamine-related behaviors of rats. J Ethnopharmacol 1990;28:329–335.

136. Gupta M, Mazumder UK, Pal DK, Bhattacharya S Anti-steroidogenic activity of methanolic extract of *Cuscuta reflexa* roxb. stem and *Corchorus olitorius* Linn. seed in mouse ovary. Indian J Exp Biol 2003;41:641–644.
137. Risa J, Risa A, Adsersen A, et al. Screening of plants used in southern Africa for epilepsy and convulsions in the $GABA_A$-benzodiazepine receptor assay. J Ethnopharmacol 2004;93:177–182.
138. Yemitan OK, Salahdeen HM. Neurosedative and muscle relaxant activities of aqueous extract of *Bryophyllum pinnatum*. Fitoterapia 2005;76:187–193.
139. Jyh-Fei L, Sung YH, Yiing-Ming J, Li-Li Y, Chieh FC. Central inhibitory effects of water extract of *Acori graminei* rhizoma in mice. J Ethnopharmacol 1998;61:185–193.

3 Plants for Chemotherapy of Neoplastic Diseases

GENERAL CONCEPT

Each year in the United States more than 1 million people are diagnosed with cancer, and about 500,000 people die from the disease. For the most part, the reason that cancer is a fatal disease is that cancer cells can invade through, and metastasize to, distant organs in the body. The hallmarks of malignant neoplastic tissue are unregulated cell proliferation, invasiveness, and metastasis to distant sites in the body. Surgery and radiotherapy can eradicate localized tumors but may fail because the cancer may have metastasized to other areas of the body; chemotherapy, if used properly, may control or eliminate metastasis. The array of drugs used for the treatment of cancer includes antimetabolites (methotrexate [Trexall®]), fluoouracil (Efudex®), mercaptopurine (Puri-Nethol®), cytarabine (Cytosar®), covalent DNA-binding drugs (nitrogen mustards, alkylating agents), noncovalent binding drugs (anthracyclines), antiestrogens, and inhibitors of chromatin function.

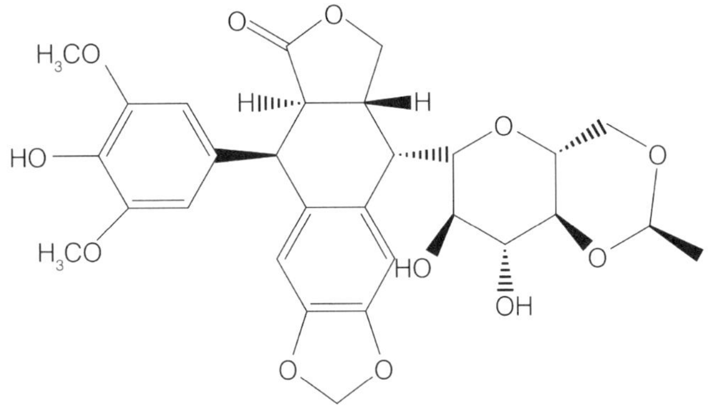

Etoposide (Vepesid®)

Examples of inhibitors of chromatin function derived from flowering plants (Fig. 80) are etoposide (lignan) and alkaloids camptothecin, *Vinca* alkaloids, and 7 epitaxol. The rhizome of *Podophyllum peltatum* L. (May apple, Berberidaceae) has been used to remove warts and to relieve the bowels from costiveness since very early times. It contains podophyllotoxin, a cytotoxic lignan from which etoposide (Vepesid®), which is used to treat lung cancer, lymphomas, and leukemias on account of its ability to inhibit the activity of

From: *Ethnopharmacology of Medicinal Plants: Asia and the Pacific*
Edited by: C. Wiart © Humana Press Inc., Totowa, NJ

topoisomerase, has been semisynthetically developed Attempts to verify the reputed antidiabetic property of *Catharanthus roseus* G. Don (periwinkle, Apocynaceae) in the 1960s led first to the observation by Canadian workers that leaf extract caused leucopenia in rats.

Researchers from Eli Lilly pharmaceuticals, (a company founded in 1876 by Colonel Eli Lilly veteran of the US Civil War), undertook further intensive phytochemical studies and characterized 60 alkaloids, of which a group of 20 binary indole alkaloids—including vincristine and vinblastine. Vinblastine sulphate (Velbe®) inhibits the polymerization of tubulin and is used to treat generalized Hodgkin's disease and chorionepithelioma, whereas vincristine sulphate (Oncovin®) is used to treat leukemia in children.

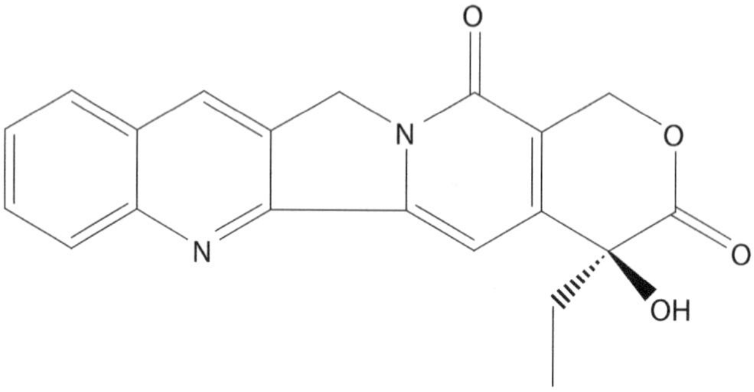

Camptothecin

Camptothecin is a monoterpenoid quinoline alkaloid that is also known to occur in the subclass Rosidae: *Camptotheca acuminata* Decsne. (family Nyssaceae, order Cornales), and *Nothapodytes fetida* (Wight.) Sleum. (family Icacinaceae, order Celastrales); and the Asteridae: *Ophiorrhiza mungos* L. (Rubiaceae). Camptothecin was found to inhibit topoisomerase and to be active against experimental tumors; however, initial clinical trials showed little response and severe cystitis, but more effective analogs were developed, such as irinotecan (Campto®). Cancer chemotherapy alone, however, is not very effective in producing long-term survival or treating the most common solid tumors, and the need for new anticancer drugs is critical.

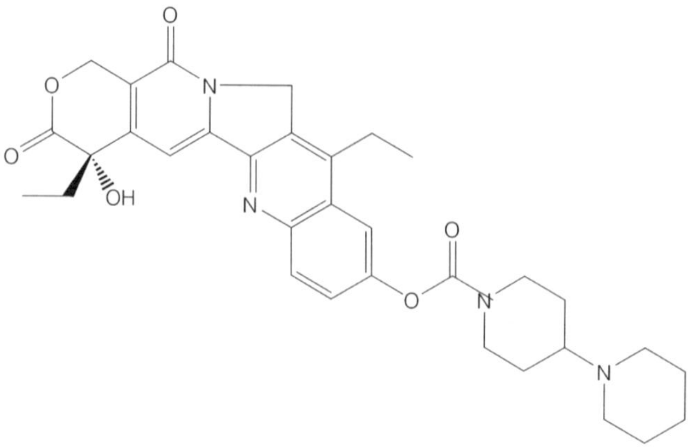

Irinotecan (Campto®)

A possible source for chemotherapeutic agents is the medicinal flora of the Asia–Pacific region. The purpose of this chapter is to provide a fundamental approach to understanding the potential of the medicinal flora of this region as a source of new anticancer drugs.

TOPOISOMERASE INHIBITORS

Topoisomerases temporarily break DNA strands and perform topological changes to selected regions of the genome available for transcription. Two main classes of topoisomerases are recognized to date: topoisomerases I and II. Topoisomerase I catalyzes the ATP-independent relaxation of DNA supercoils by transiently breaking and religating single-stranded DNA. Topoisomerase II relaxes supercoiled DNA through catalysis of a transient breakage of double-stranded DNA in an ATP-dependent manner. Examples of topoisomerase inhibitors are etoposide and camptothecin, which form a stable ternary DNA–topoisomerase II drug complex that maintains a cleaved state of DNA and interferes with DNA replication, repair, and transcription of eukaryotic cells (Fig. 80).

Medicinal Annonaceae

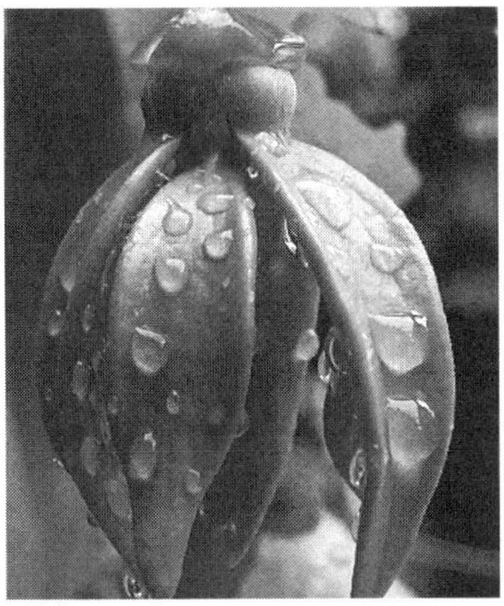

The evidence for the existence of anticancer agents in the family Annonaceae is strong and it seems likely that further research on this taxa will lead to the discovery of antineoplastic agents. Among the families of flowering plants, Annonaceae are particularly interesting in the field of oncology because this family elaborates a surprisingly broad array of secondary metabolites, which abrogate the survival of mammalian cells, including acetogenins, styryl-lactones, and isoquinoline alkaloids.

Sung et al. made the interesting observation that liriodenine, an aporphine isolated from Cananga odorata inhibited the enzymatic activity of topoisomerase II both in vivo and in vitro and caused highly catenated simian virus 40 daughter chromosomes in simian virus 40-infected CV-1 cells (1). Aporphine alkaloids from Annonaceae, but also the Magnoliidae in general, are likely to have potential as inhibitors of topoisomerase, and further investigation of flowering plants, and especially the medicinal Annonaceae of the Asia–Pacific region, as a source of cytotoxic aporphoids is encouaged.

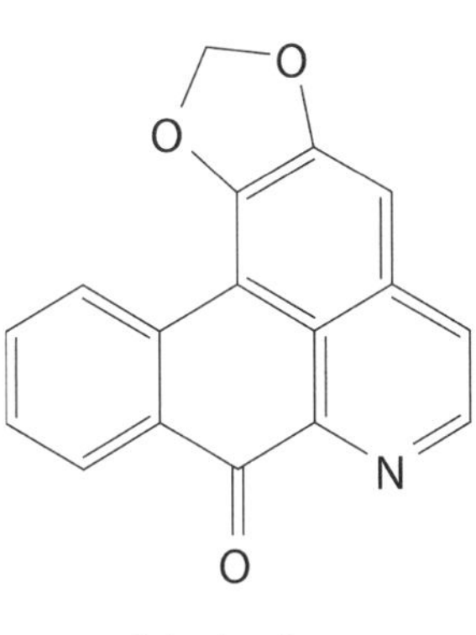

liriodenine

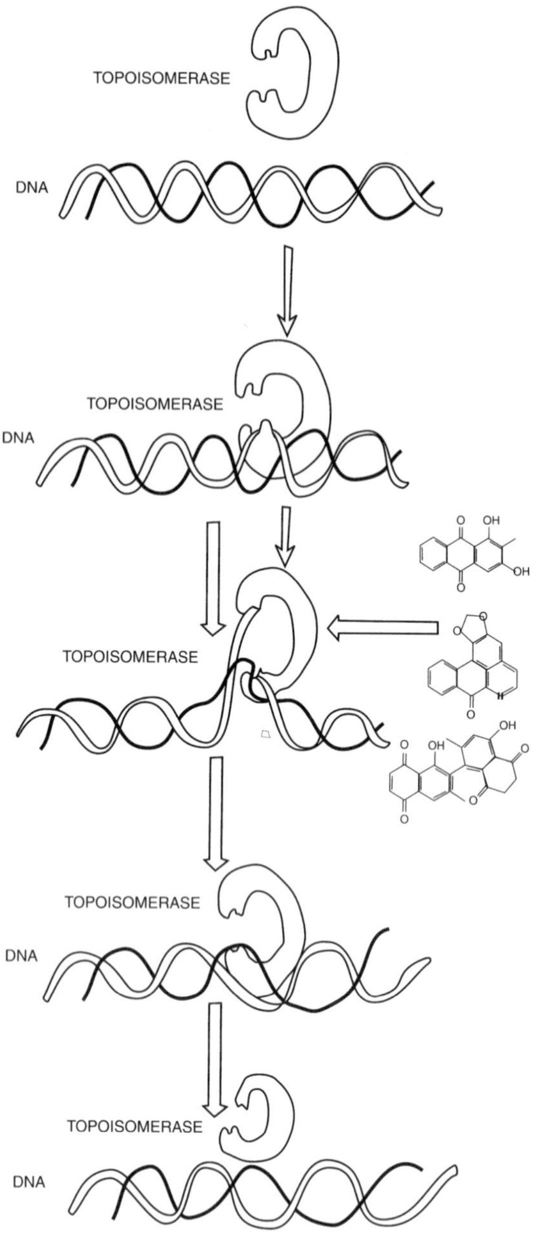

Fig. 80. DNA damage induced by inhibition of topoisomerase II.

Artabotrys suaveolens Bl., or *akar cenana* (Malay), is a woody climber that grows in the primary rainforest of Burma, Java, Moluccas, and the Philippines. The bark is blackish and smooth, and the twigs are hooked. The leaves are simple, alternate, dark green, glossy, elliptic, and 8.5 × 3.5 cm–5 × 3 cm. The fruits are green, glossy, and ellipsoid (1.4 cm × 5 mm), with ripe carpels, each containing a single seed. Indonesians drink a decoction of the leaves to treat cholera. In the Philippines, decoction of bark and roots is drunk to promote menses and to relieve childbirth exhaustion.

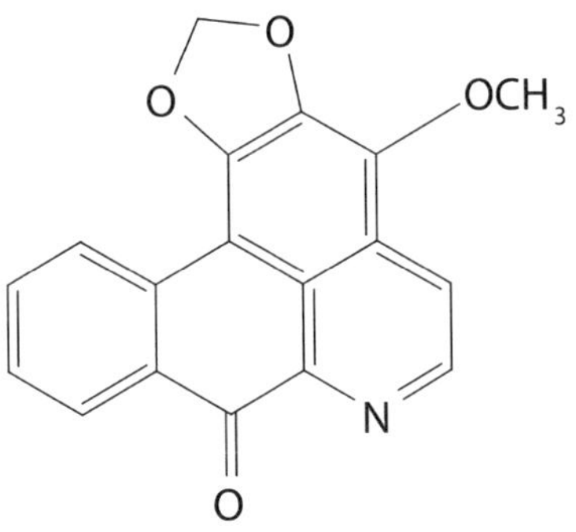

Atherospermidine

The potential properties of A. *suaveolens* Bl. has a source of topoisomerase II inhibitor is open for exploration. The plant probably elaborates aporphine alkaloids because aporphines are known to occur in the genus *Artabotrys* (2,3). Liriodenine and atherospermidine from *Artabotrys uncinatus* and artabotrine from *Artabotrys zeylanicus* abrogated the survival of cancer cells cultured in vitro (4).

Fissistigma fulgens **(Hk. f. et Th.) Merr.** (*Melodorum fulgens* Hk. f. et Th, *Uvaria fulgens* Wall.), or *pisang hutan* (Malay), is a large climber that grows in the primary rain forest of south peninsular Malaysia. The plant is easily recognized by the shining leaves with minute adpressed, tawny pubescence on the lower surface of the leaves. The stems are terete and pubescent. The leaves are simple, alternate, and exstipulate. The blade is oblong lanceolate, 7.5–15 cm × 3–5 cm, acute, the base is rounded. The blade shows 13–18 pairs of secondary nerves running out to the margin. The petiole is 7–10 mm long. The flowers have a slight sweet odor, and are terminal in a few flowered cymes. The flower pedicels are 5–10 mm long. The sepals are broadly ovate, pubescent outside, and 1–2 mm long. The petals are thick and orange; the outer petals are ovate-oblong and 1.2–1.5 cm long, and the inner petals are 7 mm long. The fruits are ripe carpels, 3–4 cm long, and 2.3 cm in diameter (Fig. 81).

In Malaysia, a paste of leaves is applied to sore legs, and a decoction of the leaves is drunk as a protective remedy given after childbirth. To date, the pharmacological potential of *F. fulgens* (Hk. f. et Th.) Merr. is unexplored. It would be interesting to learn whether further study on this medicinal plant disclose any aporphines of chemotherapeutic interest.

Friesodielsia latifolia **Hk. f. et Th.** (*Oxymitra latifolia* Hk. f. et Th.) is a climber that grows in the primary rain forest of Southeast Asia. The plant was present in Singapore in the Mac Ritchie Reservoir forest and the Botanic Garden's jungle. It is a climber that can grow to a length of 20 m. The young branches are rusty tomentose. The leaves are simple, alternate and exstipulate, and large. The blade is coriaceous,

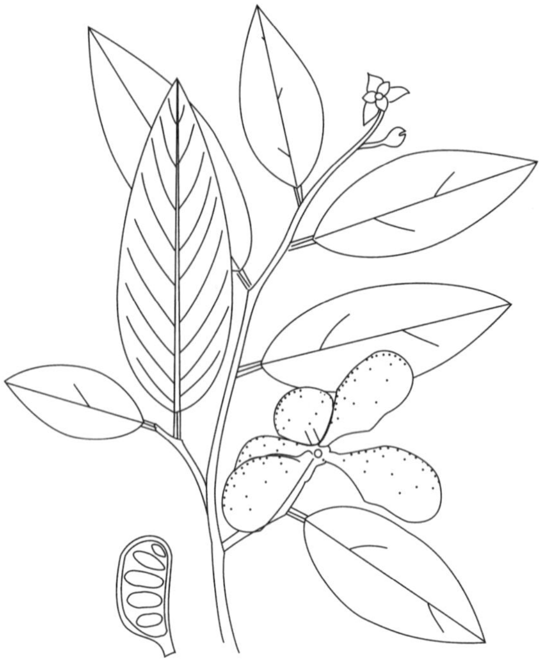

Fig. 81. *Fissistigma fulgens* (Hk. f. et Th.) Merr. Flora of Malaya. Herbarium Singapore. Field Collector: Mohd. Shah Mahmud. No 4996. Date: 7/21/1984. alt: 1200 feet. Terengganu.

dark green on top, glaucous on the bottom, glabrous (except for the midrib), glossy, broadly obovate, and 18 × 7.5 cm. The blade shows 10 pairs of secondary nerves. The petiole is 1 cm long. The flowers are solitary on 1-cm-long pedicel. The sepals are coriaceous, sub-orbicular, rusty-pubescent, and 4 mm long. The petals are creamy white turning brown, 4 cm long, inner to 2.7 cm long. The fruits are ripe carpels of about 1.5 cm in length and 7 mm diameter, oblong-ovoid, apiculate, and slightly pubescent (Fig. 82).

The plant is used by Malays to assuage body pains, and a decoction of roots is drunk as a protective remedy after childbirth. The pharmacological properties of this plant are unknown, but it is very probable that it elaborates aporphines and flavonoids as characterized in *Oxymitra velutina* (*5*).

Medicinal Lauraceae

Taxonomically close to the Annonaceae, the Lauraceae family abounds with aporphinoid alkaloids. A remarkable advance in the search for topoisomerase inhibitors from Lauraceae has been provided by Woo et al. (*6*). Using DNA-unwinding assay and structural modeling, they showed that dicentrine can attain a relatively planar conformation and molecular bulk which allow it to occupy the active site of topoisomerase II which becomes inactive. The requirement of a suboptimal conformation to achieve DNA binding appears to make dicentrine less potent against topoisomerase II than the

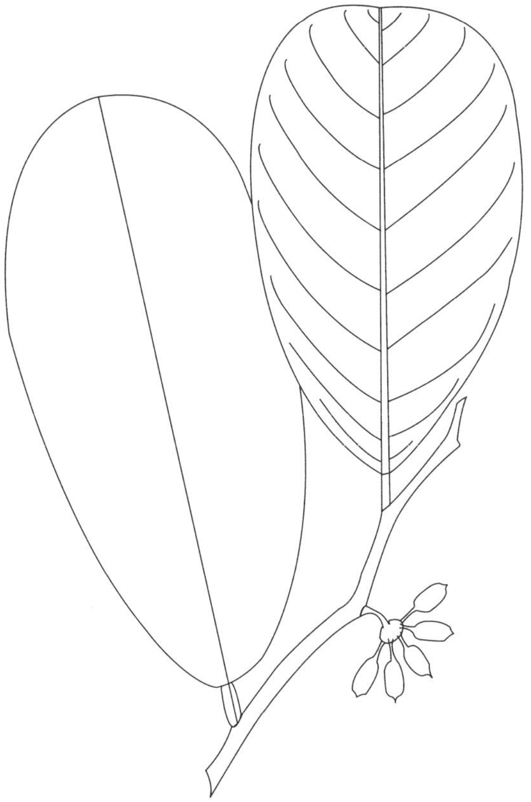

Fig. 82. *Friesodelsia latifolia*. Singapore Field No: 29434. The Botanic Gardens Singapore. 5/14/1935. Field collector: E. Corner. Botanical identification: J. Sinclair, 11/21/1953.

very planar oxoaporphine alkaloid liriodenine *(7)*. Other inhibitors of topoisomerase present in Lauraceae are diaryldimethylbutane lignans. Such compounds are found in *Persea thunbergii* (Sieb. & Zucc.) Kosterm.

***P. thunbergii* (Sieb. & Zucc.) Kosterm**. (*Machilus thunbergii* Sieb.& Zucc.), or common machilus, *tabunoki* (Japanese), is a tree native to Korea and Japan and is also found in Taiwan. The bark is smooth, fawn, and lenticelled. The leaves are spiral, simple, exstipulate-elliptic, glossy, and somewhat fleshy. In Japan and Korea, the plant affords a remedy for eczema, diseases of the spleen and stomach, and asthma.

Li et al. using bioassay-guided fractionation, isolated a number of diaryldimethylbutane lignans, of which meso-dihydroguaiaretic acid, which inhibited the enzymatic activity of topoisomerase I and II by 93.6 and 82.1%, respectively, and nectandrin B showed 79.1 and 34.3% inhibition, respectively, in vitro at a concentration of 100 mM *(8)*. Note that such lignans are present in the Myristicaceae, and one might set the hypothesis that lignans with potent topoisomerase inhibitors await discovery in the Laurales–Magnoliales group.

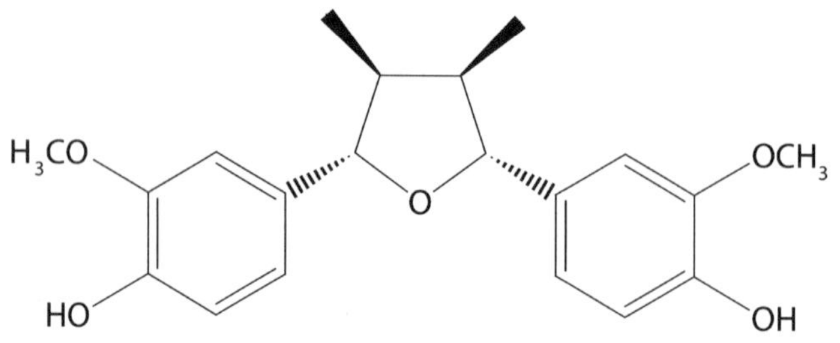

Diaryldimethylbutane lignans

Lindera tzumu Hemsl. (*Sassafras tzumu* [Hemsl.]) Hemsl, *Pseudosassafras tzumu* (Hemsl.) Lecte., *Pseudosassafras laxiflora* (Hemsl.) Nakai, *Lindera camphorata* Levl., or *cha mu, mu wang* (Chinese), is a tree that grows in China. The plant grows to 35 m tall and 2–5 m in diameter. The bark is yellow-green, smooth, and irregularly and longitudinally fissured. The wood is yellowish, finely grained, durable, and used for boat and furniture making. Leaves are simple, alternate, aggregate at apex of stems, and exstipulate. The blade is ovate or obovate and 9–18 × 6–10 cm. The fruits are subglobose, up to 10 mm in diameter, blackish-blue, and seated on a cup-shaped perianth. The wood of this tree is highly esteemed by the Chinese, who believe that a house built of this timber is never struck by lightning. The drug consists of the white inner bark, which is used as an anthelmintic, parasiticidal, antiseptic, anti-emetic, and antipyretic. The pharmacological potential of this plant is unexplored yet. Note that D-dicentrine, from the root of *Lindera megaphylla* Hemsl. abrogated the survival of a number of cancer cell lines cultured in vitro including esophageal carcinoma HCE-6, lymphoma cell lines Molt-4 and CESS, leukemia cell lines HL60 and K562, and hepatoma cell line MS-G2, and significantly inhibited the tumor incidence of leukemia cell line K562 in severe combined immunodeficient mice *(9)*.
The cytotoxic activity of dicentrine is mediated via inhibition of topoisomerase II *(6,7)*. Dicentrinone from *Ocotea leucoxylon* is closely related to dicentrine, and even more planar has shown potent topoisomerase I activity *(9)*.

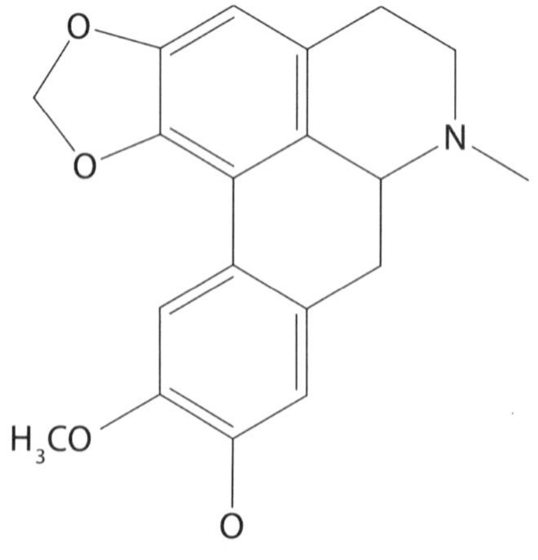

Dicentrine

***Cassytha filiformis* L.**, mentioned earlier, contains aporphine alkaloids such as actinodaphnine, cassythine, and dicentrine, which effectively bind to DNA and behave as typical intercalating agents and interfere with the catalytic activity of topoisomerases (*3,10,11*).

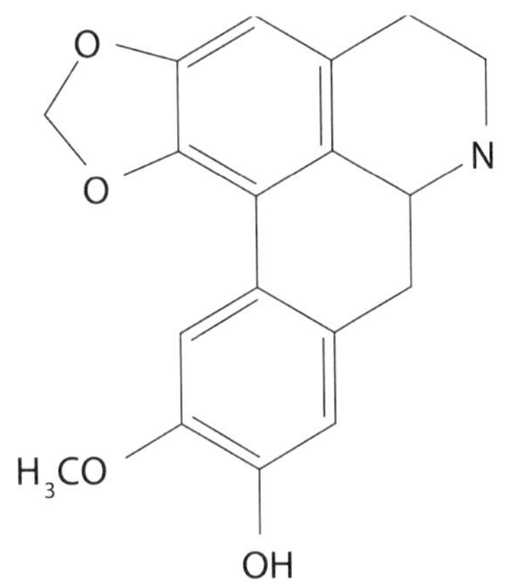

Actinodaphnine

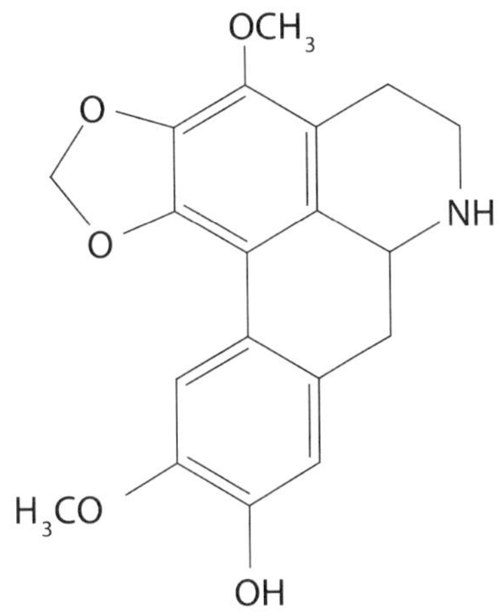

Cassythine

Medicinal Hernandiaceae

The family Hernandiaceae consists of four genera: *Hernandia*, *Illigera*, *Gyrocarpus*, and *Sparattanthelium*, and about 60 species of trees, shrubs, and woody climbers widespread in tropical regions. An example of Hernandiaceae is *Hernandia ovigera* L., which is grown as a tropical street tree. Hernandiaceae are member of the order Laurales and are known to abound with aporphines and lignans.

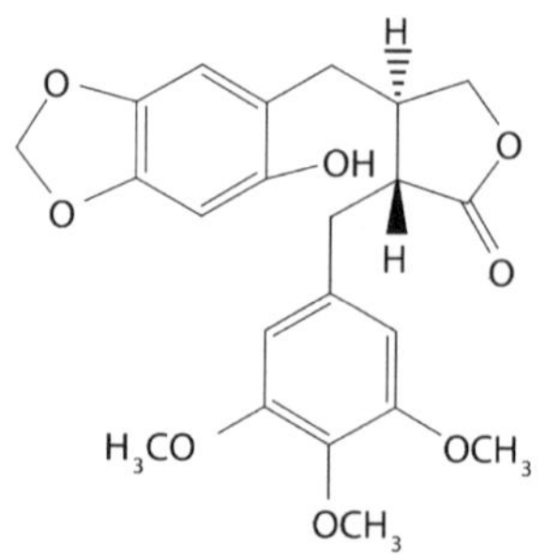

16-Hydroxyyatein

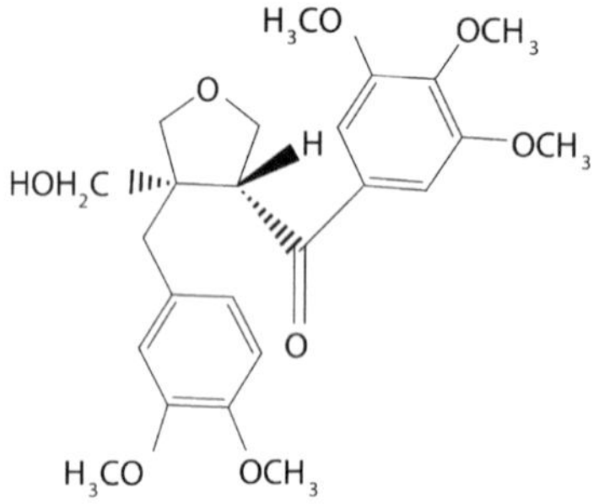

Hernone

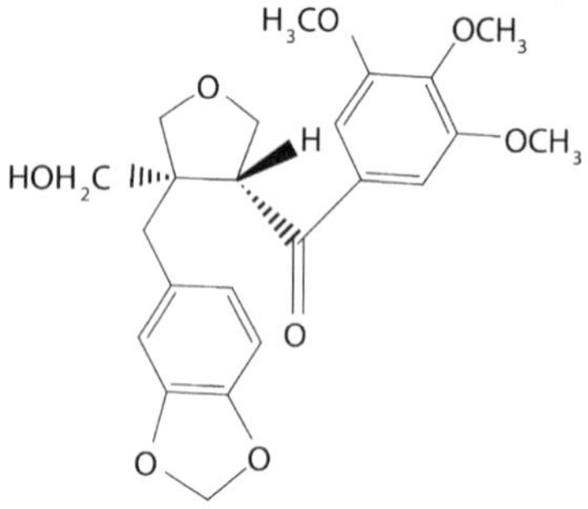

Nymphone

Lignans characterized from the bark of Hernandia nymphaeifolia: (2)-69-hydroxyyatein, (2)-hernone, and (2)-nymphone exhibited some levels of cytotoxic activities against P-388 and HT-29 cell lines with ED50 values of 0.321 and 0.740 mg/mL for (2)-nymphone; and 0.806 and 0.909 mg/mL for (2)-hernone (12). In the Asia–Pacific region, Illigera appendiculata Bl., Illigera luzonensis L., and H. ovigera L. (Hernandia peltata Meissn.) are medicinal.

***Illigera luzonensis* L.** (*Henschelia luzonensis* C. Presl., *I. luzonensis* (C. Presl.) Merr., *Henschelia luzonensis* C. Presl., *Gronovia ternata* Blanco, *Halesia ternata* Blanco, *Illigera meyeniana* Kunth ex Walpers, *Illigera pubescens* Merr., *Iligera ternata* [Blanco] Dunn.), or *tai wan qing teng* (Chinese), is a climber that grows in Taiwan, Japan (Ryuku), and the Philippines. The stems are angular. The leaves are simple, compound, and spiral. The petiole is 4–10 cm long, rough, and hairy. The folioles are ovate, rounded at base, mucronate at apex, and somewhat pubescent. The influorescences are 7–15 cm axillary cymes. The fruits bear a pair of wings.

In the Philippines, the sap expressed from the stem is drunk to alleviate headache. Using antiplatelet aggregation as a guide to fractionation, Chen et al. isolated a series of aporphines including actinodaphnine, *N*-methylactinodaphnine, launobine, dicentrine, O-methylbulbocapnine, hernovine, bulbocapnine, and oxoaporphines; dicentrinone and liriodenine were isolated from the stems of *I. luzonensis (13)*.

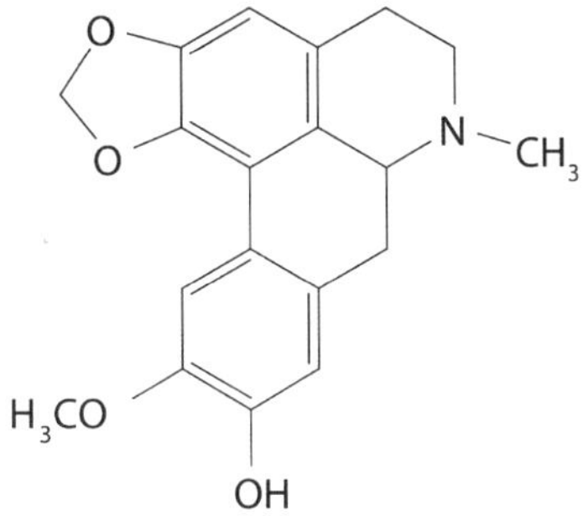

N-methyl-actinodaphnine

N-methyl-actinodaphnine possesses 5-hydroxytryptamine receptor blocking activity and a selective antagonist of α_1-adrenoceptors, selective for the α_{1B}- than for the α_{1A}-adrenoceptor subtype *(14)*. What are the activities of *N*-methyl-actinodaphnine and other aporphines of *Illigera* and *Hernandia* species against topoisomerase?

Medicinal Ebenaceae

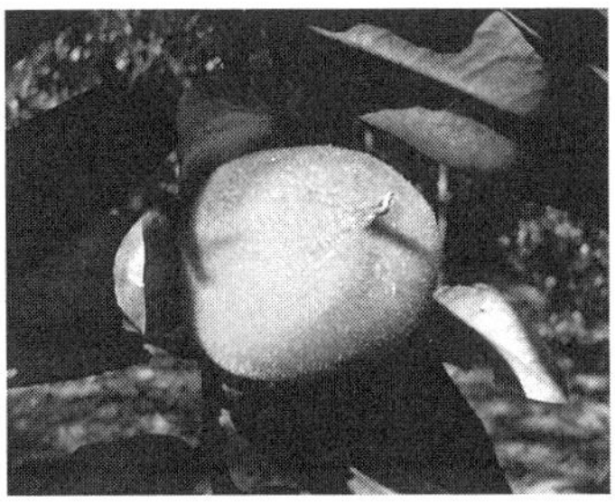

The family Ebenaceae consists of five genera and about 450 species of trees of which 20 species are used for medicinal purposes in the Asia–Pacific region. Ebenaceae and particularly *Diospyros* species have attracted a great deal of interest for their dimers and oligomers of naphthoquinones, which are antibacterial, antiviral, monoamine oxidase inhibitors, and cytotoxic. Ting et al. made the interesting observation that isodiospyrin is cytotoxic via direct binding topoisomerase I, which limits the access of the enzyme to the DNA substrate and prevents both DNA relaxation and kinase activities of topoisomerase I *(15)*. Therefore, an interesting development from Ebenaceae would be a systematic investigation of naphthoquinone for topoisomerase inhibition.

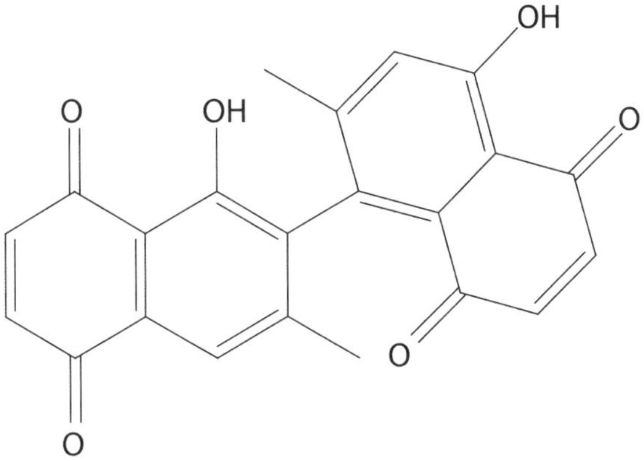

Isodiospyrin

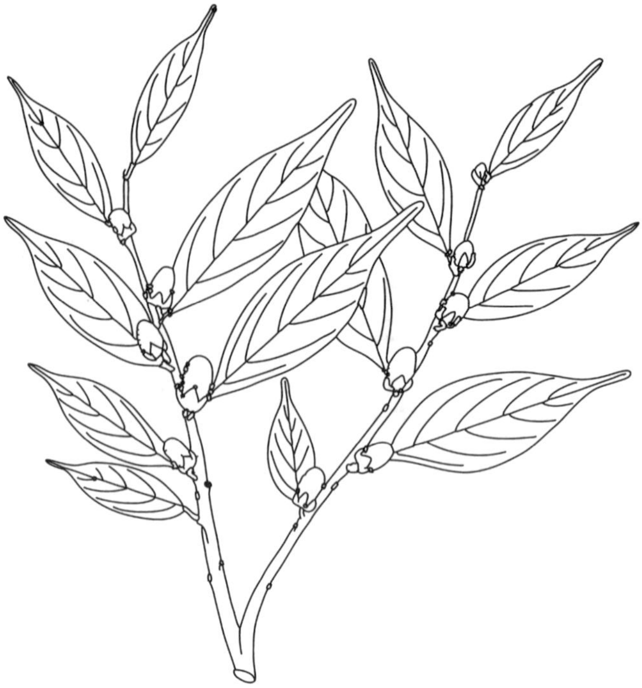

Fig. 83. *Diospyros sumatrana.* From Oxford University Department of Forestry. Forest Herbarium. T.D. Pennington. 9/11/1963. No: 7807. From: FRIM Kepong. No: 94504. Det: Ahmad.

***Diospyros sumatrana* Miq.** (*Diospyros flavicans* [Wall.] Hiern, *Diospyros dumosa* King & Gamble, *Diospyros decipiens* King & Gamble, *Diospyros tubicalyx* Ridl., *Diospyros vestita* Bakh., *Diospyros velutinosa* Bakh., *Diospyros hendersoni* Ridley.), is a tree that grows to a height of 30 m tall and a girth of 100 cm in Indonesia, Thailand, and Malaysia (Sabah, Borneo) in lowland rainforest up to 1500 m. The stems are hairy when young. The leaves are simple, elliptic, ovate, oblong, 3.5–20 × 1.2–6.5 cm, the apex is acuminate, the base is pointed, and the midrib sunken above. There are 3–11 pairs of secondary nerves. The male flowers are 5-merous in 3–10 flowered subsessile cymes, and show 16 anthers. The female flowers are four-merous, salver-shaped, and show a four-locular ovary. The fruits are globose, 1.2 × 2.4 cm, with a 2.5-cm diameter calyx (Fig. 83). Malays drink a decoction of roots as a protective remedy. The plant has not been studied for its pharmacological potentials.

***Diospyros toposioides* King & Gamble**, or *arang, kayu arang* (Malay), is a tree that grows to a height of 13 m and a girth of 60 cm in lowland rainforests of Malaysia (Borneo). The leaves are simple, oblong, oblong-ovate, 16–33 × 4–14 cm, the apex is acuminate, the base is rounded, and the midrib is sunken above; the secondary nerves are inconspicuous and loping at margin. The male flowers are in three-flowered axillary cymes and show 35–96 anthers. The female flowers are four-merous and show a eight-locular hairy ovary. The fruits are globose, 5 cm in diameter on a 3-cm-wide calyx (Fig. 84). In

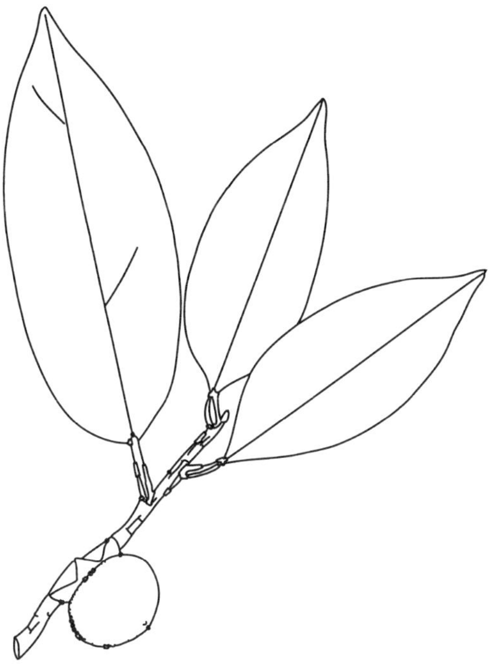

Fig. 84. *Diospyros toposioides.* Flora of Malaya. Field No 2417. Geographical localization: Chior, Perak. Field collector: 7/11/1967. K.M. Kochummen.

Malaysia, the seeds are poisonous and used to catch fish. The plant has not been studied for its pharmacological potentials. The ichthyotoxic property could involve some naphthoquinones and/or saponins.

Medicinal Rubiaceae

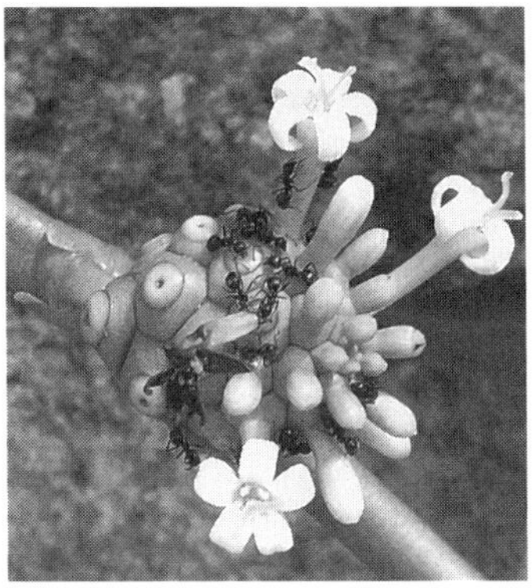

The family Rubiaceae consists of about 450 genera and 6500 species of tropical and subtropical trees, shrubs, climbers, and herbs that are known to abound with iridoid glycosides (monoterpenoid alkaloids, tannins, and anthraquinones). When looking for Rubiaceae in field collection, one is advised to look for plants with opposite simple leaves with an interpetiolar stipule, tubular flowers, which are often white, and capsules, berries, or drupes.

The contribution of Rubiaceae to Western pharmaceuticals and medicine is substantial because it is the source for *Uncaria gambier* (Hunt.) Roxb. (Catechu, *British Pharmaceutical Codex*, 1963), *Cephaëlis ipecacuanha* (Brot.) A. Rich. (*uragoga ipecacuanha*, Brazilian ipecacuanha), or *Cephaëlis acuminata* Karsten (*Cartagena ipecacuanha*) (Ipecacuanha, *British Pharmacopeia*, 1963), *Cinchona calisaya* (yellow cinchona bark), *Cinchona ledgeriana* (ledger bark), *Cinchona officinalis* (pale cinchona bark, crown or Loxa bark), and *Cinchona succirubra* (red cinchona bark) containing quinine. Classical examples of Rubiaceae are *Coffea arabica* (Arabica coffee), *Coffea liberica*, and *Coffea canephora* (Robusta coffee).

In regard to the antineoplastic potentials of Rubiaceae, some evidence has already been presented that clearly demonstrates that anthraquinones inhibit the enzymatic activity of topoisomerase II. An example of antineoplastic anthraquinones that target topoisomerase II is mitoxantrone (Novatrone®), which is currently approved for clinical use in the United States *(16)*. In the Pacific Rim, about 150 species of plants classified within the family Rubiaceae are medicinal, of which *Prismatomeris albidiflora*, *Knoxia valerianoides*, *Damnacanthus indicus*, and *Morinda umbellata* are known to produce anthraquinones. An interesting development from Rubiaceae would be to investigate its members for anthraquinones and assess them for topoisomerase inhibitors. The discovery of inhibitors of topoisomerase II of clinical antineoplastic value can be reasonably expected.

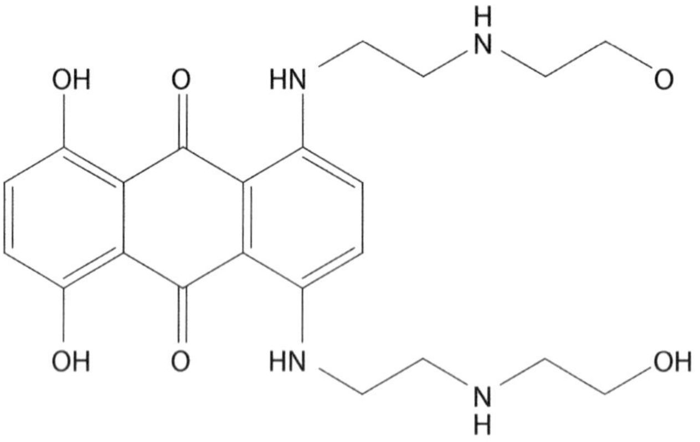

Mitoxantrone

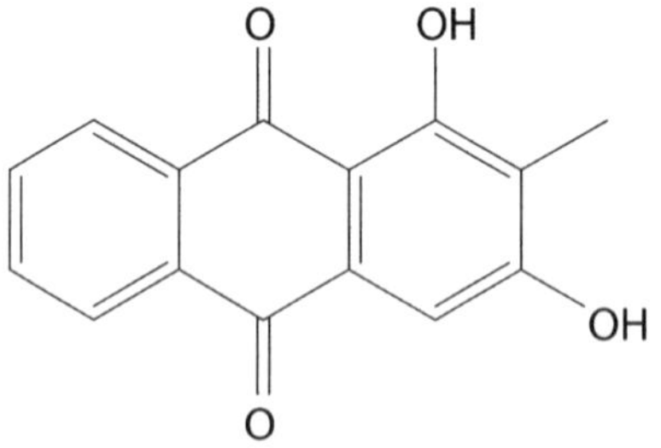

Anthraquinone

***Prismatomeris albiflora* Thaw, non King,** (*Prismatomeris tetrandra* [Roxb.] K. Sch, *Prismatomeris malayana* Ridl, *Coffea tetrandra* Roxb.), or *son kraal, duck kai dam* (Thai), is a treelet that grows to a height of 3 m in the rainforest, on rocky seashores, and in limestone rocks of Vietnam, Burma, Thailand, and Malaysia. The stems show internodes with a median longitudinal ridge ending between each pair of petioles. The leaves are simple,

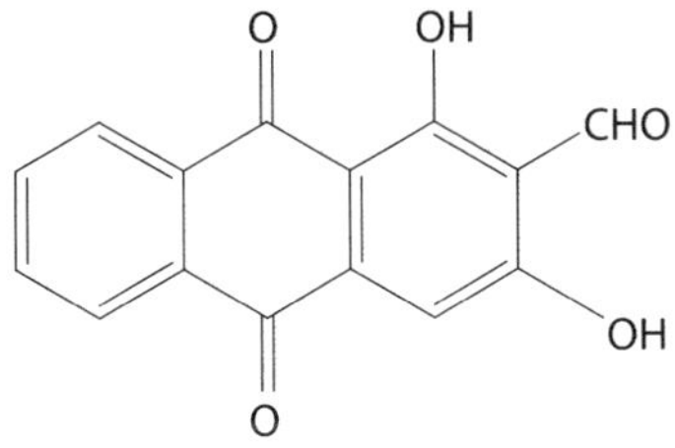

Nordamnacanthal

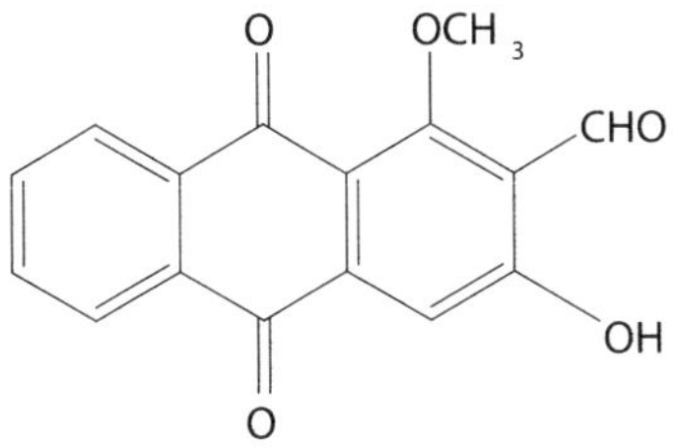

Damnacanthal

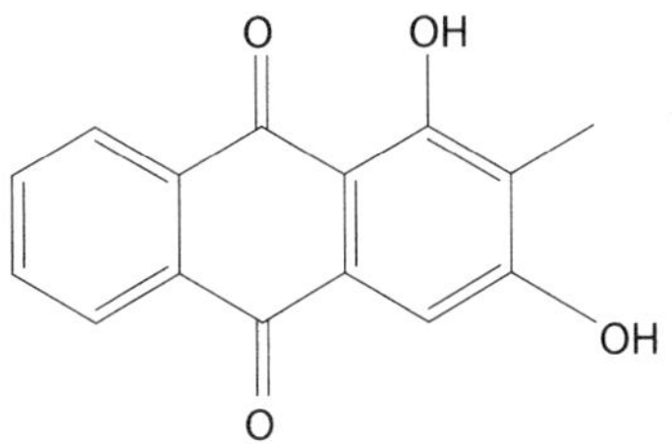

Rubiadin

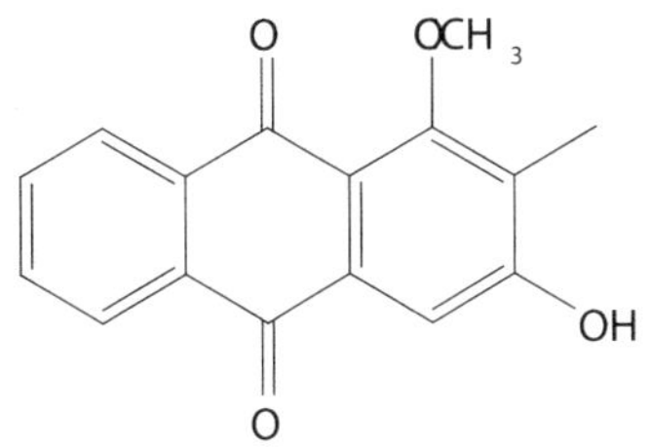

Rubiadin-1-methyl ether

Fig. 85. Cytotoxic anthraquinones of *Prismatomeris fragran.*

chartaceous decussate, and stipulate. The stipules are interpetiolar, triangular, and bifid at the apex. The blade is ovate and elliptic and shows 6–10 pairs of secondary and tertiary nerves. The influorescences are terminal and axillary clusters. The flower pedicels are 6 mm–2.1 cm long. The calyx cup is fringed. The corolla is white, tubular, and four- to five-lobed. The fruits are globose and contain one to two grooved seeds.

In Malaysia, a paste of the leaves is used to heal wounds. In Cambodia, Laos, and Vietnam, a decoction of roots is drunk to treat bronchitis, and an infusion of wood is drunk to invigorate and to expel impurities. Malays apply a paste of leaves to wounds to promote healing. The pharmacological potential of *P. tetrandra* (Roxb.) K. Schk is unexplored. Note that the plant is known to produce anthraquinones such as rubiadin *(17)*. Kanokmedhakul et al. made the interesting observation that the roots and stems of *Prismatomeris fragrans* contains a series of anthraquinones, of which nordamnacanthal, damnacanthal, rubiadin, and rubiadin-1-methyl ether abrogated the survival of exhibited cytotoxicity to the NCI-H187 cell line cultured in vitro *(18)*. It would be interesting to learn about the topoisomerase activity of these anthraquinones (Fig. 85).

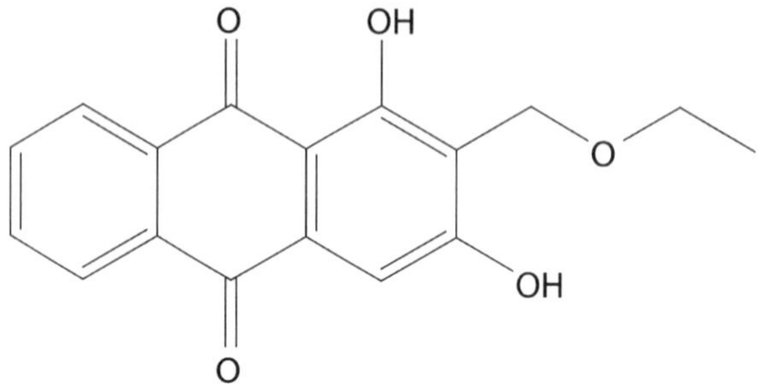

Ibericin

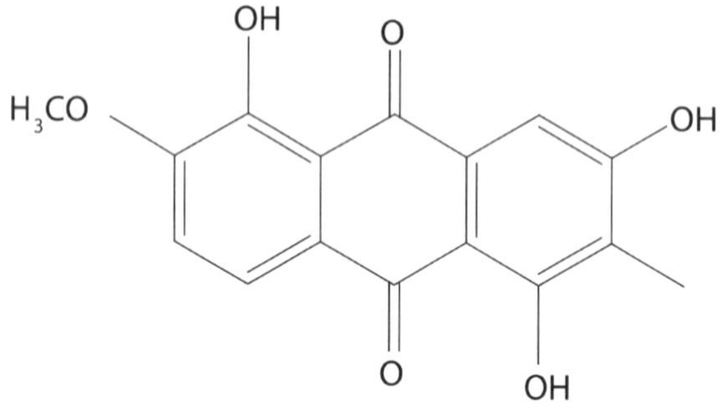

Knoxiadin

***Knoxia valerianoide* Thorel**, or knoxia root, Peking spurge root, or *Hung ya ta chi* (Chinese), is an herb that grows to a height of 60 cm in China, Cambodia, Laos, Vietnam, and North India. The roots are tuberous. The leaves are opposite and stipulate, and the blade is lanceolate and shows six to eight pairs of secondary nerves. The flowers are tubular, minute, and four-lobed (Fig. 86). In China, the plant is used to treat ailments related to excretion and to treat dropsy, but is not recommended during pregnancy. In Cambodia, Laos, and Vietnam, it is used to promote the fermentation of alcohol of rice.

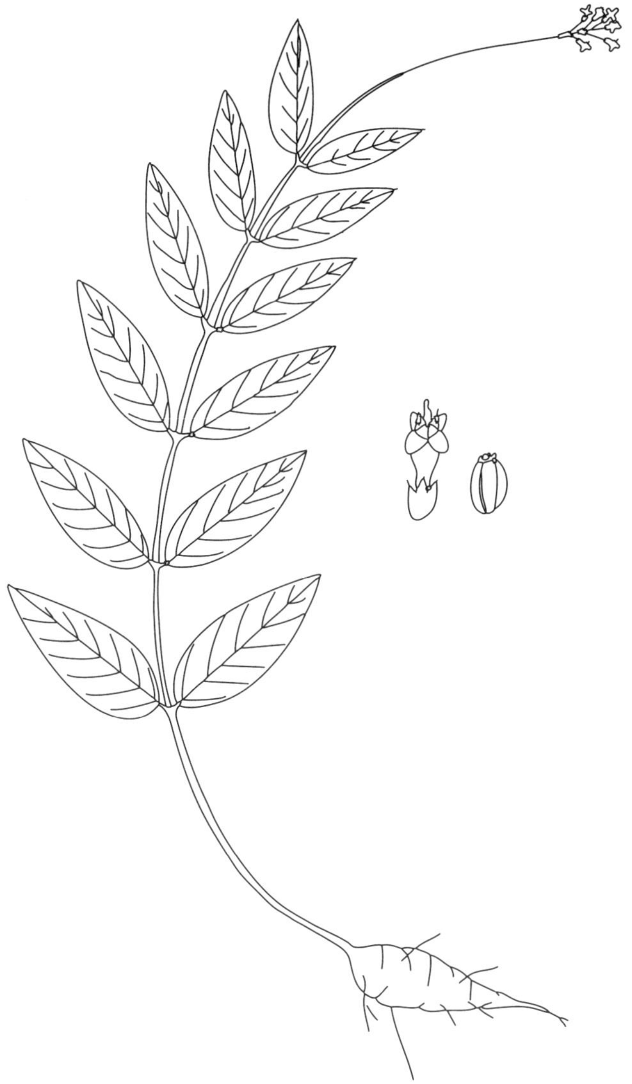

Fig. 86. *Knoxia valerianoide* Thorel.

The pharmacological property of *K. valerianoides* Thorel. is unexplored, but the plant is known to produce anthraquinones including 2-ethoxymethylknoxiavaledin, 2-formylknoxiavaledin, 2-hydroxymethylknoxiavaledin, knoxiadin, damnacanthal, nordamnacanthal;, ibericin, 3-methylalizarin, and damnacanthol *(19)*.

***D. indicus* Gaertn.** is a little shrub that grows in a geographical zone spanning from the Himalayas, North India, China, Japan, and the Philippines. The stems are terete, minutely hairy, and develop slender, interpetiolar, stipular woody thorns. The leaves are opposite and simple. The blades are broadly lanceolate, thick, dark green and glossy above, and light green below. The base of the blade is cordate and the apex is apiculate.

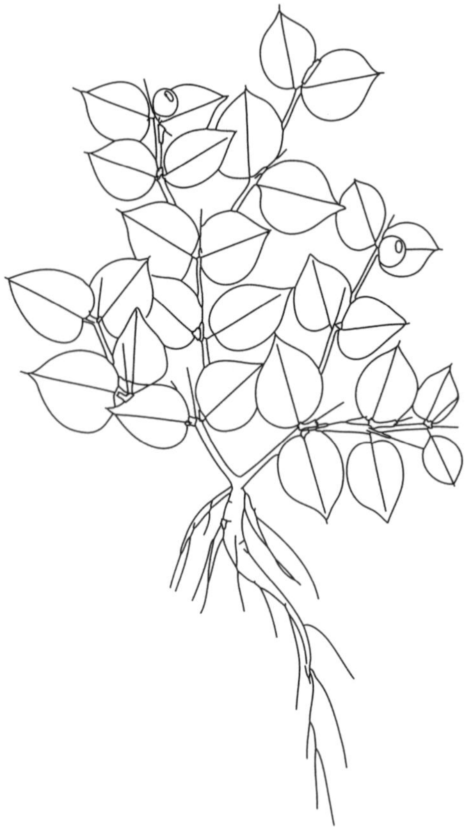

Fig. 87. *Damnacanthus indicus* Gaertn.

The flowers are white and in pairs. The fruits are red berries at axil of leaves (Fig. 87). In China, it is used to treat rheumatism, mitigate headache, and heal piles.
D. indicus Gaertn. is known to abound with anthraquinones, but its pharmacological potential remains unexplored to date *(20,21)*. Note that damnacanthal is a common component of the *Damnacanthus* species. Faltynek et al. made the interesting observation that damnacanthal inhibits the enzymatic activity of tyrosine kinase, which is involved in the propagation of metastases *(22)*. An interesting development from this observation would be to assess the topoisomerase inhibitory activity of the *Damnacanthus* species, an activity that could be associated with tyrosine kinase inhibition, hence enormous chemotherapeutic potentials.
Neonauclea pallida (Reinw. ex Havil.) Bakh f. (*Nauclea pallida* Reinw. ex Havil, *Nauclea purpurascens* sensu K. & G., *Neonauclea calycina* sensu Corner.), or hooded bur-flower tree, *bengkal batu* (Malay, Indonesian), or *krathum khao* (Thai), is a bush that grows to 2 m tall in Burma, Thailand, the Andamans, Sumatra, Java, and Borneo. In Indonesia, the leaves are used externally to promote urination. The stem is glabrous. The leaves are simple, opposite, and stipulate. The blade is glabrous, chartaceous, 16 × 8 cm, with 8–12

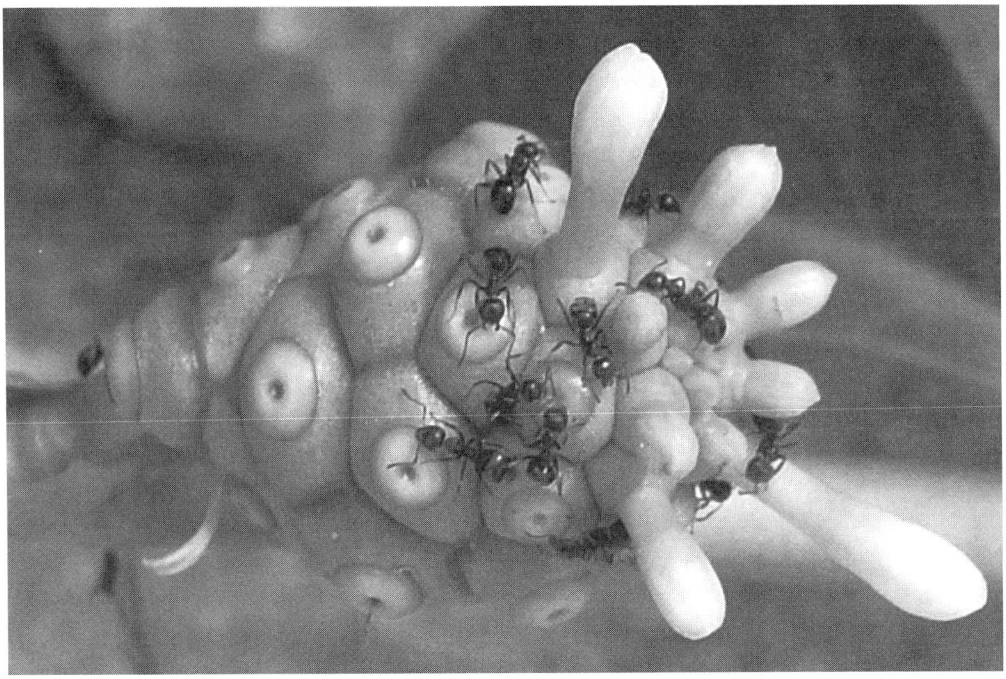

Fig. 88. Botanical hallmark of *Morinda* species: syncarps.

pairs of secondary nerves. Fruiting peduncle is axillary and terminal; the young flowering heads are enclosed in a pair of bracts. A wood extract of this plant afforded a series of anthraquinones including damnacanthal and morindone, which inhibited the enzymatic activity of topoisomerase II with IC_{50} values of 20 and 21 μg/mL, respectively *(21)*.

Morinda officinalis How, or *pa chi t'ien, ba ji tian, pa kit tian* (Chinese), *hagekiten* (Japanese), or *p'agukch'on* (Korean), is a shrub native to China, mainly the Guangdong, Guangsi, and southern Fujian provinces. Note that *Morinda* fruits are easily recognized syncarps (Fig. 88). The drug consists of the roots and is sweet and acrid in taste, fawn outside and moniliform, and purplish yellow-white inside. In China, the roots are used to treat beriberi, quiet the visceral organs, regulate urination, treat rheumatic conditions, fight sterility, and increase mental power. The roots should not be taken by pregnant or lactating women. The root of M. *officinalis* How. abounds with series of anthraquinones including rubiadin, rubiadin-1-methyl ether, 1-hydroxy- anthraquinone, 1-hydroxy-2-methylanthraquinone, 1,6-dihydroxy-2,4-dimethoxyanthraquinone, 1,6-dihydroxy-2-methoxyanthraquinone, 1-hydroxy-2- methoxyanthraquinone physcion, 2-methyl-anthraquinone, and damnacanthal *(21)*. Damnacanthal is widespread in *Morinda* species and known to inhibit the enzymatic activity of tyrosine kinase and topoisomerase *(22,23)*. Hiwasa et al. noted that human fibroblast UVr-1 cells treated with damnacanthal prior to ultraviolet irradiation presented more DNA fragmentation *(24)*. Using immunoblot analysis, they showed that pretreatment with damnacanthal followed by ultraviolet irradiation increased the levels of phosphorylated extracellular signal-regulated kinases and stress-activated protein kinases, suggesting a stimulation effect of damnacanthal on ultraviolet-induced apoptosis. In regard to the stimulant property mentioned above, it is interesting to mention that the plant extract (25–50 mg/kg) showed antidepressant properties in rats similar to clinically antidepressant drug desipramine (5–10 mg/kg *[25]*). This activity is, to date, believed to be mediated by oligosaccharides. Li et al. *(26,27)* showed that oligosaccharides (P_6) protected PC12 cells from corticosterone-induced apoptosis in a concentration- and time-dependent manner. Can we reasonably expect oligosaccharides to cross the hemato-encephalic barrier and act in the brain? Probably not.

Medicinal Rutaceae

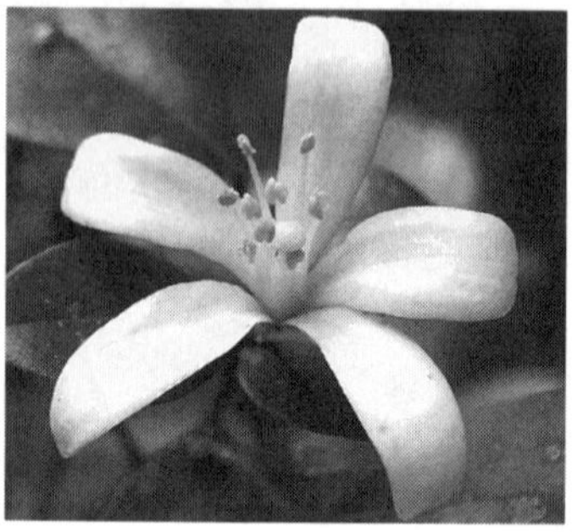

The family Rutaceae consists of 150 genera and 1500 species of treelets known to accumulate essential oils (limonene), limonoids, flavonoids (hesperidin), coumarins, and several sorts of alkaloids including, notably, carbazole and acridone alkaloids. The cardinal features to note in field collection are lemon-like aroma of crushed leaves, a blade dotted with several translucent oil glands, white flowers with retrorse petals and conspicuous globose and light green stigma, and green lemon-like fruits. The fruits of several species in this family are edible: lemon (*Citrus limon* [L.] Burm. f.), sour orange (*Citrus aurantium* L.), sweet orange (*Citrus sinensis* [L.] Osbeck), and lime (*Citrus aurantifolia* [Chaistm.] Swingle).

Western medicine has been using the essential oil of several species of Rutaceae as flavoring ingredient. The essential oil of C. *sinensis* (orange oil, *Oleum aurantii, British Pharmaceutical Codex*, 1963) has been used as a flavoring agent and in perfumery. Bergamot oil (*Oleum bergamottae, British Pharmaceutical Codex*, 1949) from *Citrus bergamia* has been used in perfumery in preparations for the hair (cologne spirit or *Spiritus coloniensis*), lemon oil (*Oleum limonis, British Pharmaceutical Codex*, 1963) from C. *limon, Citrus limonia*, and *Citrus medica* is carminative and used as a flavoring agent, and the dry peel of C. *aurantium* (*Aurantii cortex siccatus, British Pharmacopoeia*, 1963) has been used as a flavoring agent and for its bitter and carminative properties. The oil of *Ruta graveolens* L. (common rue, herb of grace) has been has been used to stop spasms, promote menses, and produce skin irritation (rue, *British Pharmaceutical Codex*, 1934).

Examples of alkaloid of relative pharmaceutical usefulness so far characterized from Rutaceae are pilocarpine from *Pilocarpus jaborandi* Holmes. This imidazole alkaloid is occasionally used to treat glaucoma.

In regard to the antineoplastic properties of Rutaceae, this family has attracted a great deal of interest for its ability to elaborate series of cytotoxic benzo[c]phenanthridine and acridin alkaloids. Examples of acridin alkaloid are pyrano-acridone and acronycine characterized from *Acronychia baueri* Scott.

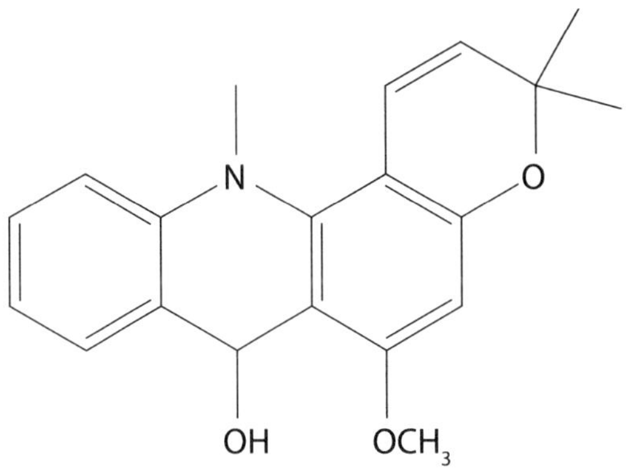

Acronycine

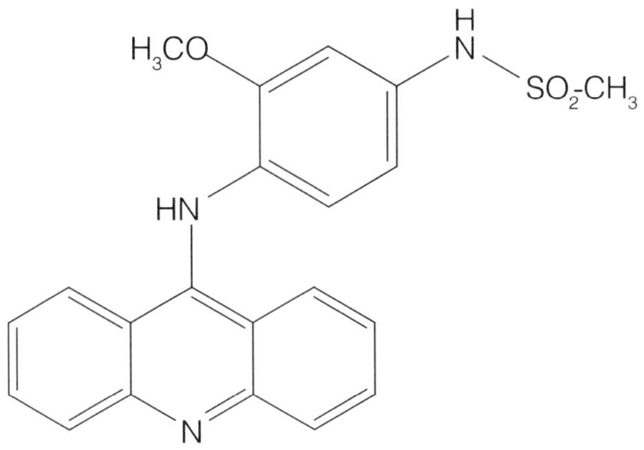

Amsacrine (Amsa P-D®)

Examples of acridin alkaloids used in therapeutics as antineoplastic agents is amsacrine (Amsa P-D®), which is used for the treatment of acute leukemia in adults and malignant lymphomas, refractory to conventional therapy. Amsacrin is an intercalating agent and topoisomerase II inhibitor.

One can reasonably envisage the family Rutaceae as a sockhouse of acridin-like alkaloids that await experimentation as inhibitors of topoisomerase and expect the discovery of antineoplastic agents of clinical value from this family. Looking for such agents, one might look into the medicinal Rutaceae of the Asia–Pacific region, which encompasses about 120 species of plants including *Zanthoxylum ailanthoides* Sieb. & Zucc, *Zanthoxylum bungei* Planch, *Zanthoxylum piperitum* (L.) DC, and *Zanthoxylum schinifolium* Sieb. & Zucc.

***Z. ailanthoides* Sieb. & Zucc.** (*Fagaras* [Sieb. & Zucc.] Engl.), or Japanese prickly ash; *karasuzanshou* (Japanese), *shih chu yii*, *yueh chiao*, or *la tzu* (Chinese), is deciduous small tree that grows to a height of 18 m in Japan, Korea, and China. The bark is grayish-brown

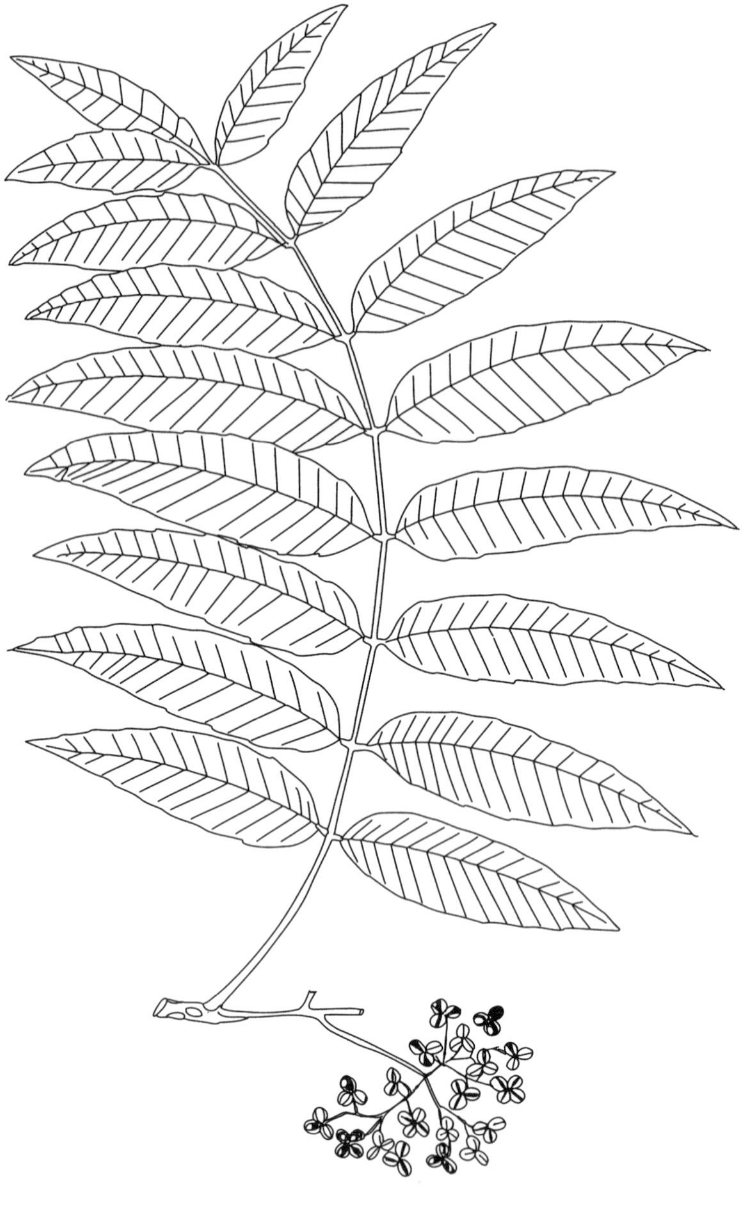

Fig. 89. *Zanthoxylum ailanthoides* Sieb. & Zucc.

and shows numerous small lenticels and is mottled with dark brown scars of thorns. The leaves are alternate, thick, and odd-pinnate. The folioles are linear-lanceolate, somewhat crenate, and show about 15 pairs of secondary nerves. The fruits are follicles, by three that open to show glossy black seeds of 5–8 mm in diameter (Fig. 89).
The follicles are green, pungent, and used as pepper. The fruits are eaten to promote digestion, as tonic, to counteract poisoning, treat sunstroke, diarrhoea, leucorrhea, and

dysentry. An infusion of leaves is drunk to treat chills and flux. The pharmacological property of this plant is as-yet unexplored. Note that the *Zanthoxylum* species are known to elaborate fagaronine and congener.

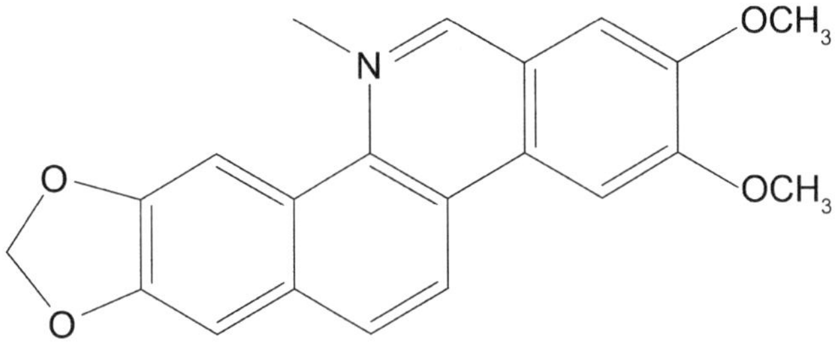

Nitidine

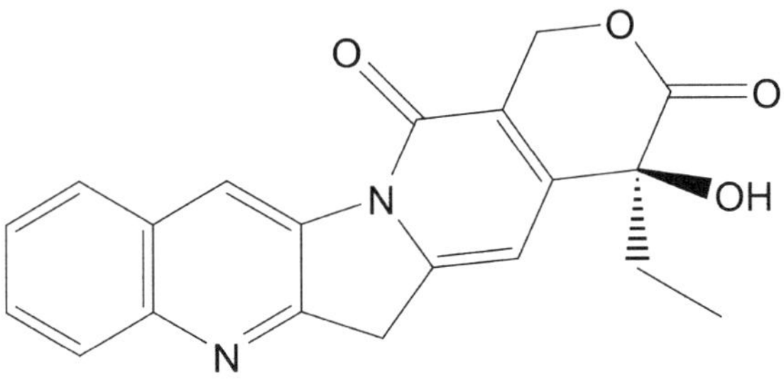

Camptothecin

Fagaronine and nitidine from *Zanthoxylum* species represent two of the more potent antitumor benzo[c]phenanthridines of Rutaceae. Both of these alkaloids have been shown to inhibit the enzymatic activity of topoisomerase in a way similar to camptothecin *(28,29)*. It would be interesting to learn whether further study on *Z. ailanthoides* Sieb. & Zucc. discloses any benzo[c]phenanthridine alkaloid of antineoplastic value.

Zanthoxylum bungei Planch. (*Zanthoxylum simulans* Hance.), or Szechuan pepper, Chinese pepper, Szechuan peppercorn, Sichuan pepper, Chinese prickly ash, *jiao mu ch'in chiao, ta chiao, hua chiao, chuan jiao* (Chinese), *sokusho* (japanese), or *ch'onch'o* (Korean), is a deciduous shrub growing to 6 m tall. The plant is native to China and Taiwan. The bark shows stout, woody, horizontal thorns. The leaves are compound-spiral and exstipulate. The blade comprises three pairs of folioles plus a terminal one. The lateral folioles are broadly elliptic, crenate, punctured with numerous oil translucent oil cells, and show four to five pairs of secondary nerves. The rachis is minutely winged. The fruits consist of 3–4-mm reddish-brown tuberculate follicles that are split open to show a black seed (Fig. 90).

The drug consists of the small, red tuberculate follicles enclosing black, round glossy seeds, which are aromatic, pungent, with a somewhat acrid aftertaste. It is a carminative and a stimulant, it promotes sweating, is an emmenagogue, astringent, and an

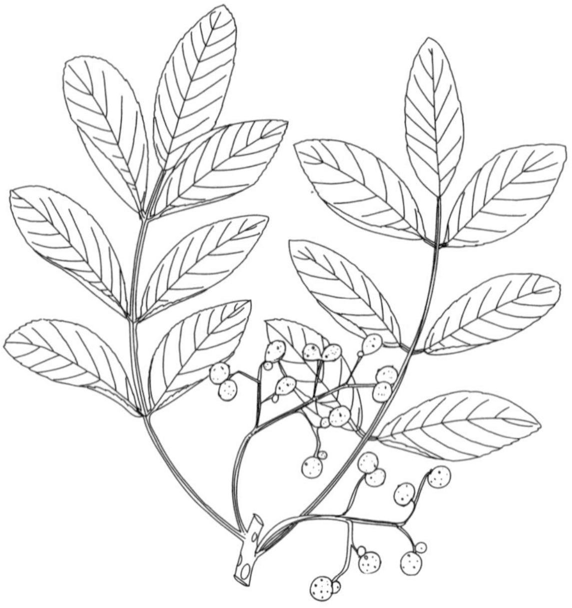

Fig. 90. *Zanthoxylum bungei* Planch.

anthelmintic, and is used as a condiment of high value for vital process. An infusion of carpels in vinegar is instilled in ears to remove insects or worms.

The plant is known to contain chelerythrine chloride, which inhibits the aggregation of rabbit platelet in vitro via inhibition on thromboxane formation and phosphoinositides breakdown *(30)*. Chelerythrine, which occurs in members of the family Papaveraceae, has been reported to inhibit the enzymatic activity of protein kinase C and to exert cell-growth inhibitory effect via the induction of apoptosis in numerous cancer cell lines *(31,32)*. What is the topoisomerase activity of chelerythrine?

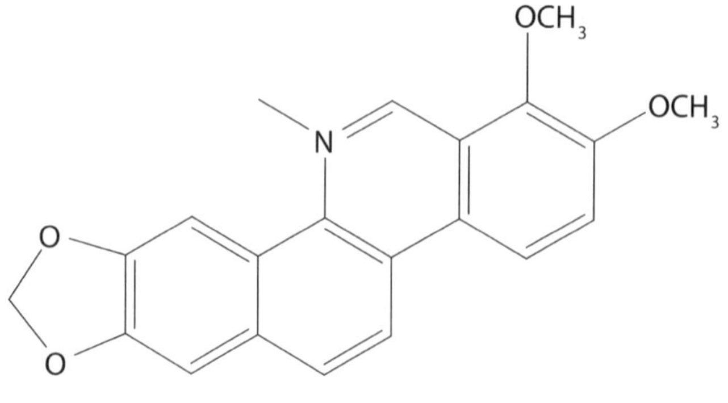

Chelerythrine

Zanthoxylum piperitum (L.) DC., or Japanese peppercorn, Japanese pepper tree, Sichuan pepper, *hajikami*, *sanshou* (Japanese), *shu chiao*, *ch'uan chiao*, or *nan chiao*

(Chinese), is a spiny, deciduous, thorny shrub that grows to 3–4 m in height in China, Japan, and Korea. The leaves are compound, spiral, and exstipulate. The blade consists of six to seven pairs of folioles, which are thick and glossy, about 3–6 cm long, elliptic-ovate, resinous, fragrant, and crenate. The rachis is thorny. The fruits are 4 mm in diameter, on terminal panicles, bright red becoming purple when ripe, and split in two to free a single, black, glossy, seed that is pungent and tastes like lemon or ginger (Fig. 91). The drug consists of the dried follicles, which are used to stimulate digestion, malaria, dysentry, spermatorrhea, galactorrhea, excessive urination, and as a tonic. The carpels are used eternally to expel parasites. The seeds are eaten to promote urination, treat dropsy, invigorate kidneys and bladder, and treat asthma. The seeds are used in China and Japan as a substitute for pepper. The pharmacological potential of this plant is unexplored.

***Zanthoxylum schinifolium* Zieb. & Zucc.** (*Zanthoxylum schinnifolium*), or Korean pepper, *yai chiao* or *yeh chiah* (Chinese), is a tree that grows in China, Japan, and Korea. The trunk is armed with broad, fattened, woody, horizontally arranged thorns. The leaves are compound, spiral, and exstipulate. The blade shows three to five pairs of folioles. The folioles are lanceolate, asymmetrical, minutely serrate, and bright green. The flowers are minute and greenish-white in panicles. The fruits are pink and split to reveal a very aromatic gray and dull seed.

The follicles are used to treat asthma and cough and to mitigate painful swollen breasts. A paste of the leave is applied to contusion. Essential oil distilled from the follicles induced apoptotic death in HepG2 human hepatoma cells in a concentration- and time-related manner, and inhibited tumor development of mice inoculated with Huh-7 human hepatoma cells *(33)*.

Medicinal Euphorbiaceae

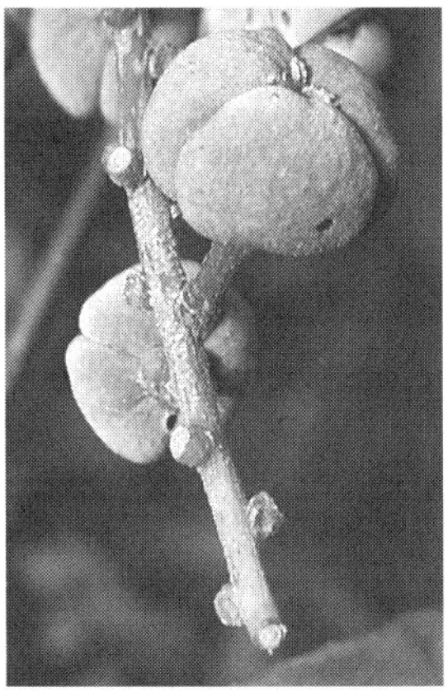

The family Euphorbiaceae contains 300 genera and about 7500 species of trees, shrubs, herbs, and climbers, about 150 species of which are of medicinal value in the Asia–Pacific region. Most of these are used to relieve the bowels from costiveness, promote urination, soothe inflammation, and promote expectoration. A cardinal feature of Euphorbiaceae, and especially *Excoecaria*, *Aleurites*, *Croton*, *Euphorbia*, *Hippomane*, *Hura*, and *Jatropha* species, is their ability to elaborate a series of complex diterpenoid esters of the tigliane, ingenane, or daphnane type, which impart drastic cathartics and ulcerating and and strongly allergizing properties. An example of such Euphorbiaceae is *Excoecaria oppositifolia*, the latex of which is a common cause of temporary blindness and anaphylactic shock in the lumberjacks of the Asia–Pacific region.

In regard to the antineoplastic potential, most of the evidence that has emerged from the last 30 years supports the fact that Euphorbiaceae represent a vast reservoir of cytotoxic agents, and one may reasonably expect the isolation of original anticancer agents from this family if enough work is done. A remarkable advance in the study of anticancer principles from Euphorbiaceae has been provided by Wada et al. *(34)*.

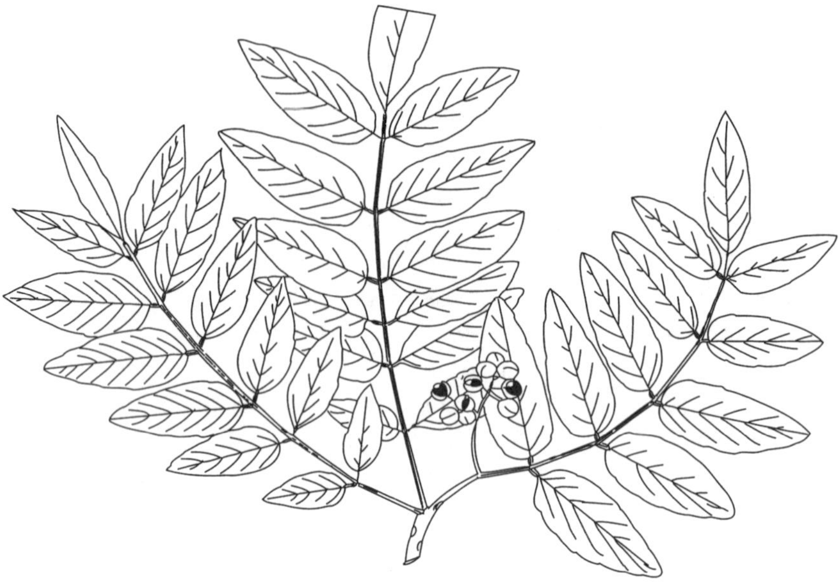

Fig. 91. *Zanthoxylum piperitum* (L.) DC.

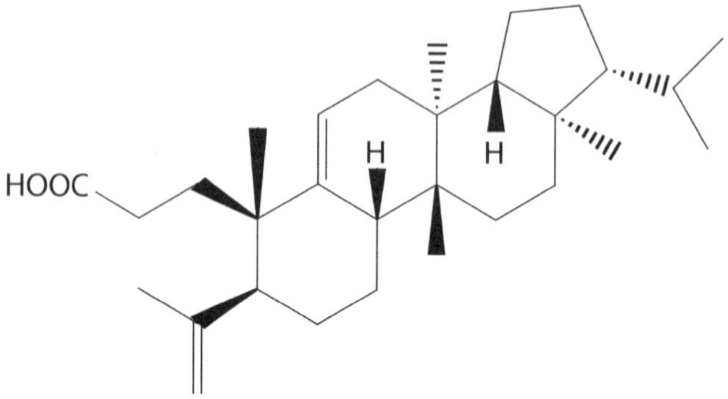

3,4-Seco-8βH-ferna-4(23),9(11)-dien-3-oic acid

3,4-Seco-8βH-ferna-4(23),9(11)-dien-3-oic acid completely inhibited the enzymatic activity of topoisomerase II at concentrations up to 25 μM dose-dependently and more potently that etoposide.

Alchornea villosa (Benth.) Muell.-Arg. is a small tree that grows to a height of 4 m in the primary rainforest of Malaysia. The stems are hairy when young and smooth. The leaves are simple, spiral, and stipulate; the stipules are linear and 5–7 mm long. The blade is hairy, lanceolate, membranaceous, 18.5 × 11.3 cm– 5 × 1.6 cm, and serrate. The fruits are capsular, bilobed, and show three stigmas at the apex that are 1.2–1.5 cm long (Fig. 92). In Malaysia, the plant is used as an antidote, and the leaves are used to calm itchiness of the skin. Indonesians have been known to drink the sap squeezed

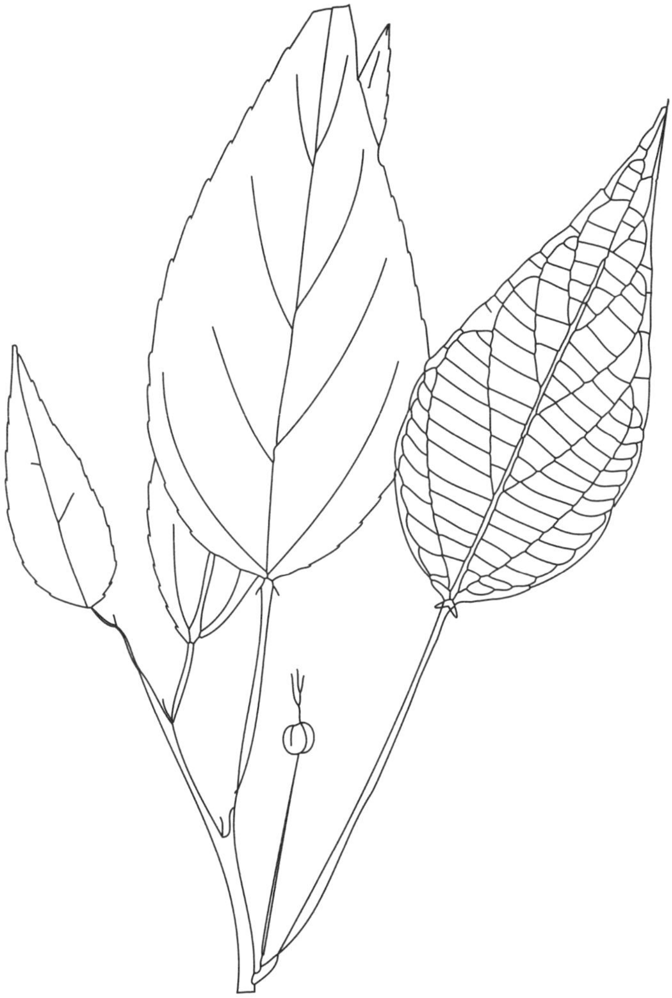

Fig. 92. *Alchornea villosa* (Benth.) Muell.-Arg. From KLU Herbarium 33970. Flora of Johore, West Malaysia. Comm. Ex. Herb. Hort. Bot. SING. Field collector & botanical identification: J.F. Maxwell. 4/10/1982. Geographical localization: Kota Tinggi Waterfalls.

from the young leaves to combat fever, and to apply a paste of leaves on the head to mitigate headaches and vertigo. The pharmacological and especially antineoplastic properties of *Alchornea villosa* (Benth.) Muell.-Arg. are, to date, unexplored. Note that seco-3,4 triterpenoids from the leaves of *Alchornea latifolia* are cytotoxic and inhibit topoisomerase II.

Seco-3,4-taraxerone and seco-3,4-friedelin 2 abrogated the survival of human hepatocellular carcinoma (Hep-G2) and human epidermoid carcinoma (A-431) cell lines cultured in vitro with IC_{50} values of 11.7 and 38.2 mM, and inhibited the enzymatic activity of topoisomerase at dose of 7 μM *(35)*.

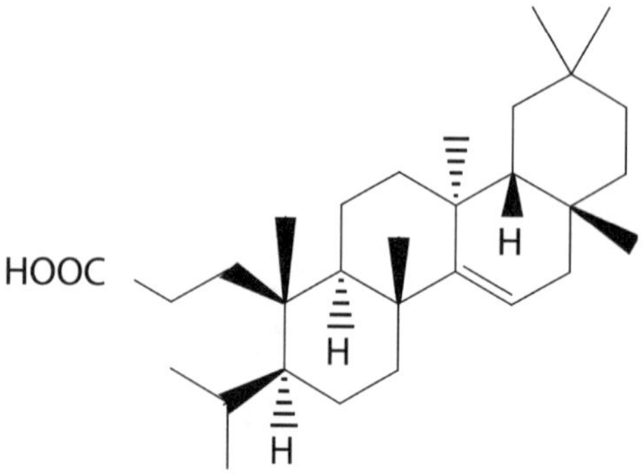

1 seco-3,4-Taraxerone

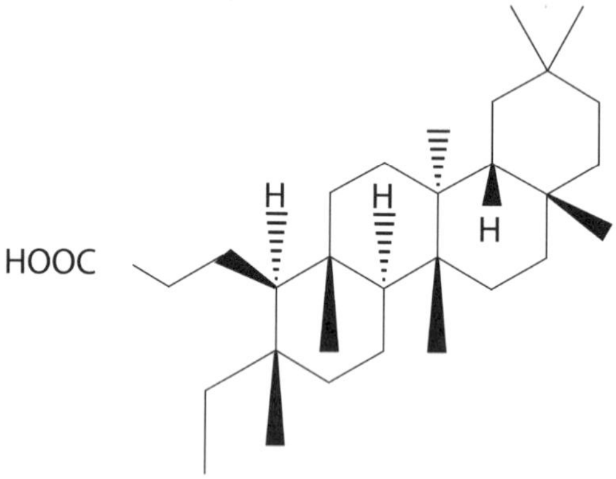

seco-3,4-Friedelin

Alchornea rugosa (Lour.) Muell. Arg (*Cladodes rugosa* Lour., *Alchornea hainanensis* Pax & K. Hoffm, *Alchornea javensis* [Endl. Ex Hassk.] M.A.) is a bush that grows up to 1.5 m tall in lowland rainforests of up to 300 m a geographical area spanning from South China, Indonesia, the Philippines, and Thailand. The leaves are simple and spiral. The blade is elliptic-lanceolate with a pair of stipels at base, hairy to scurfy below, and the margin is serrate. The fruits are up to 10 mm long. In Cambodia, Laos, and Vietnam, the seeds are eaten to relieve the bowels from costiveness. Malays use a decoction of roots and leaves to reduce fever and treat ague. The pharmacological potential of this plant is unexplored. It would be interesting to learn if further study of this plant discloses any triterpenoids of chemotherapeutic value.

Phyllanthus acidus (L.) Skeels (*Cicca acida* [L.] Merr, *Cicca disticha* L, *Phyllanthus distichus* Muell.-Arg.), or Malay gooseberry, wild plum, *mayom* (Thai), *cerme* (Indonesian), *cermai* (Malay), *thinbozihpyoo* (Burma), *kântûet* (Cambodia), *nhôm baanz* (Laos), and *chùm ruôt* (Vietnam), is a small tree that grows to a height of 9 m tall. The plant is thought to have originated in Madagascar and is now widespread in tropical Asia. The leaves are compound and consist of about 12 pairs of folioles

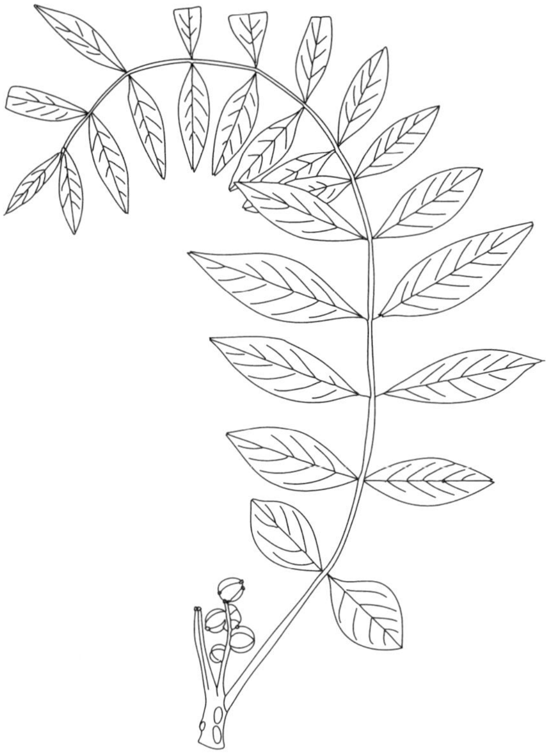

Fig. 93. *Phyllanthus acidus.* Forest Department herbarium, Brunei. Brun 5171. Geographical localization: kedayan, Cheramai. Jalan Muara, South Lumut. In old, secondary forest. 2/3/1959.

that are glaucous below and linear-lanceolate. The flowers are small, pinkish, and arranged in panicles up to 12 cm long. The fruits are cream colored, globose, six- to eight-lobed drupes of up to 2.5 cm in diameter that are palatable, apple-like in taste, sour, and containing four to six seeds (Fig. 93).

Burmese eat the fruits to promote appetite, and swallow the sap to induce vomiting and relieve the bowels from costiveness. In the Philippines, the leaves are used externally to calm itchiness, and a decoction of the bark is drunk to treat lung diseases. In Indonesia, the leaves are used as counter-irritant in sciatica and lumbago. In Malaysia, the vapors emitted when boiling the roots in water are inhaled to treat cough and headache.

The plant is known to produce norbisabolane diterpenes, including phyllanthusols A and B, which are both cytotoxic *(36)*. From the bark, pentacyclic triterpenoids, phyllanthol, and olean-12en-3β-ol (β-amyrin) have been isolated *(37)*. Note lupane- and oleanane-type triterpenoids isolated from the bark of *Phyllanthus flexuosus*, such as olean-12-en-3 β,15 α-diol, olean-12-en-3 β,15 α,24-triol, lupeol, and betulin inhibited the enzymatic activity of topoisomerase II activity with IC_{50} values in the range of 10 to 39 μM *(38)*.

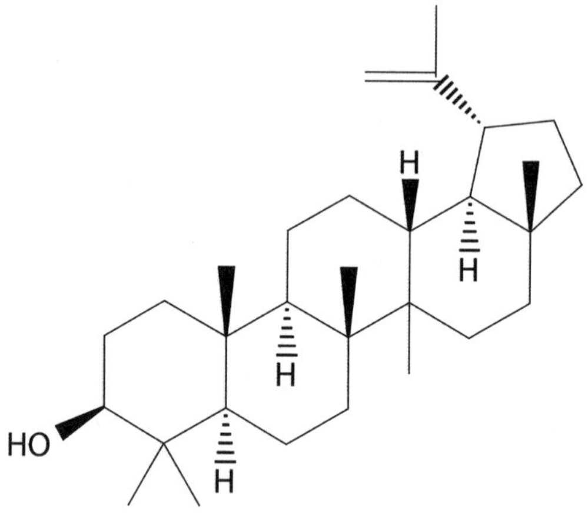

Lupeol

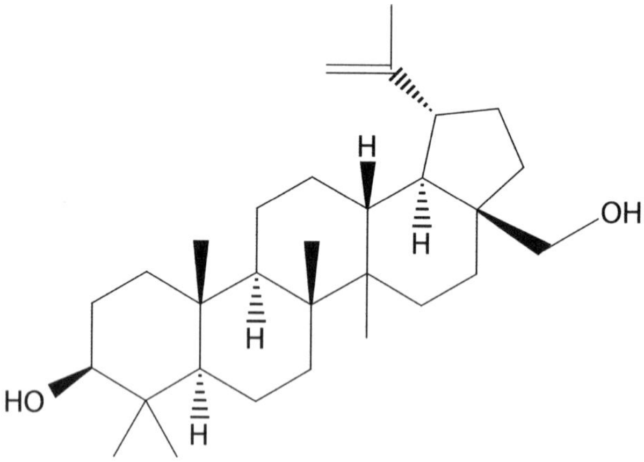

Betulin

Although the precise molecular mechanism of plant triterpenoids on topoisomerase II remains elusive, accumulated experimental evidence indicates that plant triterpenoids represent a vast potential source of antineoplastic agents. An interesting development from these results would be a massive survey of plant triterpenoids as source of topoisomerase inhibitors. Also, one might have noticed that plant triterpenoids have an affinity to phospholipase. Martelli et al. observed that during apoptosis, a phospholipase D-mediated signaling pathway operating at the nuclear level is elicited and may represent an attractive therapeutic target for the modulation of apoptotic events in human disease *(39)*.

***Macaranga triloba* (Reinw.) Muell.-Arg.**, or *mahong merah* (Malay), is a treelet that grows wild to a height of 6 m in Malaysia, Burma, Thailand in secondary forests, often gregarious, gaps, and river valleys in primary forests. The stems are hollow with ants ribbed and constricted. The leaves are simple, spiral, and stipulate. The stipules are leathery and persistent. The blades are lobed, membranaceous, with scattered yellow granular glands and conspicuous nerves below (Fig. 94).

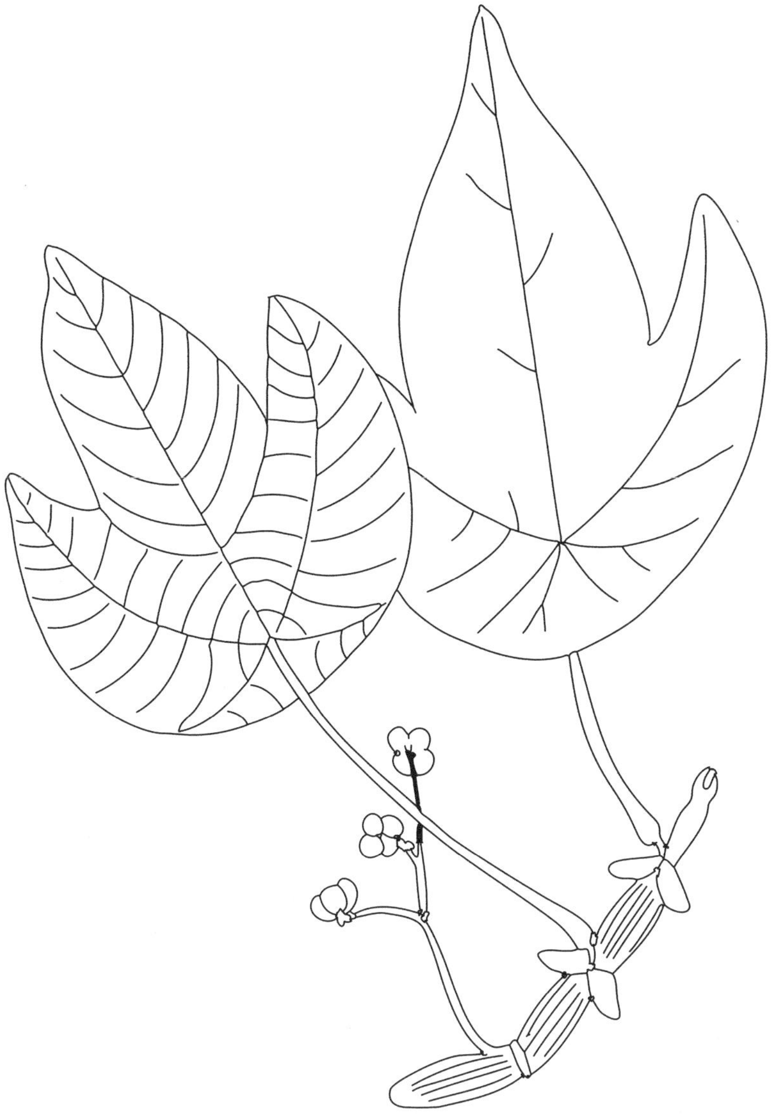

Fig. 94. *Macaranga triloba.* Flora of Malaya. FRI main road side, Kepong. Field collector: Matr. Asri.

In Malaysia, the leaves are used externally to heal boils. In Indonesia, a decoction of fruits and leaves is drunk to mitigate stomachache. The fruits are poisonous.
Activity-guided fractionation of the leaves of *Macaranga triloba* (Reinw.) Muell.-Arg. using an in vitro bioassay based on the inhibition of cyclooxygenase-2, resulted in the isolation of flavonoids, triterpenes, and of 4,5-dihydro-5′α-hydroxy-4′α-methoxy-6α,12α-dehydro-α-toxicarol *(40)*. The inhibition of cyclooxygenase 2 as an important mechanism for cancer chemoprevention has been supported by epidemiological and experimental evidence notably reported by Dannenberg et al. *(41)*.

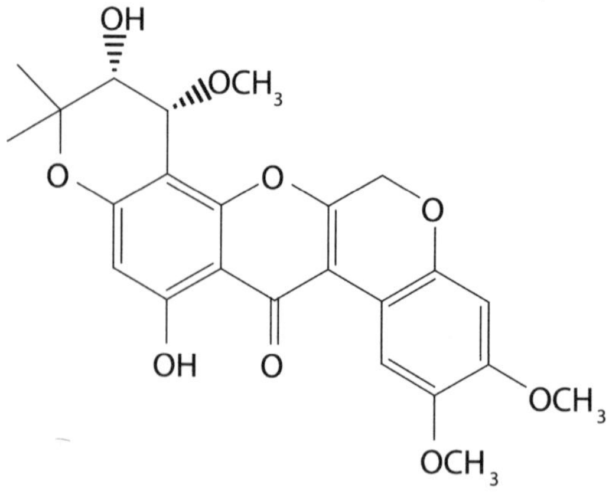

4,5-dihydro-5'α-hydroxy-4' α -methoxy-6 α,
12 α -dehydro- α -toxicarol

It would be interesting to learn whether 4,5-dihydro-5′α-hydroxy-4′α-methoxy-6α,12α-dehydro-α-toxicarol interferes with the enzymatic activity of topoisomerase. Note that taxol, a successful chemotherapeutic agent that hampers the normal microtubule machinery, has been suggested to involve additional cytotoxic pathways including p53-independent apoptosis of tumor cells and inhibition of topoisomerase II *(42)*.

Medicinal Hamamelidaceae

The family Hamamelidaceae consists of 26 genera and about 100 species of shrubs or tress known to contain tannins and iridoids. The leaves are alternate, simple, and often palmately lobed. The flowers are small and appear in spikes. The fruits are woody, capsular, and scepticidal. In Western medicine, the dried leaves of *Hamamelis virginiana* (hamamelis, *British Pharmaceutical Codex*, 1963), yielding not less that 20% of alcohol (45%)-soluble extractive, have been used as astringents for the treatment of hemorrhoids. Hamamelis water (*British Pharmaceutical Codex*, 1969) made from the stems has been used as a cooling application to sprains and bruises and as a styptic remedy. It is also used in cosmetics and as active ingredient of eye lotions.

In the Asia–Pacific region, *Altingia excelsa* Noronha (*Liquidambar altingiana* Bl.), *Altingia gracilipes* Hemsl. (*Amyris ambrosiaca* L.f.), *Liquidambar orientalis* Mill, and *Liquidambar formosana* Hance are of medicinal value. The purified basalm obtained from the trunk of *Liquidambar orientalis* Mill. or prepared storax (*British Pharmaceutical* Codex, 1969) has been used similarly as Peru basalm in the form of an ointment to treat scabies and other skin diseases, and as an ingredient of Compound Benzoin Tincture.

***Altingia excelsa* Noronha** (*Liquidambar altingiana* Bl.), or *xi qing pi* (Chinese), is a tree that grows to a height of 20 m tall in a geographical area ranging from India, Bhutan, India, Indonesia, Malaysia, Burma, and Indonesia. Leaves are simple, alternate, and stipulate; the stipules are 2–6 mm long. The petiole is slender and sparsely pubescent. The blades are aromatic with a turpentine-like aroma, ovate, 8–14 cm × 3.8–7 cm, crenate,

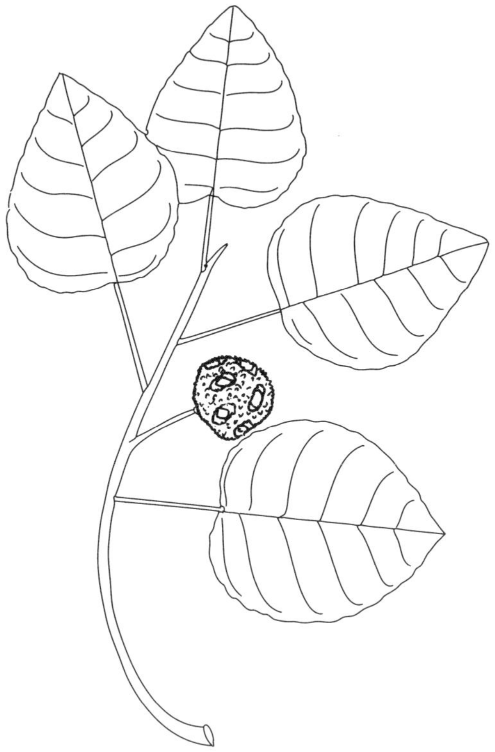

Fig. 95. *Altingia excelsa.* Plants of Indonesia. Herbarium Bogoriense—Harvard University Herbaria. Geographical localization: Bali, Timur, Tabanah 2 km west of Candi Kuning, in natural area of Kebun Raya, behind introduced Altingia forest. Alt: 1400 feet. 8° 18′S – 115° 9′E. Field collector: MacDonalds, 1961.

membranaceous, and show six to eight pairs of secondary nerves. The Infructescences are conical and 2 cm wide; and the fruits are capsules (Fig. 95).

In China, the plant affords a tonic remedy particularly recommended for chest complaints. Indonesians use the leaves medicinally because they are strongly aromatic. The pharmacological potentials of this plant are, to date, unknown. Note that 6β-hydroxy-3-oxo-lup-20(29)-en-28-oic acid and 3,11-dioxoolean-12-en-28-oic acid from the stem bark of *Liquidambar styraciflua*, as well as 25-acetoxy-3α-hydroxyolean-12-en-28-oic acid, inhibited the growth of several cancer cell lines *(43)*. What is the activity of 25-acetoxy-3α-hydroxyolean-12-en-28-oic acid against topoisomerase?

Medicinal Lamiaceae

There is an expanding body of evidence to suggest that diterpene quinone of *Salvia* species might represent a pool of potential inhibitors of topoisomerase. Diterpenoid quinones have been characterized from *Salvia officinalis* (sage, *British Pharmaceutical Codex*, 1934), *Salvia texana*, *Salvia regal*, *Salvia moorciuftiana*, and *Salvia lanata (44–47)*.

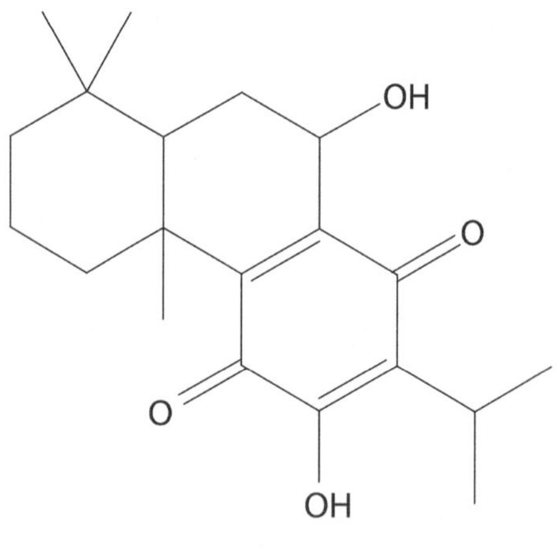

Horminone

Royleanone, horminone, and acetyl horminone isolated from the roots of *Salvia officinalis* L. abrogated the survival of colon carcinoma cell Caco-2 and human hepatoma cell HepG2, cultured in vitro with induction of DNA breaks (48).

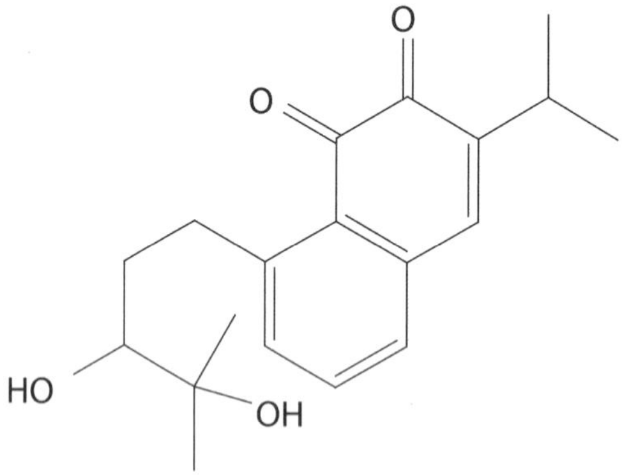

Salvicine

An other example of *Salvia quinone* is salvicine, a structurally modified diterpenoid quinone derived from *Salvia prionitis*, which is cytotoxic against multidrug-resistant cancer cell lines of topoisomerase II inhibition by trapping the DNA–topoisomerase II complex (49).

***Salvia plebeia* R.Br.** (*Salvia plebia, Lumnitzeria fastigiata* [Roth] Spreng, *Ocimum fastigiatum* Roth, *Ocimum virgatum* Thunb., *Salvia brachiata* Roxb., *Salvia minutiflora* Bunge, *Salvia plebeia* var. *latifolia* E. Peter), or *ching chich, li zhi cao* (Chinese), is an annual or biennial herb that grows in a geographical area spanning from China, Korea, Afghanistan, India, Indonesia, Japan, Korea, Malaysia, Burma, Mongolia, Thailand, Vietnam, and Australia. The stems are erect, up to 90 cm, and stout. The blade is elliptic-ovate, minutely hispid, and serrate. The influorescences are pilose. The flowers are reddish-purplish to blue, and the nutlets are ovoid and minute (Fig. 96).

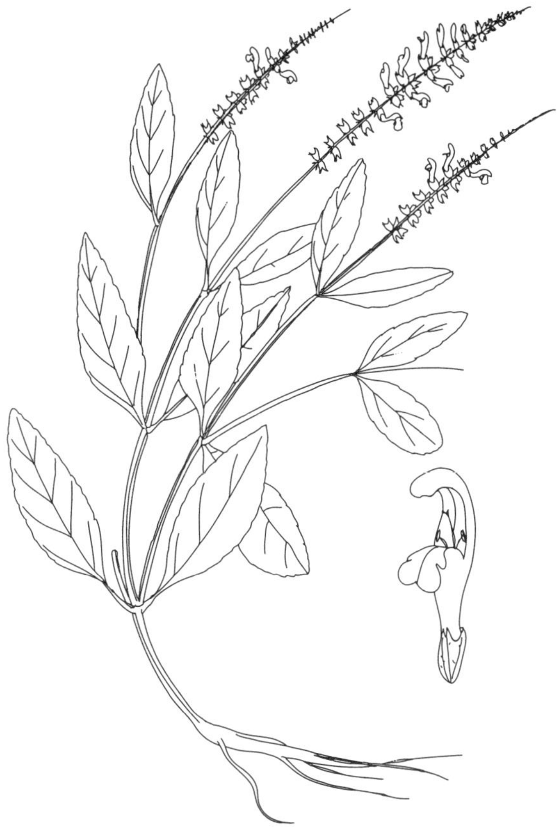

Fig. 96. *Salvia plebeia* R.Br.

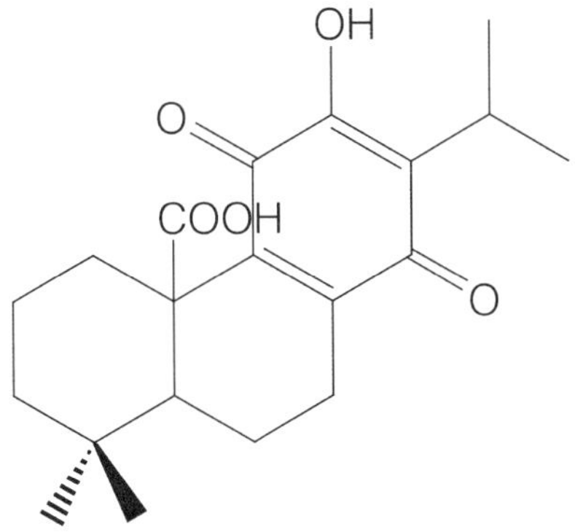

Royleanolic acid

In China, the plant is used to counteract skin putrefaction, heal boils, treat catarrh, dispel humors, and stop dysentery. In Korea, the plant is used to treat anuria and expel intestinal worms. In Cambodia, Laos, and Vietnam, the plant is used to treat colic, cholera, and dysentery.

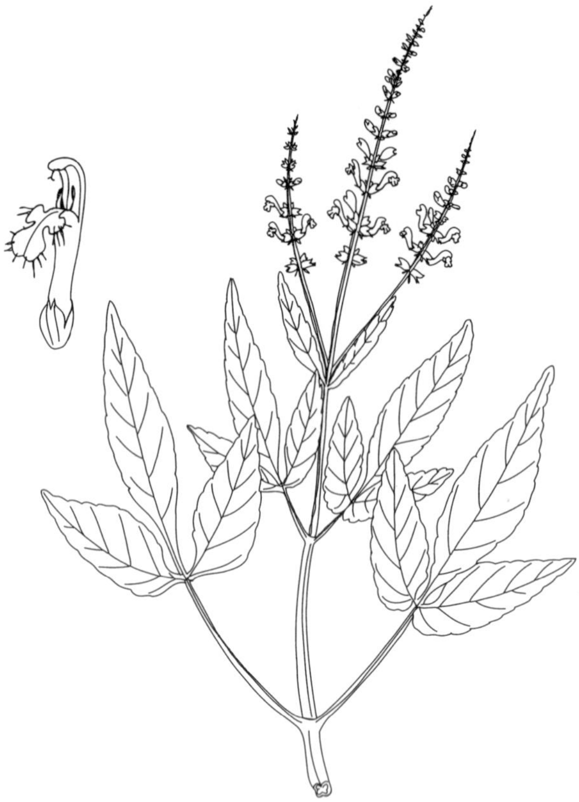

Fig. 97. *Salvia japonica* Thunb.

The plant is known to elaborate a diterpene quinone known as royleanonic acid, which is an antioxidant (50). What is the activity of royleanonic acid against topoisomerase?
***Salvia japonica* Thunb.**, or *shu wei ts'ao, wu ts'ao, shui-ch'ing, shu wei cao* (Chinese), is an annual herb that grows in marshes in China and Taiwan. The stems are erect, up to 60 cm, villous, and quadrangular. The leaves are pinnate. The petiole is 7–10 cm; the leaf blade is 6–13.5 × 5–9.5 cm; the upper stem leaves are one-pinnate. The flowers are packed in bunches on terminal racemes or panicles. The corolla is reddish to purple and 1.2 cm long. The nutlets are brown and minute (Fig. 97). The plant is used for black dye in China. The flowers and leaves are used to treat fluxes, colorless and red discharges, goiter and scrofula, ague, and dropsy. The rhizome is used for anemia, uterine hemorrhages, irregular menses, abdominal pains, inflammation, and as an antiseptic.
***Salvia miltiorrhiza* Bunge**, or red sage, *tan shen*, or *dan shen* (Chinese), is a common perennial herb of China, especially in hillsides, streamsides, and forests from 100 to 1300 m in Shensi, Shansi, Shantung, in the Peking mountains, and Japan. The leaves are hirsute. The root is red outside and purplish inside when fresh. The stems are erect, up to 80 cm tall, hirsute, and many-branched. Leaves are simple to imparipinnate and densely hirsute. The blade is circular to broadly lanceolate and crenate.

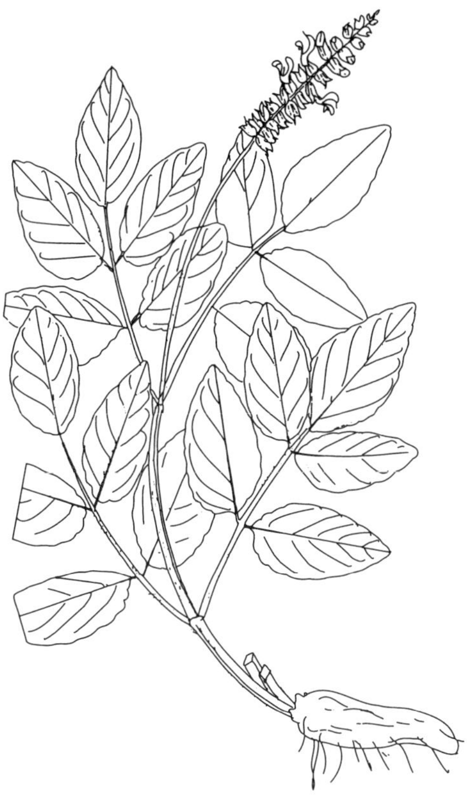

Fig. 98. *Salvia miltiorrhiza* Bunge.

The influorescences are terminal or axillary. The flowers are tubular, bilabiate, purple-blue, violet, or white, and 2–2.7 cm and pilose. The nutlets are ellipsoid and 3.2 × 1.5 mm (Fig. 98).

The drug consists of dried short pieces of roots, which are brick red-colored, with a sweet taste resembling to liquorice. This herb is regarded as one of the five astral remedies by Chinese practitioners who recommend it for the cardiovascular system and blood-related ailments, such as hemorrhages and menstruation, and to promote healing of wounds.

Extract of the plant inhibited the proliferation of $HepG_2$ cells cultured in vitro and caused apoptotosis *(51)*. Chor et al. investigated the effects of a number of Chinese medicinal herbs on cellular proliferation and apoptosis of a rat hepatic stellate cell line, HSC-T6, and found that *Salvia miltiorrhiza* has antiproliferative and pro-apoptotic activities *(52)*. The active principle involved here might be a diterpene of the tanshinone type because tanshinone IIA, from *Salvia miltiorrhiza* Bunge, is cytotoxic against various human carcinoma cell lines cultured in vitro accompanied by an increase in intracellular calcium. This triggers the release of cytochrome c, thus causing a loss of the mitochondrial membrane potential, which results in the subsequent activation of caspases, hence apoptosis *(53)*.

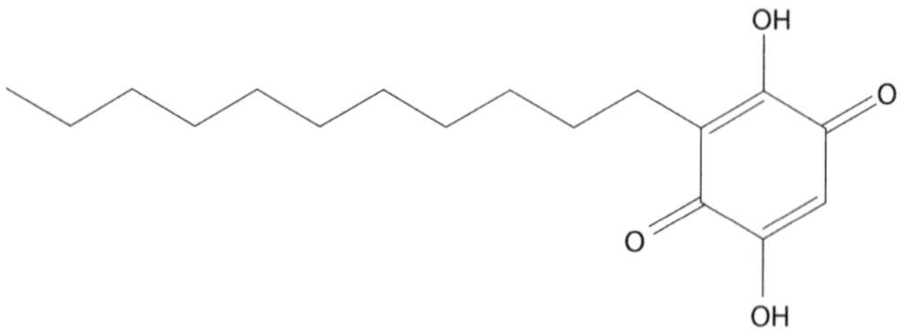

Embelin

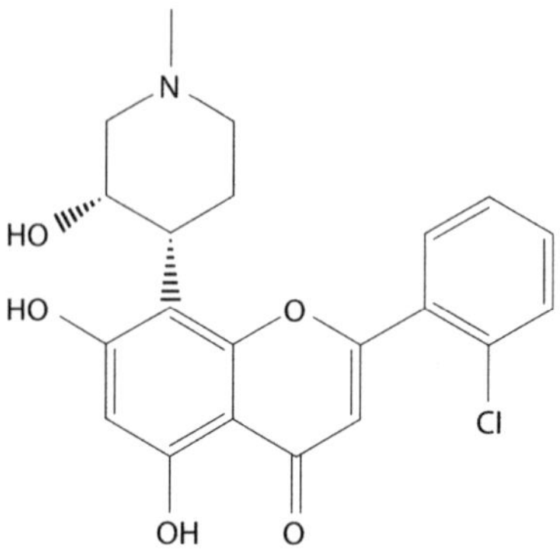

Flavopiridol

Fig. 99. Examples of natural products that interfere with apoptosis.

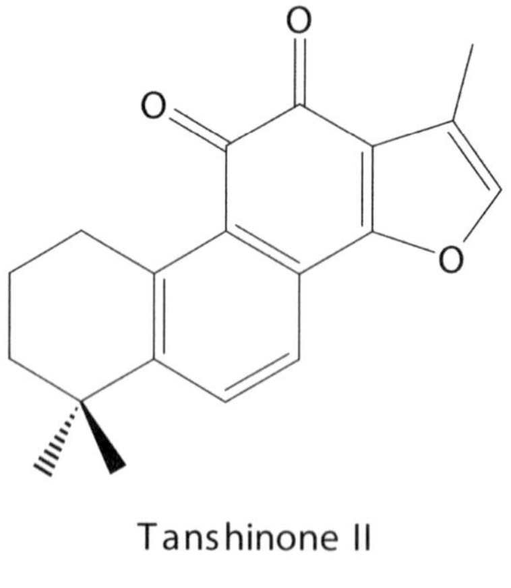

Tanshinone II

Tanshinones isolated from the dried root of *Salvia miltiorrhiza* Bunge abrogated the survival of P388 lymphocytic leukemia cells cultured in vitro. Tanshinone I and tanshinone IIA showed 86.76 and 56.05% cell inhibition, respectively, at a dose of 25 μg/mL) *(54)*. Dihydrotanshinone I and cryptotanshinone were relatively cytotoxic *(55)*. Dihydrotanshinone I induces cell growth arrest during the S phase and, subsequently, apoptosis.

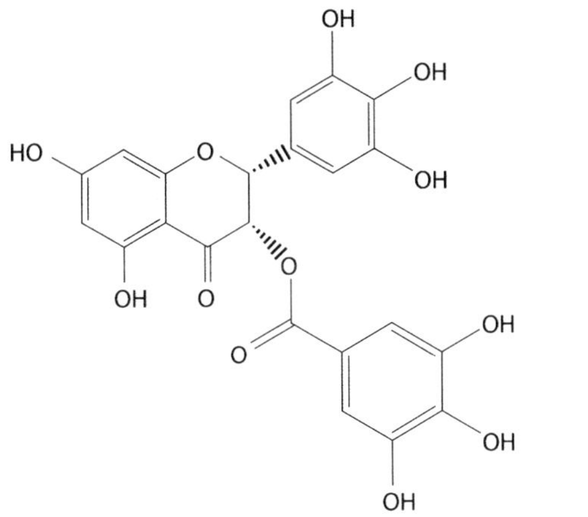

Epigallocatechin gallate

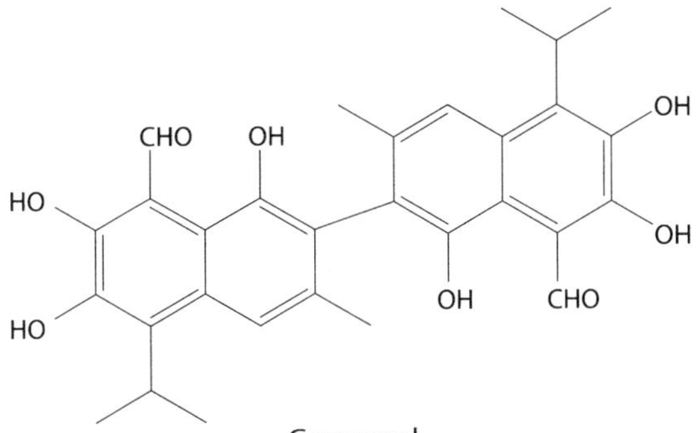

Gossypol

Fig. 100. (Continuation): Examples of natural products that interfere with apoptosis.

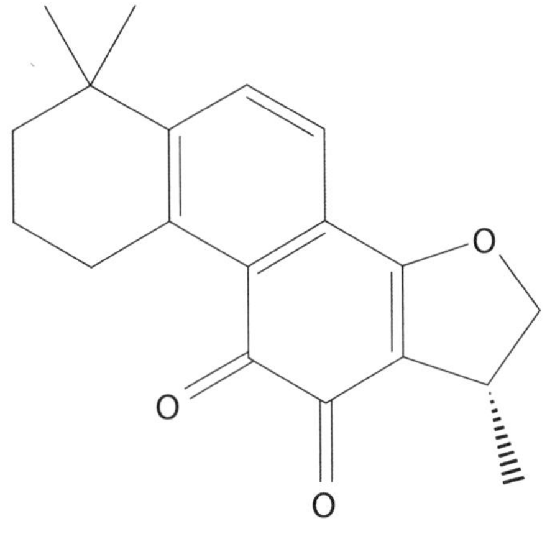

Cryptotanshinone

The evidence that emerged from the pharmacological study of *Salvia miltiorrhiza* Bunge lends strong support to the fact that tanshinone and congeners induce apoptosis. However, if the apoptotic potential of tanshinones is established, much less work has been done with the anti-topoisomerase activity of this planar compound. Further work on this topic should be encouraged, and one can reasonably expect interesting results not only in terms of antineoplastic agents but also in regard to a better understanding of the actual relationship between topoisomerase inhibition and apoptosis. What is the relationship between topoisomerase inhibitors and apoptosis induction?

APOPTOSIS

In some cells, drug treatment and other stimuli can trigger a series of complex cytoplasmic biochemical reactions that appear to constitute a cellular suicide program, culminating in the degradation and compaction of chromatin. This programmed mode of cell death is known as apoptosis, and in normal cellular conditions, it plays a considerable role in the early development of homeostasis of adult tissues. Apoptosis or literally "programmed cell death," is so far known to be triggered by three major stimuli: cell surface receptors such as FAS, mitochondrial response to stress, and cytotoxic T-cells.

The Fas receptor (CD95) mediates apoptotic signaling by Fas ligand expressed on the surface of other cells. Binding of FAS to Fas ligand activates apoptotic signaling through activation of a series of cytoplasmic enzymes called caspases. Caspases are cysteine proteases that convey the apoptotic signal by cleaving and activating other caspases, which then degrade DNA. Caspase-8 is the initial caspase involved in response to receptors with a death domain such as FAS. The mitochondrial stress pathway begins with the release of cytochrome *c* from mitochondria, which then interacts with Apaf-1, causing self-cleavage and activation of caspase-9, which activates caspase-3, -6 and -7, which act themselves to cleave cellular targets. One mechanism used by cytotoxic T-cells to kill tumor cells and virus-infected cells is the release of perforin and granzyme proteins. Granzyme B and perforin proteins released by cytotoxic T-cells induce apoptosis in targeted cells, forming transmembrane pores, and trigge apoptosis through cleavage of caspases. For the past two decades, there has been a considerable amount of research of agents that interfere with apoptosis, and natural products, most of which are elaborated in Asian plant species, are being scheduled for clinical trials, such as theaflavins from tea, flavonoid derivative flavopiridol, epigallocatechin gallate, gossypol, and embelin (Figs. 99, 100) *(56–60)*.

Embelin, which is common in the family Myrsinaceae in plants such as *Embelia ribes* Burm f., is of particular interest because it binds to the BIR3 domain of X-linked mammalian inhibitor of apoptosis protein (XIAP) and competes with caspase-9. Embelin inhibits cell growth, induces apoptosis, and activates caspase-9 in prostate cancer cells with high levels of XIAP, but has a minimal effect on normal prostate epithelial and fibroblast cells with low levels of XIAP and represents a promising lead compound for designing an entirely new class of anticancer agents that target the BIR3 domain of XIAP.

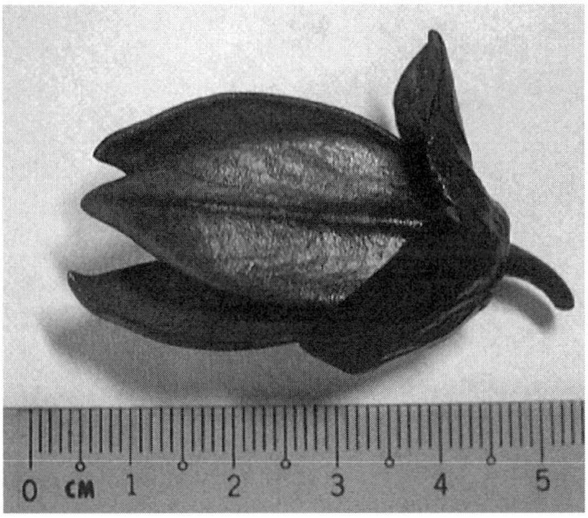

Fig. 101. Typical flower of *Goniothalamus* (*Goniothalamus scortechinii* King). The figure shows the veined petals and sepals.

One might have noticed that most of these natural products are of a phenolic nature and we can reasonably expect, in light of the complexity of apoptosis and the broad spectrum of cytotoxic agents elaborated from flowering plants, the discovery of lead apoptotic–antineoplastic agents in the relatively near future. When looking for such agents, one could investigate the medicinal flora of the Asia–Pacific region.

Medicinal Annonaceae

The evidence currently available strongly suggests that members of the family Annonaceae hold some potential as sources of proapoptotic agents. Of particular interest in this regard is the genus *Goniothalamus*. The main macroscopically botanical characteristics to look for in field collection of *Goniothalamus* are treelets or shrubs with smooth, thin, and fibrous bark; aromatic wood; simple, alternate, and exstipulate leaves, with long glossy blades, and without obvious secondary nerves; a triangular thalamus or receptacle; and a perianth, which consists of a calyx, and two series of three greenish petals that are veined and somewhat woody (Fig. 101). Lens examination of the corolla shows that the inner whorl of the petal is smaller than the outer one and is fused in a vault above the androecium. The fruits are one- to two-seeded ripe carpels that are olive green and smooth.

Within the Annonaceae, *Goniothalamus* species are thought to have evolved from the tribe Uvariae, from which they have possibly inherited the ability to elaborate styryl-lactones and acetogenins, the former possibly being present in several other genera in the tribe Annoneae and known to occur in other Magnoliidae, including the Laurales and Piperales.

***Goniothalamus* species.** Six *Goniothalamus* species are used in the traditional medicinal Asian system, and most of these have been used in Malaysia in connection with

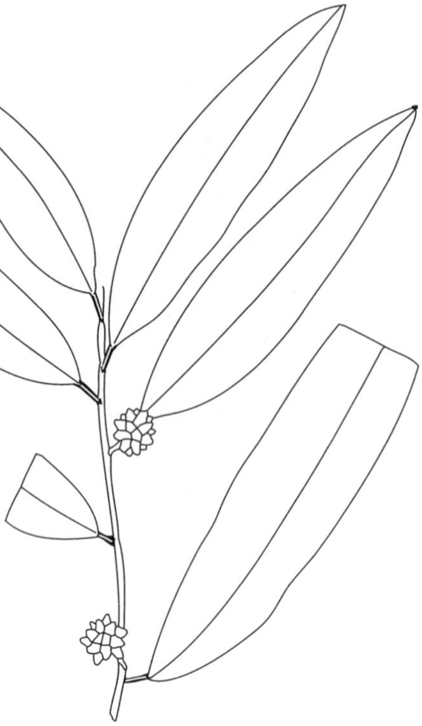

Fig. 102. *Goniothalamus macrophyllus* (Bl.) Hook. f. & Thoms.

abortion and childbirth since very early times. The leaves of *Goniothalamus macrophyllus* Hook. f. & Thoms. are used to abrogate fever, and a decoction of the roots is given as a postpartum remedy and to cause abortion. The roots of *Goniothalamus giganteus* Hook. f. & Thoms. (Fig. 102) are used to abort and treat colds, and the heated leaves are applied to swellings. A decoction of *Goniothalamus scortechinii* King is given as a postpartum protective remedy. The roots of *Goniothalamus tapis* Miq. (Fig. 103) are used as an abortifacient during early months of pregnancy. In Indonesia, an infusion of the roots is used to treat typhoid fever. In Taiwan, the seeds of *Goniothalamus amuyon* Merr. are used to treat scabies. In the Philippines, the seeds are used to treat rheumatism and tympanites, and the fruit is stomachic. None of the uses mentioned here has been substantiated yet via pharmacological experimentation; however, these species are well-known for their phytochemical constituents, as all six have been phytochemically investigated. Most phytochemical reports found so far on *Goniothalamus* species deal with the chemical constituents of *Goniothalamus giganteus* Hook. f. & Thoms. Phytochemical studies on *Goniothalamus* species have resulted, so far, in the isolation of two major classes of lipophilic secondary metabolites: acetogenins and styryl-lactones, both possessing complex stereochemistry and existing in different stereoisomeric forms with varying levels of toxicity toward several human tumor cell lines.

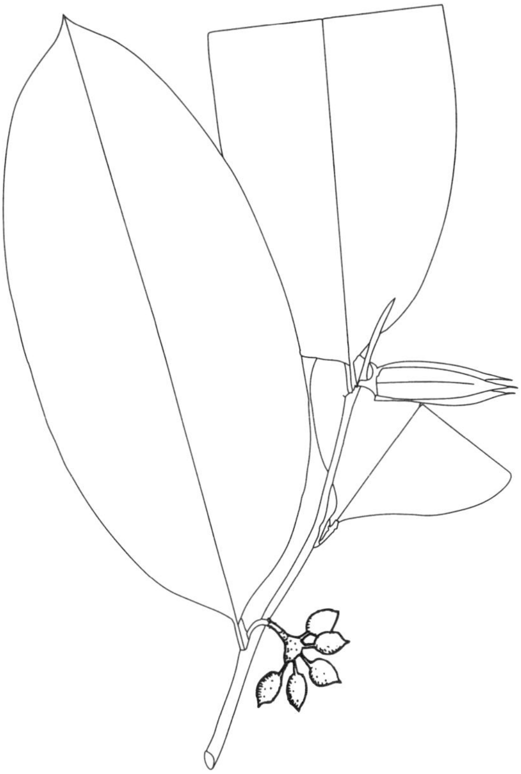

Fig. 103. *Goniothalamus tapis.* From Flora of Malaya. FRI No 19803. Geographical localization: Le Song F.R. Pahang, low undulating seasonal swamp primary forest, alt: 100 feet. Det: Y. C. Chan.

Irrespective of the presence of a large variety of cytotoxic acetogenins and styryl-lactones in the genus *Goniothalamus*, only 19 species out of 160, or 12%, of species have been phytochemically investigated to date, namely *Goniothalamus amuyon* Merr., *Goniothalamus andersonii* J.Sincl., *Goniothalamus arvensis* Scheff, *Goniothalamus borneensis* Mat-Salleh, *Goniothalamus cardiopetalus* Hook. f. & Thoms., *Goniothalamus cheliensis.* Hu, *Goniothalamus donnaiensis* Finet & Gagnep., *Goniothalamus gardneri* Hook. f. & Thoms., *Goniothalamus giganteus* Hook. f. & Thoms, *Goniothalamus griffithii* Hook. f. & Thoms, *Goniothalamus leiocarpus* (W.T.) Wang P.T.Li, *Goniothalamus malayanus* Hook. f. & Thoms, *Goniothalamus montanus* J.Sincl., *Goniothalamus scortechinii* King, *Goniothalamus sesquipedalis Hook. f. & Thoms.*, *Goniothalamus tapis* Miq., *Goniothalamus thwaitesii* Hook. f. & Thoms, *Goniothalamus uvaroides* King., and *Goniothalamus velutinus* Airy Shaw.

Note that both acetogenins and styryl-lactones are cytotoxic for mammalian cells, as the result of distinct biochemical pathways, which, however, have their molecular origin near or in the mitochondrial membrane and/or the mitochondrial respiratory system *(61,62)*. Acetogenins were first characterized as the active principles responsible for

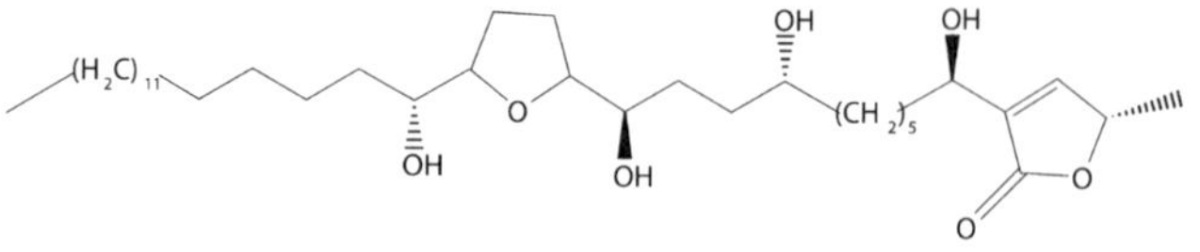

Goniotetracin

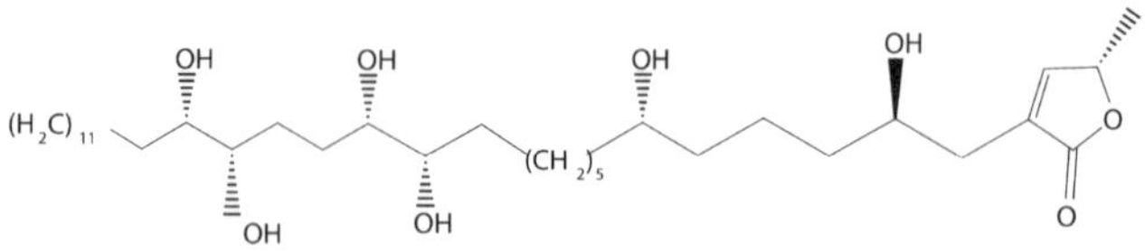

Gardnerilin A

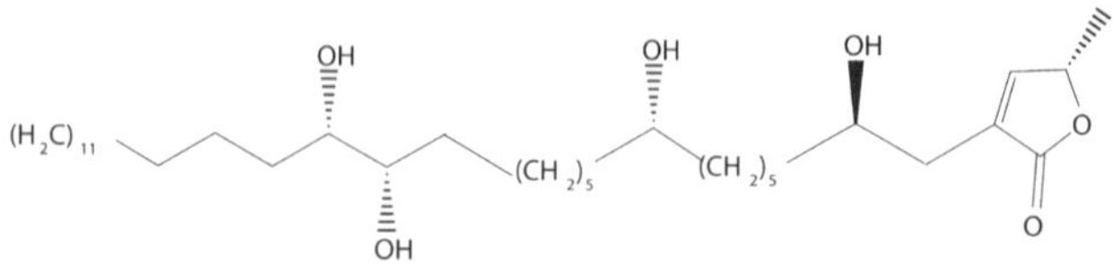

Gardnerilin B

Fig. 104. Examples of cytotoxic acetogenins from *Goniothalamus* species.

shrimp lethality from the bark of *Goniothalamus giganteus* Hook. f. & Thoms. collected from Thailand. Extract of the bark showed toxicity in the brine shrimp test and showed murine cytotoxicity in the 3PS (P388) leukemia bioassay *(63)*.

From the crude ethanol of the bark of *Goniothalamus giganteus* Hook. f. & Thoms., a series of cytotoxic acetogenins were isolated, including giganin, goniothalamicin, annonacin, gigantriocin, gigantetrocin, gigantrionenin, giganenin and gonionenin, goniodenin, asimilobine, gigantecin, bullatalicin, bullatalicinone *cis*-giantrionenine, 4-acetylgigantetrocin A and gigantransenins A, B, and C, pyranicin and pyragonicin, goniotrionin, goniotetracin, and 2,4-*cis*- and *trans*-gonioneninone *(64–71)*.

Gigantransenins A, B, and C showed selective inhibitory effects on the human breast tumor cell line (MCF-7) comparable with the potency of adriamycin *(68)*. Pyranicin and pyragonicin were selectively cytotoxic against the pancreatic cell line (PACA-2) in a panel of six human solid tumor cell lines, with pyranicin showing 10 times the potency of adriamycin, whereas goniotrionin was more potent against MCF-7. Both goniotetracin and 2,4-*cis*- and *trans*-gonioneninone are selectively and significantly cytotoxic to the human pancreatic tumor cell line (PACA-2).

Goniodonin and 34-*epi*-goniodonins were isolated from *Goniothalamus donnaiensis* Finet & Gagnep. collected from Guangxi Province, China *(72)*. Gardnerilins A and B from *Goniothalamus gardneri* Hook. f. & Thoms. collected from DiaoLo mountain, Hainan Province, China, gave cytotoxic IC_{50} values against Bel 7402 human tumor cell lines of 3.6 and 8.5 μg/mL, respectively (Fig. 104; refs. *73–75*).

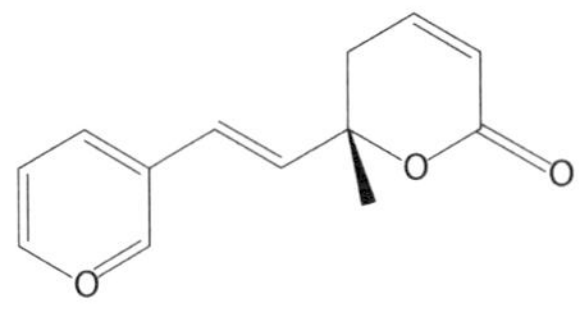

Goniothalamin

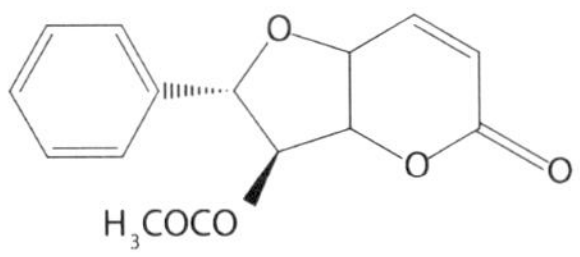

3 acetylaltholactone

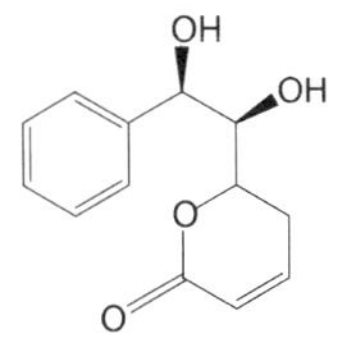

Goniodiol

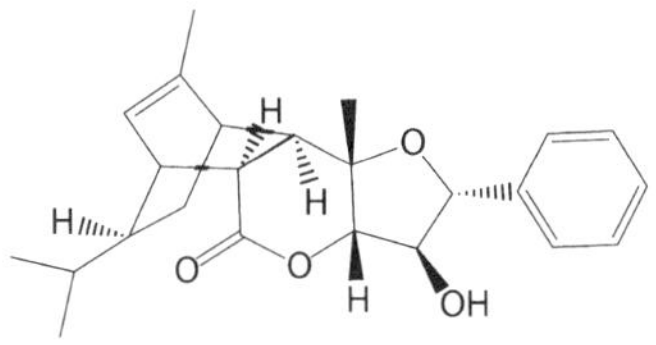

Cardiopetalolactone

Fig. 105. Examples of cytotoxic styryl-lactones from *Goniothalamus* species.

In regard to the precise molecular mode of action of acetogenins, there is an expanding body of evidence to suggest that both tetrahydrofuran or tetrahydropyran rings and/or hydroxy groups, which are hydrophilic, and the hydrocarbon chains, which are hydrophobic, moor the molecules by anchoring the mitochondrial membrane outside and inside, respectively. The pharmacophores, i.e., the lactones, are therefore secured and interact with the complex I (nicotinamide adenine dinucleotide [NADH]-ubiquinone oxidoreductase) in the mitochondrial electron transport system and abrogate the survival of cancer cells by asphyxiation *(61)*.

Jewers et al. first reported goniothalamin (Fig. 105) as the active constituent of the bark of *Goniothalamus andersonii* J. Sincl., *Goniothalamus macrophyllus* Miq., and *Goniothalamus malayanus* Hook. f. & Thoms. collected in the peat swamp of Sarawak, Malaysia *(75)*. Styryl-lactones such as goniothalamin have since attracted a great deal of interest on account of their ability to inhibit the mitochondrial respiratory chain and to induce apoptosis *(76–83)*. An additional example of an apoptogenic styryl-lactone is altholactone characterized from *Goniothalamus arvensis* Scheff. collected in the

National Park of Variant in the central province of Papua New Guinea, and from the *Goniothalamus borneensis* Mat-Salleh collected in Malaysia (*84*).

An additional example of a cytotoxic styryl-lactone is cardiopetalolactone characterized from the stem bark of *Goniothalamus cardiopetalus* Hook. f. & Thoms. collected from the Palaruvi forest in Kerala, India, with altholactone, goniopypyrone, cardiobutanolide, goniothalamin, goniodiol, goniofufurone, and goniofupyrone (*85,86*). 8-Acetylgoniofufurone, 7-acetylgonio-pypyrone, 5-acetylgonio-pypyrone, goniofu-furone, goniopypyrone, goniothalamin, goniothalenol, (+)-isoaltholactone, goniodiol, 7-acetylgoniodiol, goniotriol, 8-acetylgoniotriol, and 9-deoxygoniopypyrone were isolated from the roots of *Goniothalamus griffithii* Hook. f. & Thoms. (*87*). An isomer of altholactone, (+)-isoaltholactone was isolated from stem bark of *Goniothalamus malayanus* Hook. f. & Thoms, from the leaves of *Goniothalamus montanus* J. Sincl., and the roots of *Goniothalamus tapis* Miq. (*88*). Goniolactones A through F were identified from the roots of *Goniothalamus cheliensis* Hu, among which was goniolactone B, exhibiting significant cytotoxicity against A2780, HCT-8, and KB cells with IC_{50} values of 7.40, 4.43, and 7.23 μM, respectively (*89*).

Digoniodiol, deoxygoniopypyrone A, goniofupyrone, goniothalamin, deoxygoniopypyrone A, gonodiol-8-monoacetate, and gonotriol were characterized from the aerial parts of *Goniothalamus amuyon* Merr. collected in the southern part of Taiwan near the coastal regions (*90,91*). The petroleum ether extract of the stem bark of *Goniothalamus sesquipedalis* Hook. f. & Thoms. collected in Bangladesh afforded goniothalamin, isogoniothalamine oxide, 5-acetoxygoniothalamine, and 5-acetoxygoniothalamine oxide (*92*). 5-Acetyl goniothalamin was characterized from *Goniothalamus uvaroides* King collected in Bangladesh (*93*).

Altholactone is apoptogenic in HL-60 promyelocytic leukemia cells via oxidative stress (*94*). Goniothalamin is cytotoxic against the HepG2 cancer cell line, with IC_{50} values in the range of 0.19 to 0.64 μg/mL, and abrogates the survival of cancerous (HGC-27, MCF-7, PANC-1, HeLa) and non-cancerous (3T3) cell lines time- and dose-dependently (*82,95*). Goniothalamin induces apoptosis in Jurkat T-cells by the activation of the enzymatic activities of effector caspases-3 and -7 (*82*). Current paradigms of apoptosis suggest that the loss of mitochondrial transmembrane potential occurs earlier in the commitment phase of apoptosis, which results in the release of mitochondrial apoptogenic proteins—and possibly inhibition of the respiratory chain—including cytochrome c, which in the presence of ATP, interacts with Apaf-1, resulting in the activation of caspases 9 (a cysteine proteinase). This, in turn, activates effector caspases such as caspases-3 or -6, hence cell death. Note that styryl-lactones inhibit the mitochondrial respiratory chain in mammalian cells.

A critical factor for *Goniothalamus* use as a medicinal herb is its content of styryl-lactones, which promote apoptosis in mammalian cells. One might set the hypothesis that the abortifacient and/or postnatal and anti-inflammatory traditional uses of *Goniothalamus*

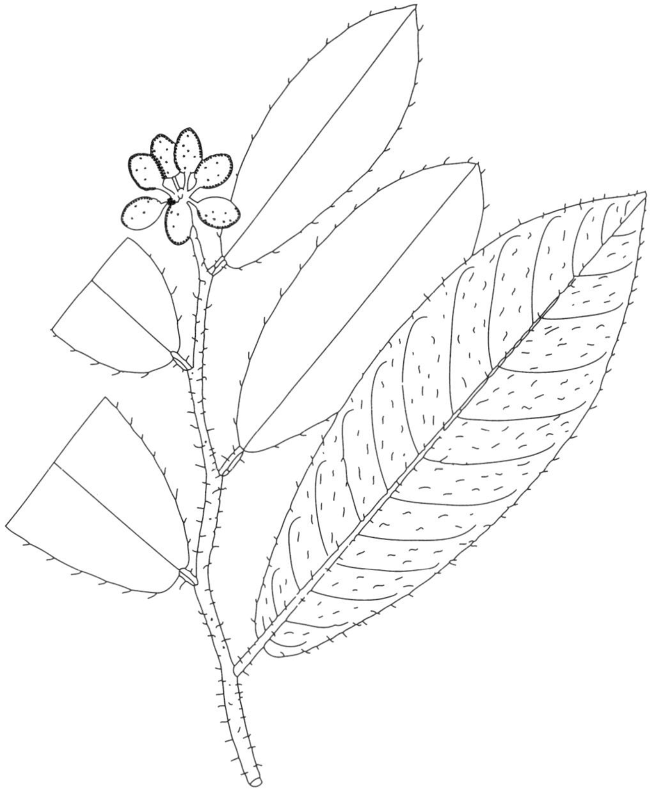

Fig. 106. *Pseudouvaria setosa.* Herb Hort. Bot. Sing. Geographical localization: Raub Pahang. Date: 4/19/1932. Field collector: Osman. Det: J. Sinclair 2/8/1949.

species might involve styryl-lactones because apoptosis is known to play a crucial role in trophoblasts of patients with recurrent spontaneous abortion of unidentified cause, and in T-cells in the human decidua as defense mechanism against rejection of fetal allograft by the maternal immune system (96,97).

***Pseudouvaria setosa* (King) J. Sinclair** (*Orophea setosa* King) is a small tree that grows wild in the primary rainforests of Thailand and the northern part of peninsular Malaysia. The young stems, petioles, leaf margin, lower midrib, and secondary nerves are covered with irritating hairs. The leaves are simple, exstipulate, and alternate and membranaceous, 11–16 cm × 4.5–7 cm. The blade is oblong to oblong-oblanceolate and shows 12–13 pairs of secondary nerves prominent beneath. The flowers are solitary on a 1.8–2-cm-long pedicel. The sepals are minute and suborbicular. The corolla consists of two series of petals which are white with pink bases, ovate, and pubescent. The inner petals are 6 mm long, and united iat apex into a vault. The fruits are one to six globose, ripe carpels that are grayish-yellow and tomentose and up to 2 cm in diameter (Fig. 106).

The roots are chewed by Malays to treat cough. The roots are boiled then reduce into a powder form, which is applied externally to reduce fever. The leaves are part of a mixture eaten with *sireh* to promote libido. The pharmacological properties of *Pseudouvaria setosa* (King) J. Sincl., and of the genus.

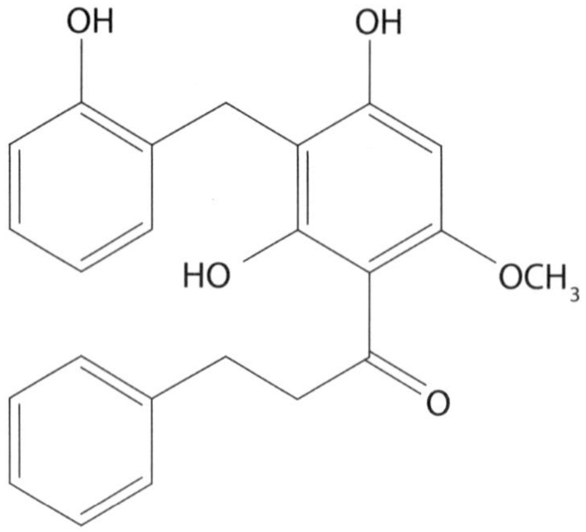

Uvaretin

Pseudouvaria in general, is unknown. Note that the *Pseudouvaria* species, and Uvariae in general, have the interesting tendency to elaborate C-benzylated chalcones, which induce apoptosis. Examples of such flavonoids are triuvaretin and isotriuvaretin, uvaretin, isouvaretin, diuvaretin, and angoluvarin from *Uvaria leptocladon* and *Uvaria angolensis* *(98–100)*. Uvaretin and diuvaretin from *Uvaria acuminata* abrogated the survival of human promyelocytic leukemia HL-60 cells cultured in vitro with chromatin degradation and condensation arrest of cells in G1 phase and activation of caspase-3 *(101,102)*.

Medicinal Asteraceae

Rivero et al. studied the cytotoxic effects tatridin A, tamirin, reynosin, and ineupatorolide A on the myeloid leukemia cell lines HL-60 and U937, and made the interesting observation that ineupatorolide A, isolated from *Allagopappus viscosissimus*, induced apoptosis accompanied by both the activation of caspase-3 and the fragmentation of poly(ADP-ribose) polymerase-1 and an early release of cytochrome *c* from the mitochondria *(103)*. The evidence for the existence of proapoptotic sesquiterpene lactones in the family Asteraceae is therefore strong, and it seems likely that further study in this field might result in the discovery of antineoplastic agents of clinical value.

An exciting area of potential for proapoptotic agents would be the medicinal flora of the Asia–Pacific region, which encompasses about 250 species of medicinal Asteraceae awaiting pharmacological exploration.

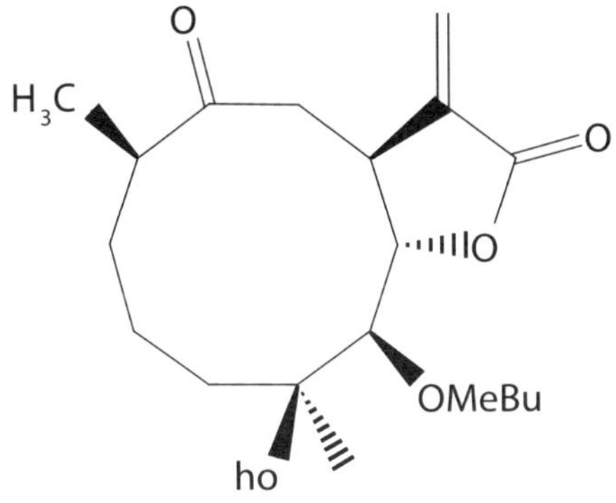

Ineupatorolide A

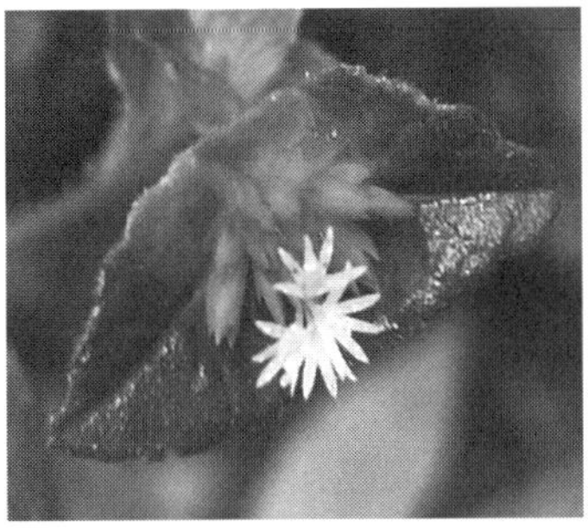

Elephantopus mollis Kunth. (*Elephantopus cernuus* Vell, *Elephantopus martii* Graham, *Elephantopus scaber* L, *Elephantopus sericeus* Graham, *Elephantopus serratus* Blco.), or elephantopus, elephant's foot, soft elephant's foot, *jangli tambaku* (Fiji), *papago vaca, papago halom tano* (Guam), or *lata hina* (Tonga), is an erect herb that grows to a height of 1 m. The plant is native to Central America but has invaded the tropical belt. The stems are pilose, slender, somewhat corymbose, and grayish to bluish-green. The leaves are simple, spiral, grouped in rosette near the roots and cauline along the stem. The blade is pilose, elliptic-oblong or up to 15 cm long, serrate, and lobed. The influorescences are globose heads of minute white or pinkish flowers that are 4 mm long (Fig. 107).

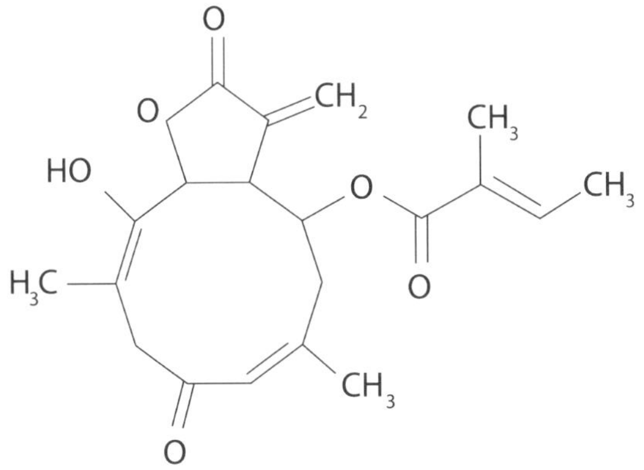

Molephantinin

In Burma, a decoction of the aerial parts is drunk to treat irregular menses. In China, the plant is eaten as a salad and is a believed to improve general health. In several Southeast Asian countries the plant is used to break fevers and prompt urination. In

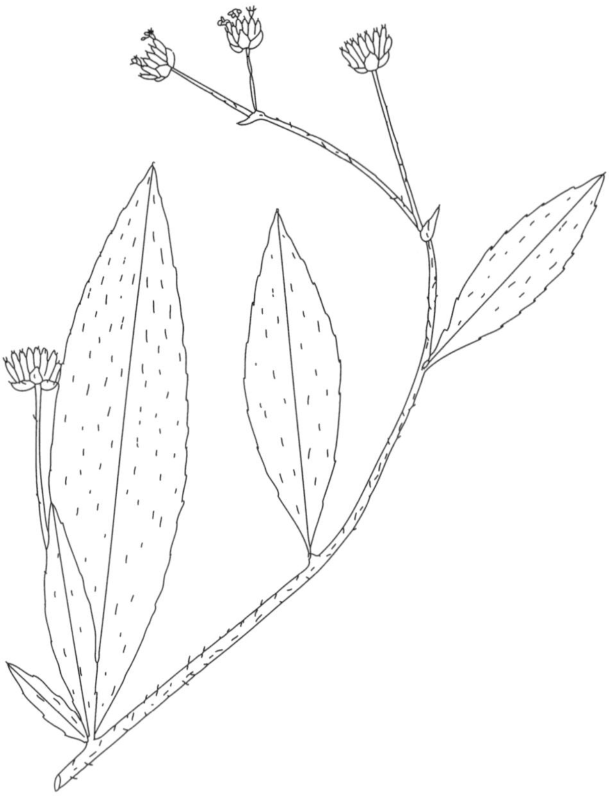

Fig. 107. *Elephantopus mollis*. Flora of Malaya. FRI No 2171. Geographical localization: Fraser's Hill Pahang. Hillside near a stream. 10/15/1966. RM Kochummen. Det: 7/1974, Leiden.

the Philippines, a decoction of the plant provides an emollient remedy. In Guam, the plant is used to treat asthenia fever.

Elephantopus mollis is interesting because it elaborates a series of cytotoxic antitumor germacranolides including molephantinin and phantomolin, which are cytotoxic in vitro and in vivo against Ehrlich ascites carcinoma and Walker 256 carcinosarcoma in rodents *(104,105)*. Molephantinin mitigates DNA and protein synthesis in Ehrlich ascites carcinoma cells and DNA synthesis. What is the activity of molephantinin on apoptosis *(106)*?

Blumea riparia **(Bl.) DC.** (*Blumea pubigera* [L.] Merr., *Blumea chinensis* DC.) is a sprawling herb that grows to 3 ft high in Malaysia, Taiwan, and Indonesia. The stems are terete and finely ribbed. The leaves are simple, spiral, and exstipulate. The blade is lanceolate, elliptic, and serrate and shows five to eight pairs of secondary nerves. The influorescences are conical heads (Fig. 108). In Taiwan, the plant is used externally to assuage headaches. Malays drink a decoction of roots to treat colic. In Indonesia, the plant is used to treat beriberi and gynecological disturbances. The plant is known to contain protocatechuic acid *(107)*.

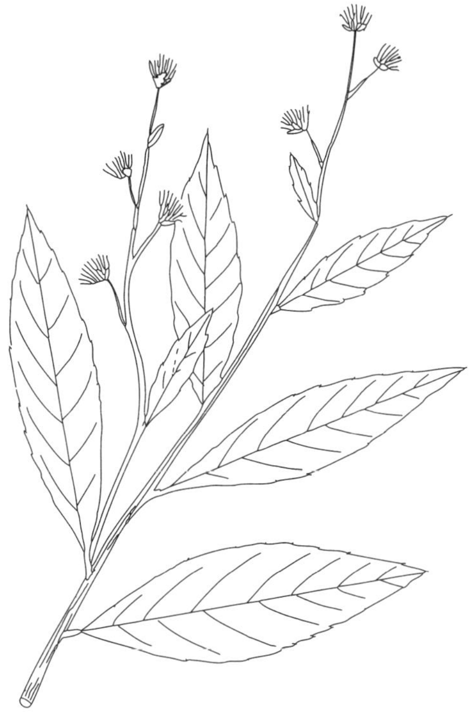

Fig. 108. *Blumea riparia* (Bl.) DC. Distributed from The Herbarium Botanic Gardens Singapore. No HMB: 2589. 7/17/1961. Coll. & Det.: Burkill. Geographical localization: Gunong Pulai. Exposed on rock. Alt: 1200 ft.

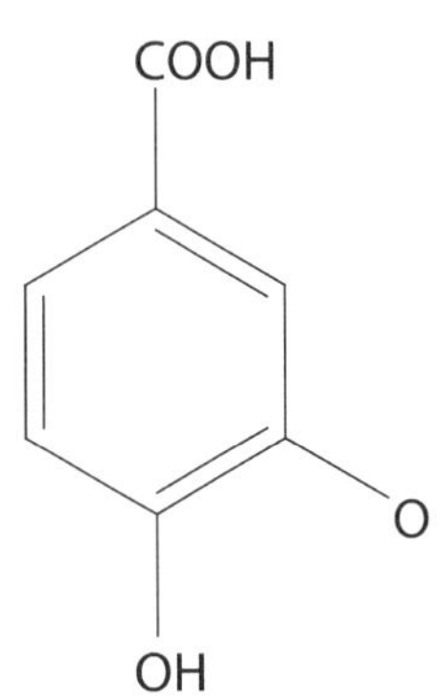

Protocatechuic acid

Kampa et al. made the interesting observation that protocatechuic acid, which is found in grapes and red wine from *Vitis vinifera* (Vitaceae), showed a time- and dose-dependent inhibitory effect on cell growth of T47D human breast cancer cells at low concentrations *(108)*. The phenolic compound is a potent inhibitor of topoisomerase I *(109)*. The plant likely contains some germanacrolides because these sesquiterpenes are known

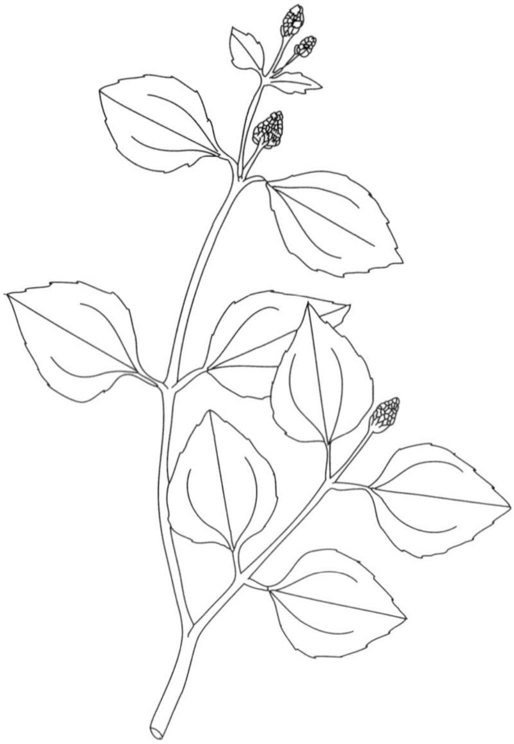

Fig. 109. *Spilanthes paniculata.* From Flora of Singapore, Comm. Ex. Herb. Heort. Bot. Sing. Geographical localization: Geylang Singapore. 7/27/1934. Field collector: Teruya No: 2526. Det. Sri S. Tjitrosvedirjo 7/27/1998.

to occur in members of the genus *Blumea*, the apoptotic property of which is open for exploration *(110)*.

Spilanthes paniculata Wall. ex DC (*Spilanthes acmella* [L.] Murr,), or para cress, toothache plant, *heukala* (Burmese), *pokok getang kerbau*, *kerabu*, *galang*, *gutang* (Malay), *biri* (Philippino), *herbe de Malacca*, *cresson des Indes* (French), or *cuc ao*, *ngo ao* (Vietnamese), is a tropical, branched, annual and herb that grows in the wild to a height of 15–30 cm in open waste places, old clearings, at low and medium altitudes. The stems are glabrous, fleshy, and purplish. The leaves are simple, without stipules, and opposite. The petiole is 2–7 mm long. The blade is 1.5–3 cm long, deltoid, and shows a single pair of secondary nerves. The influorescences consist of conical capitula, which are on 2.5–7-cm-long pedicels. The fruits consist of triquetous or compressed achenes (Fig. 109).

The plant is used in Cambodia, Laos, and Vietnam to treat dysentery and scorbut. The plant is used externally in Malaysia to assuage toothache and headaches, and a decoction is drunk to treat leukemia. In Indonesia, the capitula are chewed to promote salivation. In the Philippines, the roots are used to relieve the bowels from costiveness, and an infusion of the plant is drunk to promote urination. In Papua New Guinea, the

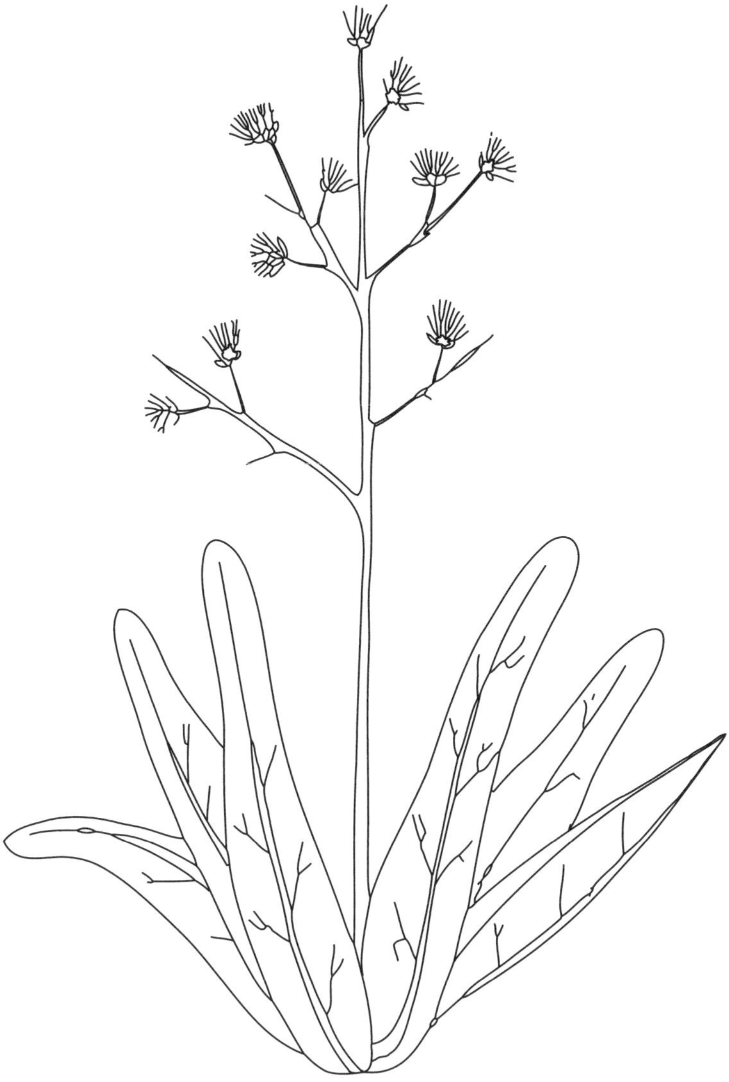

Fig. 110. *Lactula indica.* Flora of Malay Peninsula. Geographical localization: Expt. Plantation Kepong. Date: 6/12/1927. No 11786. Field collector: Ranger.

roots are chewed to mitigate toothaches. It would be interesting to learn whether further experiments on this plant confirm the antileukemic property mentioned previously. Is apoptosis involved here?

***Lactuca indica* L.** (*Lactula brevirostris* Champ.) is an herb that grows in a geographical area spanning from North Asia to Papua New Guinea (Fig. 110). In China, the leaves are eaten as salad to facilitate digestion, and a decoction is drunk to break fever. In Taiwan, the plant is used to break fever, and it is used externally to soothe swellings. In Cambodia, Laos, and Vietnam, the plant is used to invigorate, promote digestion, and it yields a paste used externally to soothe inflammation. The latex of the plant is known to induce narcosis. In Papua New Guinea, the seeds are chewed for social purposes.

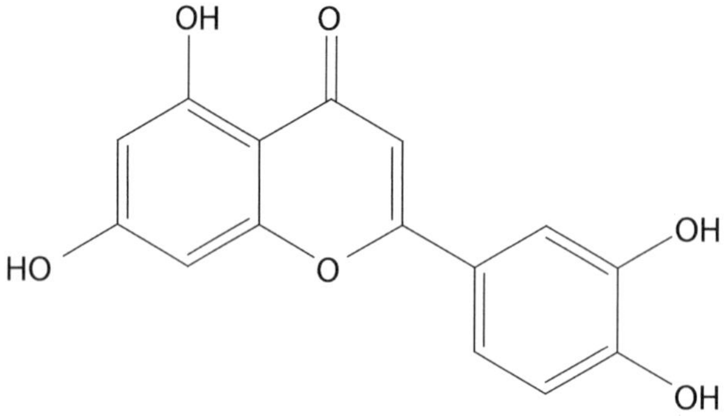

Luteolin

An extract from *Lactuca indica* showed significant free radical scavenging activity, and protected phix174 supercoiled DNA against strand cleavage and reduced oxidative stress in human promyelocytic leukemia HL-60 cells. On account of protocatechulic acid, methyl *p*-hydroxybenzoate, caffeic acid, 3,5-dicaffeoylquinic acid, luteolin 7-O-β-glucopyranoside, and quercetin 3-O-β-glucopyranoside are the major antioxidative constituents (*111*).

Note that luteolin, a naturally occurring flavonoid, induces apoptosis in various cancer cell lines through death receptor (DR) 5 upregulation. Luteolin induced the expression of DR5, along with Bcl-2-interacting domain cleavage and the activation of caspase-8, -10, -9, and -3. In addition, suppression of DR5 expression with siRNA efficiently limited luteolin-induced caspase activation and apoptosis. Human recombinant DR5/Fc also abrogated luteolin-induced apoptosis (*112*).

SUMMARY AND FUTURE PROSPECTS

A massive body of evidence has already been presented clearly indicating that the medicinal plants of the Pacific Rim elaborate a broad array of cytotoxic substances. Most of these have been characterized using experimental procedures designed to examine the cytotoxicity of natural products against human tumor cell lines. These procedures involve in vitro screening where the viability of cultured cells after exposure to an extract or a purified substance is measured.

However, one might take the time to think back and to ask if the extensive use of such techniques might not have failed to characterize important lead compounds from plants, and especially medicinal plants. As a matter of fact, a molecule inactive in vitro might, after metabolic transformation in vivo, be effective in abrogating metastasis. The opposite is true, and promising in vitro results have often led to disappointing clinical trials.

In terms of pharmacokinetics, many host factors, such as the route of administration, the metabolism, the catabolism and clearance will considerably determine the antineoplastic success of a drug. One major difficulty with the clinical effectiveness of chemotherapy of neoplastic diseases is the requirement that it kill malignant tumor cells at doses that allow cells in the patient's vital organs to survive so that the recovery can occur. In other words, it is to obtain a reasonably safe therapeutic index favoring introduction into clinical practice.

Ideally, future antineoplastic drug discovery should be based on a more rational, botanical, chemical, and pharmacological approach. A possible way to test the antineoplastic effects of compounds would be to use some semi in vitro–in vivo models. A more rational approach in antineoplastic research, combined with the enormous chemodiversity of flowering plants, will lead to the discovery of several molecules of clinical value.

The ability of natural products to inhibition of topoisomerase and precipitate apoptosis mentioned in this chapter are two abilities among several others, of which inhibition of microtubule formation, inhibition of DNA polymerase, protein kinases, protein phosphatase and aromatase, and the use of cytokines, interleukins, and tumor necrosis factor and yet uncovered cellular targets.

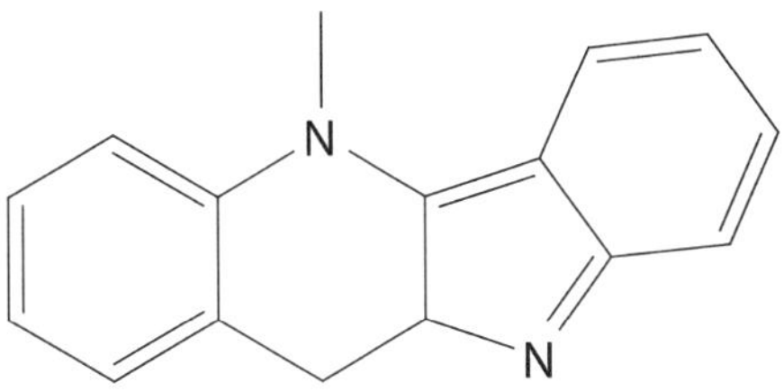

Cryptolepine

An interesting development from the study of the precise pharmacomolecular mechanism of natural products is to bring further light to cellular targets and synergistical cytotoxic mechanisms. One such study has been carried out by Dassonneville et al. They made a careful study of the cytotoxic effects of cryptolepine from the roots of an Asclepiadaceae *Cryptolepis sanguinolenta* and showed that the alkaloids intercalate into DNA and interfere with the enzymatic activity of topoisomerase II, inducing cleavage of poly(ADP-ribose) polymerase and the release of cytochrome c from the mitochondria *(113)*.

In regard to the inhibitors of tubulin polymerization, Shi et al. showed that a flavonoid such as 5,3′-dihydroxy-3,6,7,8,4′-pentamethoxyflavone from a medicinal Capparaceae of the Asia–Pacific region—*Polanisia dodecandra*—abrogated the survival of a surprisingly broad array of cancer cell lines, including central nervous system cancer (SF-268, SF-539, SNB-75, U-251), nonsmall-cell lung cancer (HOP-62, NCI-H266, NCI-H460, NCI-H522), small-cell lung cancer (DMS-114), ovarian cancer (OVCAR-3, SK-OV-3), colon cancer (HCT-116), renal cancer (UO-31), a melanoma cell line (SK-MEL-5), and leukemia cell lines (HL-60 [TB], SR), and inhibited tubulin polymerization with an IC_{50} value of 0.83 μM *(114)*.

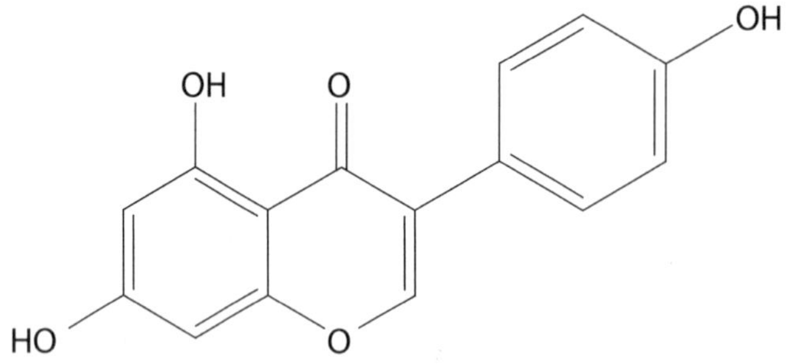

Genisteine

An example of flavonoid of interest is genistein (4′5, 7-trihydroxyisoflavone). Perhaps no other flavonoid has aroused more interest in the field of oncology that genistein, a flavonoid found notably in soybean (*Glycine max* [L.] Merr, from the family Fabaceae). Genistein has been suggested to lower the incidence of tumor formation, inhibit protein tyrosine skinase activity, and augment the efficacy of radiation for breast and prostate carcinomas, and underwent phase I/II clinical trials. Several biotechnological firms in Japan, Australia, and in the United States manufacture genistein as food supplement in multimillions of US dollars in yearly benefits.

A definitive conclusion regarding the clinical applicability of natural products would seem premature at this time. In fact, the question remains controversial. The hope for a spectacular cancer cure has not materialized, and there are a few cases where natural products alone seem to yield better results than conventional forms of therapy. The use of a logical approach could bring some change to this rather pessimistic picture. Meanwhile, the medicinal plants of the Asia–Pacific region remain in the stage of "potent source of antineoplastic drugs awaiting discovery."

REFERENCES

1. Sung HW, Reynolds MC, Nan JS, Cassady JM, Snapka RM. Inhibition of topoisomerase II by liriodenine. Biochem Pharmacol 1997;54:467–473.
2. Sagen AL, Sahpaz S, Mavi S, Hostettmann K. Isoquinoline alkaloids from *Artabotrys brachypetalus*. Biochem Syst Ecol 2003;31:1447–1449.
3. Wu YC, Chen CH, Yang TH, et al. Cytotoxic aporphines from *Artabotrys uncinatus* and the structure and stereochemistry of artacinatine. Phytochemistry 1989;28: 2191–2195.
4. Wijeratne EMK, Gunatilaka AAL, Kingston DGI, Haltiwanger RC, Eggleston DS. Artabotrine: a novel bioactive alkaloid from *Artabotrys zeylanicus*. Tetrahedron 1995;51:7877–7882.

5. Achenbach H, Hemrich H. Alkaloids, flavonoids and phenylpropanoids of the West African plant *Oxymitra velutina*. Phytochemistry 1991;30:1265–1267.
6. Woo SH, Sun NJ, Cassady JM, Snapka RM. Topoisomerase II inhibition by aporphine alkaloids. Biochem Pharmacol 1999; 57:1141–1145.
7. Makhey D, Gatto B, Chiang Y, Liu A, Liu LF, LaVoie EJ. Coralyne and related compounds as mammalian topoisomerase I and topoisomerase II poisons. Bioorg Med Chem 1996;4:781–791.
8. Li G, Lee CS, Woo MH, Lee SH, Chang HW, Son JK. Lignans from the bark of *Machilus thunbergii* and their DNA topoisomerases I and II inhibition and cytotoxicity. Biol Pharm Bull 2004;27:1147–1150.
9. Huang RL, Chen CC, Huang YL, et al. Anti-tumor effects of D-dicentrine from the root of *Lindera megaphylla*. Planta Med 1998;64:212–215.
10. Zhou BN, Johnson RK, Mattern MR, et al. Isolation and biochemical characterization of a new topoisomerase I inhibitor from *Ocotea leucoxylon*. J Nat Prod 2000;63:217–221.
11. Hoet S, Stevigny C, Block S, et al. Alkaloids from *Cassytha filiformis* and related aporphines: antitrypanosomal activity, cytotoxicity, and interaction with DNA and topoisomerases. Planta Med 2004;70:407–413.
12. Chen IS, Chen JJ, Duh CY, Tsai IL. Cytotoxic lignans from formosan *Hernandia nymphaeifolia*. Phytochemistry 1997;45:991–996.
13. Chen KS, Wu YC, Teng CM, Ko FN, Wu TS. Bioactive alkaloids from *Illigera luzonensis*. J Nat Prod 1997;60:645–647.
14. Guh JH, Ko FN, Yu SM, Wu YC, Teng CM. Pharmacological evaluation of *N*-methyl-actinodaphnine, a new vascular α-adrenoceptor antagonist, isolated from *Illigera luzonensis*. Eur J Pharmacol 1995;279: 33–41.
15. Ting CY, Hsu CT, Hsu HT, et al. Isodiospyrin as a novel human DNA topoisomerase I inhibitor. Biochem Pharmacol 2003;66:1981–1991.
16. Hande KR. Clinical applications of anticancer drugs targeted to topoisomerase II. Biochim Biophys Acta1998;1400(1-3):173–184.
17. Lee HH. Colouring matters from *Prismatomeris malayana*. Phytochemistry 1969;8: 501–503.
18. Kanokmedhakul K, Kanokmedhakul S, Phatchana R. Biological activity of anthraquinones and triterpenoids from *Prismatomeris fragrans*. J Ethnopharmacol 2005;100:284–288.
19. Zhou Z, Jiang SH, Zhu DY, Lin LZ, Cordell GA. Anthraquinones from *Knoxia valerianoides*. Phytochemistry 1994;36:765–768.
20. Yang YJ, Shu HY, Min ZD. Anthraquinones isolated from *Morinda officinalis* and *Damnacanthus indicus*. Yao Xue Xue Bao 1992;27:358–364.
21. Li S, Ouyang Q, Tan X, Shi S, Yao Z. Chemical constituents of *Morinda officinalis* How. Zhongguo Zhong Yao Za Zhi 1991;11:675–676.
22. Faltynek CR, Schroeder J, Mauvais P, et al. Damnacanthal is a highly potent, selective inhibitor of p56lck tyrosine kinase activity. Biochemistry 1995;34: 12,404–12,410.

23. Tosa H, Iinuma M, Asai F, et al. Anthraquinones from *Neonauclea calycina* and their inhibitory activity against DNA topoisomerase II. Biol Pharm Bull 1998;21:641–642.
24. Hiwasa T, Arase Y, Chen Z, et al. Stimulation of ultraviolet-induced apoptosis of human fibroblast UVr-1 cells by tyrosine kinase inhibitors. FEBS Lett 1999;444: 173–176.
25. Zhang ZQ, Li Y, Ming Y, Luo ZP, Zhao YM. The effect of *Morinda officinalis* How, a Chinese traditional medicinal plant, on the DRL 72-s schedule in rats and the forced swimming test in mice. Pharmacol Biochem Behav 2002;72:39–43.
26. Li YF, Zheng HG, Ming Y, Yi MZ, Zhi PL. Inhibition of the oligosaccharides extracted from *Morinda officinalis*, a Chinese traditional herbal medicine, on the corticosterone induced apoptosis in PC12 cells. Life Sci 2003;72:933–942.
27. Li YF, Liu YQ, Ming Y, et al. The cytoprotective effect of inulin-type hexasaccharide extracted from *Morinda officinalis* on PC12 cells against the lesion induced by corticosterone. Life Sci 2004;75: 1531–1538.
28. Wang LK, Johnson RK, Hecht SM. Inhibition of topoisomerase I function by nitidine and fagaronine. Chem Res Toxicol 1993;6:813–818.
29. Larsen AK, Grondard L, Couprie J, et al. The antileukemic alkaloid fagaronine is an inhibitor of DNA topoisomerases I and II. Biochem Pharmacol 1993;46:1403–1412.
30. Ko FN, Chen IS, Wu SJ, Lee LG, Haung TF, Teng CM. Antiplatelet effects of chelerythrine chloride isolated from *Zanthoxylum simulans*. Biochim Biophys Acta 1990;1052:360–365.
31. Chmura SJ, Dolan ME, Cha A, Mauceri HJ, Kufe DW, Weichselbaum RR. In vitro and in vivo activity of protein kinase C inhibitor chelerythrine chlorise induces tumor cell toxicity and growth delay in vivo. Clin Cancer Res 2000;6:737–742.
32. Kemény-Beke A, Aradi J, Damjanovich J, et al. Apoptotic response of uveal melanoma cells upon treatment with chelidonine, sanguinarine and chelerythrine. Cancer Lett 2005, in press.
33. Paik SY, Koh KH, Beak SM, Paek SH, Kim JA. The essential oils from *Zanthoxylum schinifolium* pericarp induce apoptosis of HepG2 human hepatoma cells through increased production of reactive oxygen species. Biol Pharm Bull 2005;28: 802–807.
34. Wada S, Reiko T, Akira I, Shunyo M. In vitro inhibitory effects of DNA topoisomerase II by fernane-type triterpenoids isolated from a *Euphorbia* genus. Bioorg Med Chem Lett 1998;8:2829–2832.
35. Setzer WN, Xiaoming S, Bates RB, et al. A Phytochemical investigation of *Alchornea latifolia*. Fitoterapia 2000;71:195–198.
36. Vongvanich N, Kittakoop P, Kramyu J, Tanticharoen M, Thebtaranonth Y. Phyllanthusols A and B, cytotoxic norbisabolane glycosides from *Phyllanthus acidus* Skeels. J Org Chem 2000;65:5420–5423.
37. Sengupta P, Mukhopadhyay J. Terpenoids and related compounds—VII: triterpenoids of *Phyllanthus acidus* Skeels. Phytochemistry 1966;5:531–534.
38. Wada S, Iida A, Tanaka R. Screening of triterpenoids isolated from *Phyllanthus flexuosus* for DNA topoisomerase inhibitory activity. J Nat Prod 2001;64:1545–1547.

39. Martelli AM, Bortul R, Bareggi R, et al. The pro-apoptotic drug camptothecin stimulates phospholipase D activity and diacylglycerol production in the nucleus of HL-60 human promyelocytic leukemia cells. Cancer Res 1999;59:3961–3967.
40. Jang DS, Cuendet M, Pawlus AD, et al. Potential cancer chemopreventive constituents of the leaves of *Macaranga triloba*. Phytochemistry 2004;65: 345–350.
41. Dannenberg AJ, Altorki NK, Boyle JO, et al. Cyclo-oxygenase 2: a pharmacological target for the prevention of cancer. Lancet Oncol 2001;2:544–551.
42. Kniss DA, Garver CL, Perkins DJ, Zimmerman PD, Fertel RH. Taxol enhances macrophage tumoricidal activity via suppression of PGE_2 biosynthesis. J Soc Gynecol Invest 1996;3:377A.
43. Sakai K, Fukuda Y, Matsunaga S, Tanaka R, Yamori T. New cytotoxic oleanane-type triterpenoids from the cones of *Liquidamber styraciflua*. J Nat Prod 2004;67: 1088–1093.
44. Mukherjee KS, Ghosh PK, Mukherjee RK. Diterpenoid quinones of *Salvia lanata*. Phytochemistry 1983;22:1296–1297.
45. Simões F, Michavila A, Rodríguez B, Maria C, Alvarez G, Hasan M. A quinone methide diterpenoid from the root of *Salvia moorciuftiana*. Phytochemistry 1986;25: 755–756.
46. Hernández M, Esquive Bl, Cárdenas J, Rodríguez-Hahn L, Ramamoorthy TP. Diterpenoid abietane quinones isolated from *Salvia regla*. Phytochemistry 1987;26: 3297–3299.
47. González AG, Aguiar ZE, Luis JG, Ravelo AG, Domínguez X. Quinone methide diterpenoids from the roots of *Salvia texana*. Phytochemistry 1988;27: 1777–1781.
48. Slamenova D, Masterova I, Labaj J, et al. Cytotoxic and DNA-damaging effects of diterpenoid quinones from the roots of *Salvia officinalis* L. on colonic and hepatic human cells cultured in vitro. Basic Clin Pharmacol Toxicol 2004;94:282–290.
49. Meng LH, Zhang JS, Ding J. Salvicine, a novel DNA topoisomerase II inhibitor, exerting its effects by trapping enzyme–DNA cleavage complexes. Biochem Pharmacol 2001;62:733–741.
50. Gu L, Xinchu W. Antioxidant activity and components of *Salvia plebeia* R. Br—a Chinese herb. Food Chem 2001;73:299–305.
51. Liu J, Shen HM, Ong CN. *Salvia miltiorrhiza* inhibits cell growth and induces apoptosis in human hepatoma $HepG_2$ cells. Cancer Lett 2000;153:85–93.
52. Chor SY, Hui AY, To KF, et al. Anti-proliferative and pro-apoptotic effects of herbal medicine on hepatic stellate cell. J Ethnopharmacol 2005;100:180–186.
53. Yang LJ, Jeng CJ, Kung HN, et al. Tanshinone IIA isolated from *Salvia miltiorrhiza* elicits the cell death of human endothelial cells. J Biomed Sci 2005;12: 347–361.
54. Mosaddik MA. In vitro cytotoxicity of tanshinones isolated from *Salvia miltiorrhiza* Bunge against P388 lymphocytic leukemia cells. Phytomedicine 2003;10:682–685.
55. Lee D-S, Lee SH. Biological activity of dihydrotanshinone I: effect on apoptosis. J Biosci Bioeng 2000;89:292–293.
56. Leone M, Zhai D, Sareth S, Kitada S, Reed JC, Pellecchia M. Cancer prevention by tea polyphenols is linked to their direct inhibition of antiapoptotic Bcl-2-family proteins. Cancer Res 2003;63:8118–8121.

57. Parker BW, Kaur G, Nieves-Neira W, et al. Early induction of apoptosis in hematopoietic cell lines after exposure to flavopiridol. Blood 1998;91:458–465.
58. Hayakawa S, Saeki K, Sazuka M, et al. Apoptosis induction by epigallocatechin gallate involves its binding to Fas. Biochem Biophys Res Commun 2001;285: 1102–1106.
59. Adlakha RC, Ashorn CL, Chan D, Zwelling LA. Modulation of 4′-(9-acridinylamino)methanesulfon-m-anisidide-induced, topoisomerase II-mediated DNA cleavage by gossypol. Cancer Res 1989;49:2052–2058.
60. Nikolovska-Coleska Z, Xu L, Hu Z, et al. Discovery of embelin as a cell-permeable, small-molecular weight inhibitor of XIAP through structure-based computational screening of a traditional herbal medicine three-dimensional structure database. J Med Chem 2004;47:2430–2440.
61. Motoyuki T, Kaoru K, Hironori N, Akira T, Hajime I, Hideto M. Definition of crucial structural factors of acetogenins, potent inhibitors of mitochondrial complex I. Biochim Biophys Acta 2000;1460:302–310.
62. Inayat-Hussain SH, Osman AB, Din LB, Ali AM, Snowden RT, MacFarlane M, Cain K. Caspases-3 and -7 are activated in goniothalamin-induced apoptosis in human Jurkat T-cells. FEBS Lett 1999;456: 379–383.
63. Alkofahi A, Rupprecht J, Smith DL, Chang CJ, McLaughlin JL. Goniothalamin and annonacin: bioactive acetogenins from *Goniothamalus giganteus* (Annonaceae). Experientia 1988;44:83–85.
64. Alkofahi A, Rupprecht J, Liu YM, Chang CJ, Smith DL, McLaughlin JL. Gigantecin: a novel antimitotic and cytotoxic acetogenin, with non adjacent tetrahydrofurane rings, from *Goniothalamus giganteus* (Annonaceae). Experientia 1990;46:539–541.
65. Fang XP, Anderson JE, Smith DL, Wood KV, McLaughlin JL. Gigantetronenin and gigantrionenin: novel cytotoxic acetogenins from *Goniothalamus giganteus*. J Nat Prod 1992;55:1655–1663.
66. Gu ZM, Fang XP, Zeng L, et al. Gonionenin: a new cytotoxic annonaceous acetogenin from *Goniothalamus giganteus* and the conversion of mono-THF acetogenins to *bis*-THF cetogenins. J Org Chem 1994;59:3472–3479.
67. Lu Z, Yan Z, Qing Y, Gouen S, Kan H, McLaughlin JL. *cis*-Gigantrionenin and 4-acetyl gigantetrocin A, two new bioactive annonaceous acetogenins from *Goniothalamus giganteus*, and the stereochemistries of acetogenin 1,2,5-triols. Bioorg Med Chem 1996;4:1271–1279.
68. Lu Z, Yan Z, McLaughlin JL. Gigantransenins A, B, and C, novel mono-THF acetogenins bearing trans-double bonds, from *Goniothalamus giganteus* (Annonaceae). Tetrahedron Lett 1996;37:5449–5452.
69. Feras QA, Lingling R, Yan Z, McLaughlin JL. Unusual bioactive annonaceous acetogenins from *Goniothalamus giganteus*. Tetrahedron 1998;54:5833–5844.
70. Feras QA, Yan Z, Lingling R, McLaughlin JL. Mono-tetrahydrofuran acetogenins from *Goniothalamus giganteus*. Phytochemistry 1998;49:761–768.
71. Xin PF, Rong S, Zhe-ming G, et al. A new type of cytotoxic annonaceous acetogenin: Giganin from *Goniothalamus giganteus*. Bioorg Med Chem Lett 1993;3:1153–1156.

72. Jiang Z, Chen Y, Ruo-Yun CH, De-Quan Y. Mono-tetrahydrofuran ring acetogenins from *Goniothalamus donnaiensis*. Phytochemistry 1997;46:327–331.
73. Ying C, Zhong J, Ruo RC, et al. Two linear acetogenins from *Goniothalamus gardneri*. Phytochemistry 1998;49:1317–1321.
74. Seidel V, Bailleul F, Waterman PG. Goniothalamusin, a linear acetogenin from *Goniothalamus gardneri*. Phytochemistry 1999;52:1101–1103.
75. Jewers K, Davis JB, Dougan J, et al. Goniothalamin and its distribution in four *Goniothalamus* species. Phytochemistry 1972;11:2025–2030.
76. El-Sharkawi S, Yusuf Z, Pihie AHL, Ali AM. Metabolism of goniothalamin in animal and microbial systems. Bull Chim Farmaceutica 1996;135:35–40.
77. Ali AM, Umar-Tsafe N, Mohamed SM, et al. Apopotosis induction in CEM-SS T-lymphoblastic leukemic cell line by goniothalamin. J Biochem Mol Biol Biophys 2001;5:253–261.
78. Pihie AHL, Stanslas J, Din LB. Non-steroid receptor-mediated anti-proliferative activity of styrylpyrone derivative in human breast cancer cell lines. Anticancer Res 1998;18:1739–1743.
79. Ali AM, Mackeen MM, Hamidi M, et al. Cytotoxicity and electron death cell induced by goniothalamin. Planta Med 1997;63:81–83.
80. Lee ATC, Azimahtol HLP, Tan AN. Styrylpyrone derivatives (SPD) induces apopotosis in caspases-7-dependent manner in the human breast cancer cell line MCF-7. Cancer Cell Int 2003;3:1–8.
81. Inayat-Hussain SH, Osman AB, Din LB, et al. Caspase-3 and -7 are activated in goniothalamin-induced apopotosis in human Jurkat T-cells. FEBS Lett 1999;456: 379–383.
82. Inayat-Hussain SH, Annuar BO, Din LB, Ali AM, Ross D. Loss of mitochondrial transmembrane potential and caspase-9 activation during apoptosis induced by the novel styryl-lactone goniothalamin in HL-60 leukemia cells. Toxicol In Vitro 2003; 17: 433–439.
83. Lee ATC, Azimahtol HLP. Styrylpyrone derivative (SPD) induces apoptosis through the up-regulation of bax in the human breast cancer cell line MCF-7. J Biochem Mol Biol 2003;36:269–274.
84. Almudena B, Amparo BM, Rao SK, Cortes D. Styryl-pyrones from *Goniothalamus arvensis*. Phytochemistry 1998;47:1375–1380.
85. Hisham A, Toubi M, Shuaily W, Ajitha MDB, Fujimoto Y. Cardiobutanolide, a styryl-lactone from *Goniothalamus cardiopetalus*. Phytochemistry 2003;62:597–600.
86. Hisham A, Harassi A, Shuaily W, Shizue E, Fujimoto Y. Cardiopetalolactone: a novel styryllactone from *Goniothalamus cardiopetalus* Tetrahedron 2000; 56:9985–9989.
87. Mu Q, Tang WD, Liu RY, et al. Constituents from the stems of *Goniothalamus griffithii*. Planta Med 2003;69:826–830.
88. Steven MC, Laily BD, Abdul L, et al. (+)Isoaltholactone: a furanopyrone isolated from *Goniothalamus* species. Phytochemistry 1990;29:1701–1704.
89. Wang S, Zhang YJ, Chen RY, Yu DQ. Goniolactones A–F, six new styrylpyrone derivatives from the roots of *Goniothalamus cheliensis*. J Nat Prod 2002;65:835–841.

90. Lan YH, Chang FR, Liaw CC, Wu CC, Chiang MY, Wu YC. Digoniodiol, deoxygoniopypyrone A, and goniofupyrone A: three new styryl-lactones from Goniothalamus amuyon. Planta Med 2005;71:153–159.
91. Wu YC, Fang-Rong C, Chang-Yih D, Shang-Kwei W, Tian-Shung W. Cytotoxic styrylpyrones of *Goniothalamus amuyon*. Phytochemistry 1992;31:2851–2853.
92. Hasan CM, Mia MY, Rashid MA, Connolly JD. 5-Acetoxyisogoniothalamin oxide, an epoxystyryl lactone from *Goniothalamus sesquipedalis*. Phytochemistry 1994;37: 1763–1744.
93. Fasihuddin BA, Wan AT, Siraj O, Atan MS. 5-Acetyl goniothalamin, a styryl dihydropyrone from *Goniothalamus uvaroides*. Phytochemistry 1991;30:2430–2431.
94. Inayat-Hussain SH, Annuar BO, Laily BD, Naoyuki T. Altholactone, a novel styryllactone induces apoptosis via oxidative stress in human HL-60 leukemia cells. Toxicol Lett 2002;131:153–159.
95. Peris E, Estornell E, Cabedo N, Cortes D, Bermejo A. 3-Acetylaltholactone and related styryl-lactones, mitochondrial respiratory chain inhibitors. Phytochemistry 2000;54:311–315.
96. Jerzak M, Kasprzycka M, Wierbicki P, Kotarski J, Gorski A. Apoptosis of T cells in the first trimester human deciduas. Am J Reprod Immunol 1998;40: 130–135.
97. Vadillo OF, Avila VMA, Guerrero HC, Arechavaleta VF, Montoya BJ. Apoptosis in trophoblast of patients with recurrent spontaneous abortion of unidentified cause. Ginecol Obstet Mex 2000;68: 122–131.
98. Nkunya MH, Weenen H, Bray DH, Mgani QA, Mwasumbi LB. Antimalarial activity of Tanzanian plants and their active constituents: the genus UvariaPlanta Med 1991;57:341–343.
99. Hufford CD, Babajide O. Oguntimein Dihydrochalcones from *Uvaria angolensis*. Phytochemistry 1980;19:2036–2038.
100. Mayunga HH, Weenen H, Renner C, Waibel R, Achenbach H. Benzylated dihydrochalcones from *Uvaria leptocladon*. Phytochemistry 1993;32: 1297–1300.
101. Fall D, Duval RA, Gleye C, Laurens A, Hocquemiller R. Chamuvarinin, an acetogenin bearing a tetrahydropyran ring from the roots of *Uvaria chamae*. J Nat Prod 2004;67:1041–1043.
102. Nakatani N, Ichimaru M, Moriyasu M, Kato A. Induction of apoptosis in human promyelocytic leukemia cell line HL-60 by C-benzylated dihydrochalcones, uvaretin, isouvaretin and diuvaretin. Biol Pharm Bull 2005;28:83–86.
103. Rivero A, Quintana J, Eiroa JL, et al. Potent induction of apoptosis by germacranolide sesquiterpene lactones on human myeloid leukemia cells. Eur J Pharmacol 2003;482:77–84.
104. Lee KH, Ibuka T, Huang HC. Letter: Antitumor agents XIV: molephantinin, a new potent antitumor sesquiterpene lactone from *Elephantopus mollis*. J Pharm Sci 1975;64:1077–1078.
105. Lee KH, Ibuka T, Furukawa H, Kozuka M, Wu RY, Hall IH, Huang HC. Antitumor agents XXXVIII: Isolation and structural elucidation of novel germacranolides and triterpenes from *Elephantopus mollis*. J Pharm Sci 1980;69:1050–1056.

106. Hall IH, Liou YF, Lee KH. Antitumor agents LII: The effects of molephantinin on nucleic acid and protein synthesis of Ehrlich ascites cells. J Pharm Sci 1982;71: 687–690.
107. Xie PD, Sang T, Gong XZ. Determination of protocatechuic acid in *Blumea riparia* (Bl.) DC. by RP-HPLC. Zhongguo Zhong Yao Za Zhi 2000;25: 227–229.
108. Kampa M, Alexaki VI, Notas G, et al. Apoptotic effects of selective phenolic acids on T47D human breast cancer cells: potential mechanisms of action. Breast Cancer Res 2004;6:R63–R74.
109. Stagos D, Kazantzoglou G, Magiatis P, Mitaku S, Anagnostopoulos K, Kouretas D. Effects of plant phenolics and grape extracts from Greek varieties of *Vitis vinifera* on mitomycin C and topoisomerase I-induced nicking of DNA. Int J Mol Med 2005;15: 1013–1022.
110. Pandey UC, Ram PS, Palaniappan K, Herz W. Isoalantolactone derivatives and germacranolides from *Blumea densiflora*. Phytochemistry 1985;24: 1509–1514.
111. Wang SY, Chang HN, Lin KT, Lo CP, Yang NS, Shyur LF. Antioxidant properties and phytochemical characteristics of extracts from *Lactuca indica*. J Agric Food Chem 2003;51:1506–1512.
112. Horinaka M, Yoshida T, Shiraishi T, et al. Luteolin induces apoptosis via death receptor 5 upregulation in human malignant tumor cells. Oncogene 2005;24:7180–7189.
113. Dassonneville L, Lansiaux A, Wattez N, et al. Cytotoxicity and cell cycle effects of the plant alkaloids cryptolepine and neocryptolepine: relation to drug-induced apoptosis. J Nat Prod 2001;64:134–135.
114. Shi Q, Chen K, Li L, et al. Antitumor agents, 154. Cytotoxic and antimitotic flavonols from *Polanisia dodecandra*. J Nat Prod 1995;58:475–482.

Index

B–C

D

E

F–G

H

I–K

T

U–V

W–Z